REHABILITATION MANAGEMENT OF RHEUMATIC CONDITIONS

This volume is one of the series,
Rehabilitation Medicine Library,
Edited by John V. Basmajian

New books and new editions published, in press or in preparation for this series:

BANERJEE: Rehabilitation Management of Amputees
BASMAJIAN: Therapeutic Exercise, third edition*
BISHOP: Behavioral Problems and the Disabled: Assessment and Management
BROWNE, KIRLIN AND WATT: Rehabilitation Services and the Social Work Role: Challenge for Change
CHYATTE: Rehabilitation in Chronic Renal Failure
HAAS ET AL.: Pulmonary Therapy and Rehabilitation: Principles and Practice
INCE: Behavioral Psychology in Rehabilitation Medicine: Clinical Applications
JOHNSON: Practical Electromyography
KHALILI: Management of Spasticity with Peripheral Phenol Nerve Blocks
LEHMANN: Therapeutic Heat and Cold, third edition*
LONG: Prevention and Rehabilitation in Ischemic Heart Disease
REDFORD: Orthotics Etcetera, second edition*
ROGOFF: Manipulation, Traction and Massage, second edition*
SHA'KED: Human Sexuality in Rehabilitation Medicine

* *Originally published as part of the Physical Medicine Library, edited by Sidney Licht.*

Rehabilitation Management of Rheumatic Conditions

Edited by

GEORGE E. EHRLICH,

M.D., F.A.C.P.

Professor of Medicine,
Director of the Division of Rheumatology,
Hahnemann Medical College and Hospital;
Formerly Professor of Medicine and Professor of Rehabilitation Medicine,
Temple University School of Medicine;
Arthritis Center,
Albert Einstein Medical Center and
Moss Rehabilitation Hospital
Philadelphia, Pennsylvania

WILLIAMS & WILKINS
Baltimore/London

Made in the United States of America

Reprinted 1981

Library of Congress Cataloging in Publication Data

Main entry under title:

Rehabilitation management of rheumatic conditions.

(Rehabilitation medicine library)
Includes index.
1. Rheumatism. 2. Arthritics—Rehabilitation. I. Ehrlich, George E. II. Series.
RC927.R394 616.7'2 79-22564
ISBN 0-683-02791-3

Composed and printed at the
Waverly Press, Inc.
Mt. Royal and Guilford Aves.
Baltimore, Md. 21202, U.S.A.

To the memory of my father
whose erudition encouraged emulation

and

to my mother who served as catalyst
during my formative years

Series Editor's Foreword

Rheumatic conditions include a variety of disabilities beyond arthritis. Therefore, when I was seeking an editor for a new edition of Sidney Licht's *Arthritis* I sought a clinician of outstanding and broad clinical experience with a proved editorial ability. Dr. Ehrlich fills these criteria. In turn he has assembled an outstanding group of authors with both special knowledge and a broad view of rheumatic conditions.

From the concerns of social workers through transportation problems, nursing problems, surgery, and medical approaches, the chapters touch on and examine all the significant problems and solutions. Because of the completely new nature of this book it is not a second edition of *Arthritis*. That excellent volume served its time well and was a credit to the late Sidney Licht. Along with his authors he gave us a book that for a time was unrivalled. Now this book in the new *Rehabilitation Medicine Library* series should capture a very prominent place in both the rheumatology and the general rehabilitation fields. Professionals in many adjacent fields (e.g., nursing, social work, etc.) will find most of the book speaks directly to them as well.

JOHN V. BASMAJIAN, M.D.

Preface

Rehabilitation is a philosophical concept, one that is peculiarly contemporary. It suggests that anyone flawed by disease, injury, congenital defects, and loss of an organ or part or of the function thereof can have the deficits filled in to create as normal a life as possible. Normality in this instance is defined as the full rights and space and enjoyment that life has to offer. Restoration is not enough; for some, who have never participated fully in the pursuit of happiness, rehabilitation is the first introduction rather than a restoration. Thus, teaching Helen Keller to read and to communicate with others and to discover the wideness of the world is a shining example of the application of the concept; helping the aphasic paralyzed victim of an automobile accident return to his full function is another. In most instances, rehabilitation is not a major project, and probably goes unrecognized for what it is. Recovery from an acute illness or from a minor injury is relatively quick and complete, and the counsel that helps restore vigor, the medicines and operations, and even the increasingly longer out-of-bed orders are all part of the rehabilitative process. Strangely, while these aspects of every day health care go unrecognized as being rehabilitative, other matters, such as helping the adult or child from a deprived background to achieve work, family, housing, and self-respect, are now classified under the heading of rehabilitation.

Not only are rehabilitation hospitals supposed to wield their magic with strokes, emphysema, amputations, heart attacks, and arthritis, the prisons are supposed to rehabilitate the criminal. City planners rehabilitate neighborhoods. Classes euphemistically mislabeled rehabilitate recalcitrant learners. The broadening of the concept creates it own ennui. The term is heard but easily bypassed. Any concept so broad ceases to be a paradigm and becomes instead a cliche. Rehabilitation, the cliche, can still command fiscal backing (who can be against motherhood?) but attracts the interest and study of few who should be concerned. Yet rehabilitation and comprehensive medical care are almost synonymous. Rehabilitation is more than gadgetry, more than physical medicine, more than something that is done elsewhere; it is a pervasive concept that all who care for the sick and the injured need to master.

Basic to rehabilitation is *prognosis*. What is the outlook for someone with a given problem? If nothing is done. If medication is given. If the medication reacts adversely. If the medication works better than expected. If an operation is required. If the operation is accepted and goes well. If the operation fails. If the operation is rejected. If the subject needs attendants during the recovery period. If there is a supportive family or if there is not. If there are private means or if public monies need to be obtained. If there are time limits. If the home has stairs or if it does not. If adequate nutrition is likely or if it is not. If assistive devices and other aids will be needed. If private transportation is available or if public transportation needs to be used. If public transportation is available. If the deficit does not preclude getting into a stock car. If one can drive oneself or if one becomes a passenger only.

Each question creates at least a binary answer system. One can easily postulate the algorithms of the decision-making process, but the majority of practitioners in the health professions will rapidly find themselves beyond the limits of their expertise. That is because the simplicity of the solution when the technology is fully developed, as Lewis Thomas has pointed out, permits easy answers, rapid mastery, and little expense. In most chronic illness, in most instances where the rehabilitation process is the biggest challenge, only a partial technology exists, requiring many hands and minds, different disciplines, and far heavier expense. Generally, the more complex problems now require teams of professionals, and the contents of these teams are not exclusive memberships.

Take arthritis, for example, the subject of this volume. Joint function is inhibited. Inflammation is a remote or immediate cause, and inflammation can often be contained by medication. In gout and a few other forms of arthritis, inflammation is acute, relatively short-lived, and severe. It fulfills the clinical definition of inflammation, namely a condition that produces localized heat, redness, swelling, pain, and loss of function. Many of the molecular and cellular events that lead to this have been identified, and in some instances, specific antagonists are available. Antiinflammatory compounds are reasonably successful in combating such inflammation. They stop the gouty attack, and they can subdue the acute inflammatory attacks that punctuate more chronic inflammation as well. But chronic inflammation is a different story. Heat and redness are sometime events. Swelling has many causes other than the acute inflammation. Pain tends to be modest but long lasting. The chronicity of the pain is the threat: it was there yesterday, it is there today, it will be there tomorrow. Not its intensity but its persistence makes it unbearable. And so function is not totally abolished either, only inhibited most of the time. But symptoms feed on each other, and soon a querulousness develops and a depression and personality changes which, with limited mobility, lead to a shrinking of life space and life content. Such chronic inflammation is where the emphasis now lies, where rehabilitation is most needed.

Drug management is part of the solution. Removal of symptoms can at least make life more bearable. Subduing the progression of disease can improve the outlook for the future. Even just removing the secondary consequences, as by suppressing the secondary inflammation in osteoarthritis, can bring symptoms to a level that many are willing to tolerate. Orthotic devices can improve function, if compliance can be achieved. Programs of joint conservation and joint protection will enhance diminished function. Various surgical procedures can improve or restore function as well, and at the same time ameliorate the pain that use of the joint has provoked. Heat and cold delivered in various ways sedate taut muscles and reduce pain. Exercises improve movement. Appreciation that disease occurs in the patient and the patient in the community permits a definition of the person involved and perhaps some help with social and societal deficits. On balance, these various measures help more often than not, although they are subject to failure as well, sometimes of disastrous proportion. But there are still design and architectural barriers to overcome, transportation to be arranged, not just for medical attention or for dental or eye care, but for social needs as well. The ramifications of chronic disease extend their pseudopods into the entire fabric of society. Ultimately, hardly anyone escapes being part of the solution, part of the team that permits the patient with chronic ills, the patient with arthritis, to gain and regain a place in the sun.

Rehabilitation has not always been of particular concern, to the profession of medicine or to society. Like consumer activism, it is a relatively recent phenomenon. Before that, the halt, the lame, and the blind received no special consideration. As a matter of fact, life was deliberately made harder for them. In medieval times, the blind would grope their way from place to place, usually following a leader who had a staff with which to test the ground ahead. Limbs were replaced, if at all, with wooden pegs which fit roughly. To be crippled by a deficit or disability was to become an object of derision. If there was no family to look after those who were disabled, they begged, went hungry, and froze. Their life was nasty, brutish, and short. No particular grace was thought to descend upon them, and no consideration was given to their ability of access or use of public and private facilities. Even those who were disabled in military service were not rewarded especially, and when captured by the enemy could expect no mercy.

Hospitals are relatively recent additions to health care, barely a few centuries old, and in some parts of the world, only introduced in this century. They formerly were places to die in. Only recently have they been identified as possibly giving rise to life, and adding content to life. Most of the professions dealing with the sick are even more modern. There is scant history and shorter tradition to fall back on. This has taken legislation, enacted in the last 20 years in most countries that have it (and there are still few of these), to address the civil rights of the disabled population. Exclusion from work and school and even from society were commonplace before that.

The concept that there is some inherent human right to happiness and to health is also a very recent one. Yet where rehabilitation exists, that concept has been accepted, as it is at the basis of rehabilitation itself. The expanding teams are necessary to deal with the total picture and to bring into focus the totality of life. They support the recognition that patient is a role played by a person when ministered to by health professionals; this same person has other roles to play: father and mother, son and daughter, employer and employee, and so on.

The past is history. The present is described in this book, which may raise as many questions as it provides answers. The state of the art of removing handicap from disability, which also defines rehabilitation, has been refined by the various professionals of many disciplines whose contributions follow. All who wrote for this book had practical experience in rehabilitation in their disciplines. All have themselves contributed to emerging concepts of what their roles might be. All are qualified to advise where we are, and to speculate where we might be going. All have confronted the definition of handicap as the social consequence of disability, which itself is the functional consequence of disease. Disability does not preclude full participation in the world, but handicap imposes the additional burden that makes this participation difficult, if not impossible.

In the sense in which it is used, we are all handicapped in one way or another, and in learning to overcome our handicaps, the ones that have been imposed as barriers for us, we also learn how to help others overcome handicaps. A positive attitude is helpful, accompanied by laughter and pride in accomplishment, but despite the claims of some capable polemicists who think themselves recovered from crippling illnesses, including arthritis, it does take more than willpower to achieve such goals. However, willpower is important and should not be downgraded. All assessments of goals for the patient (even when the patient is included in the decision-making process, which is not always the case) takes into account the desire of the individual to improve and the level to which such an individual can aspire.

The fruits of laboratory research are not far from application these days. The recently discovered analgesic substances of the brain, the endorphins, may lead us to revise our concept of pain, for example. We may have to view it as the subtraction of self-analgesia rather than the addition of a new sensation. In other words, pain may be a byproduct of the functioning of many of our parts, dulled by internal secretions that make us unaware of the discomfort. When these internal secretions diminish or are inactivated, for some reason, pain may come to the fore. That may explain why pleasant environmental events can cause pain to diminish, even if it is seemingly intractable, whereas other environmental events that provoke stresses and tensions exacerbate pain.

This concept, for which more and more evidence accrues, should lead to a revision of our understanding of pain and the treatment that we bring to it. As pain is the chief reason that health professionals are consulted, its abolition also becomes one of the chief tasks of the health professions. Some deal with it through medication, some through surgical ablation, some through resting of the part, some through environmental manipulation, and some through removing potential contributors to pain, such as malalignment, weakness of muscle, or externally imposed barriers in design. Improvement of function is the chief aim of working together, because pain control is the individual task of one or another specialty. Only functional improvement requires interdisciplinary teams, and if that is not one of the goals in patient care, then rehabilitation plays no part in the treatment of that particular individual.

Arthritis is a multiplicity of disorders masquerading under a single expression. Because nature is economical in its ways, insults to joints from whatever cause express themselves similarly. Acuteness implies inflammation, whether it is primary or secondary. Chronicity of the process is the fate of all joints once they are insulted. Perhaps mere changes should not be regarded as diseases. The spurs one finds adjacent to joints in osteoarthritis are there probably to splint the joint and to reduce its range of motion. We identify this reduced range of motion as a functional deficit and seek to cure it. But, in reality, it is an attempt on the part of nature to combat chronic inflammation, which, as everyone knows, splinting can do. Therefore, some earlier inflammation is implied, an inflammation that set up the changes that led to spurs. Included among these changes is loss of cartilage and inflammation incited by debris. While roentgenologic descriptions of joints, including the disc spaces of the back, feature such terms as *degenerative*, implying some inevitable alteration in form and reduction in function, and *osteoarthrosis*, denying the inflammation that preceded and at time accompanies these changes, the symptoms may well derive from some other source. The mere presence of an abnormality, or better, of a change, does not confirm that the change is responsible for even appropriate symptoms. In other words, back pain may be situational far more often than it is the result of disc narrowing and treatments that regard it as a consequence of an organic change are usually doomed to failure. Therefore, many operations on the spine or the nerves fail to work as well as desired.

Folk wisdom is often just that; a pain in the neck and an aching back are recognized for what they are, and it is people and events, not structural changes, that are obviously blamed. Rehabilitation in any condition, particularly in the arthritic disorders in which life's quality, not its quantity, is threatened must become cognizant of all these factors to achieve success. And success may not mean that all people are made alike, and that someone with a deficit will totally lose that deficit. Success may require a more modest goal. However, the many quadriplegic victims of accidents and the ankylosed or flail-jointed victims of virulent arthritis who compose music, write books, and paint, even by holding brushes or pens in the mouth, may achieve more success and gratification in such limited achievements than many unencumbered individuals. The acquisition of deficits can be neutralized, as the rheumatoid arthritic Renoir and Raoul Dufy and the sclerodermatous Paul Klee proved, not to mention the many other artists who suffered from other, nonrheumatic, disorders (the deaf Beethoven, the blind Homer, and so ad infinitum). If we are what we accomplish, then each step forward improves mankind. There are not many professions that can vie with rehabilitation in that.

And last, but most important, rehabilitation is education. It is that concept that gives normative impetus to the book that follows. Despite tugs in both directions, we have attempted to keep a balance between the solipsistic ways of immunologists, who bid fair to take over rheumatology, and the antinomian professional rehabilitationists. In the middle ground lies education for the professional and for those ministered to as well. Legislative attempts to remedy ills can best achieve their aims by addressing education primarily. A succinct summary of the results has it that one thus progresses from yearning to learning to earning.

While not all areas of rehabilitation of arthritis are as fully covered in this book as others, this volume is meant to compliment my earlier book Total Management of the Arthritic Patient, although it can certainly stand alone.

GEORGE E. EHRLICH, M.D.

Acknowledgments

When a book finally appears, all the effort that went into it seems worthwhile, but only the editor and his authors share the credit for the completed work. Many others labored to make it possible, and I hereby cite John Basmajian, who encouraged and commissioned this work; James Sangston, who took over as in-house editor in midstream and patiently awaited completion; to Diana Welch, Production Editor, and Carol Eckhart, Production Coordinator, for their efforts throughout the production of the book; Mrs. Janet VanArtsdalen, my Administrative and Executive Secretary, who kept order; and Patricia Ochs, who had the thankless task of typing and retyping. Miss Marcia Poland, formerly my Administrative Secretary, started it all. My wife put up with the ill temper that delays can bring, and the contributors were good-humored in the face of my importuning and my editorial suggestions and revisions. Dr. Ved Gupta, for years my associate, added to his schedule to lighten mine. A parade of Fellows through the years eased my burden as well: Doctors David Bevan, Victor Labbate, Alan Mallace, George Wineburgh, Mori Schwartzberg, Robert Freed, Moshe Revach, Norman Brodsky, Michael Perilstein, Sallyann Bowman, Mark Keeley, Bernard Rubin, and Eileen Moynihan; and Naomi Kaplinsky, back for a reprise during a year of study leave. To my students and colleagues who were the testing ground for some of these concepts, my thanks as well.

GEORGE E. EHRLICH, M.D.

Contributors

Steven L. Abrams
Political Consultant
Philadelphia, Pennsylvania

Warren L. Benson
Executive Director
Arthritis Foundation
Southern Arizona Chapter
Community Liaison
Southwest Arthritis Center
University of Arizona
Tucson, Arizona

Michael H. Boblitz, O.T.R.
Assistant Professor
Department of Orthopedics and Rehabilitation
University of Virginia School of Medicine
Charlottesville, Virginia

Mary P. Brassell, R.N., B.S.
Rehabilitation Arthritis Nurse Specialist
Arthritis Center
Moss Rehabilitation Hospital
Philadelphia, Pennsylvania

John A. Downey, M.D., D. Phil. (Oxon)
Simon Baruch Professor and Chairman
Department of Rehabilitation Medicine
College of Physicians and Surgeons
Columbia University
New York, New York

Judy L. Erfling, M.S.W.
Social Service Department
Rose Medical Center
Denver, Colorado

Hanna Gruen, B.S., O.T.R.
Private Practice and Consultation
Essex House
Essex Square
Apt. 1506
Pittsburgh, Pennsylvania

Mark S. Kauffman, M.D.
Former Assistant Clinical Professor
Orthopedic Surgery and Physical Medicine
Temple University
School of Medicine
Sarasota Memorial Hospital
Sarasota, Florida

Colleen Cavanah Miller, R.N., M.S.N.
Arthritis Clinical Nurse Specialist
Rose Medical Center
Denver, Colorado
Clinical Senior Instructor
University of Colorado
Health Sciences Center
Denver, Colorado

Pauline H. E. Neubauer, M.C.P.A.
Director of Physiotherapy Services
The Arthritis Society B. C. Division
Vancouver, Canada

Janice Smith Pigg, R.N., B.S.N.
Nurse Consultant Rheumatology
Rheumatic Disease Program
Columbia Hospital
Milwaukee, Wisconsin

Jean Porta, M.S., Ph.D.
Division of Biometry and Health Information Systems
University of Minnesota
Minneapolis, Minnesota

Evelyn Rossky, O.T.R.
Occupational Therapy Department
Moss Rehabilitation Hospital
Philadelphia, Pennsylvania

Richard D. Roth, D.P.M.
Assistant Professor, Department of Medicine
Pennsylvania College of Podiatric Medicine
Philadelphia, Pennsylvania
Former Podiatric Fellow in Clinical Rheumatology
Albert Einstein Medical Center
Northern Division
Philadelphia, Pennsylvania

Sanford H. Roth, M.D.
Director of the Phoenix Arthritis Center
Chairman of the Rheumatology Section
St. Luke's Hospital
Phoenix, Arizona
Honorary Chairman of the Antiinflammatory
Drug Study Group (American Rheumatism Association)
International Consulting Editor of *Drugs* (Published by ADIS)
Phoenix, Arizona

Philip Spergel, Ed. D.
Director of Psychological Services
Moss Rehabilitation Hospital
Assistant Clinical Professor of Rehabilitation Medicine
Temple University Medical School
Philadelphia, Pennsylvania

Robert L. Swezey, M.D., F.A.C.P.
Medical Director
The Arthritis & Back Pain Center, Inc.
Santa Monica, California
Clinical Professor of Medicine
UCLA School of Medicine

CONTENTS

1

Arthritis Rehabilitation: Staff, Facilities, and Evaluation

ROBERT L. SWEZEY

Staff—Who Does It? (The Arthritis Health Care Team—Why Are We Where We Are?)

Rehabilitation management of the arthritic patient is a medical Humpty Dumpty. By the time "rehabilitation" penetrates the consciousness of the arthritis patient's physician, the "great fall" has occurred and Humpty Dumpty is a fragmented and multifaceted mess. The setting for arthritis rehabilitation should, and often does, begin in the primary physician's office. The complexities of some rheumatic diseases, their chronicity, and the extent of their impact on the patient-family-economic interfaces tend to overwhelm the primary physician. Lack of experience with the spectrum of therapeutic strategies and limited resources available to the primary physician generate a "band-aide" palliative approach consisting of: some antiinflammatory therapy, advice to "take it easy" and to "keep those joints from 'freezing up,'" coupled with haphazard exercise recommendations and little, if any, constructive guidance. The primary physician can effectively implement a rehabilitation program for his arthritic, neck or back pain patient by carefully monitoring both his diagnostic and therapeutic strategies and moving rapidly to consultative "back-up" by rheumatology, orthopaedics, psychiatry, physiatry, and social and psychological counseling where available. These professional resources are not, however, always available and if available are not commonly found integrated in an organized facility. Therefore, referral to a facility that has such organization and is prepared to provide comprehensive therapy for rheumatic diseases may be required. It cannot be emphasized too strenuously or too often that early comprehensive planning for catastrophic disorders (any disorder that necessitates a meaningful change or a patient's perception of such a change in his life style) is the key to a healthy adjustment and to a satisfactory therapeutic outcome.

Just as the primary physician may be limited or handicapped in his sophistication or his access to resources needed to cope with any unrelenting rheumatological problem, his consultants may also be unable to sort out adequately either the diagnostic specifics or therapeutic strategies essential to a desirable resolution of a given patient's problem. The *rheumatologist* may be able to identify and categorize the nature of an inflammatory joint disorder, but is all too often reliant on pharmacological therapies with increasing spectra of toxicities for his treatment program. Alternatively, or simultaneously, he may refer a patient for physical therapy to a therapist who has little understanding of rheumatic diseases and perhaps less specific knowledge about their rehabilitative management. The arthritis patient may then be treated as though he had suffered either a stroke or recent trauma—to no avail.

Psychiatric problems (depression, anxiety, and iatrogenic and organic difficulties) may compound the picture. Unless the consulting *psychiatrist* is aware of the rheumatological vagaries, sensitive to the need for short-term directive psychiatric intervention, and is available for close coordination of psychiatric-medical-surgical-social management, the hoped-for benefits from psychiatric referral may not be realized. The *orthopaedic* consultant must be experienced in the management of rheumatic diseases and related musculoskeletal disorders. He must be aware of the role for and proper application of nonsurgical therapy, the limitations of and indications for surgical interventions, and he must have the sophistication to judge the appropriate timing and sequencing of indicated surgeries. He must be highly experienced in the surgical techniques he uses or capable of critically evaluating and assessing any innovative procedures he may select—there are currently more than fifty different total knee operations! The *physiatrist* must be experienced in the management of arthritic conditions. The coordination of therapy regimens with other health care "team" members must be closely supervised to assure that nonsurgical "orthopaedic" measures are appropriately instituted, carried out, and reassessed.

The bottom line is that a coordinated, comprehensive treatment or rehabilitation program for the arthritic patient must consist of more than a series of referrals to "appropriate" specialists—it must consist of a smoothly coordinated constellation of interactions directed by a responsible physician in concert with needed consultants who have specialized knowledge, experience, and judgment in their respective disciplines and in the treatment of the arthritic disorders per se.

The *allied health professional "team"* consists of physical (physio) therapists, occupational therapists, psychologists, social workers, nurses, patient educators, vocational counselors, podiatrists, orthotists, dietitian-nutritionists and all other professionals and paraprofessionals who may at a given time interact with the arthritis patient. Even when all of these disciplines are housed under one roof, it becomes extremely unwieldly and expensive to coordinate and integrate their activities. Timing of appointments, inflexibilities of departmental scheduling, personality conflicts, territoriality of health professions within institutions, and economic constraints all conspire to disassemble organizational efforts to make the "team approach" work (1–3).

The sum may be less than the total of its parts. Unfortunately even where there is teamwork, a lack of sophistication about arthritic diseases and the specifics of their management may make the best intended and coordinated effort come to naught. Very few of our allied health professionals have had more than one or two lectures on arthritic diseases in their undergraduate training. Rarely are these lectures given by persons who are knowledgeble about rehabilitation therapies, and even more rarely are highly specific rehabilitation therapies for the arthritis patient taught—let alone learned (4). From the standpoint of rheumatological rehabilitation some of the more glaring problems in the various allied health professions are the following.

PHYSICAL THERAPY

A lack of knowledge about the type, frequency, intensity of exercise therapies, and regimens for specific problems, e.g., how many repetitions of a given range of motion exercise (and what is the basis for selection of that exercise) for a moderately contractured shoulder associated with biceps tendinitis is optimal 1. to maintain range of motion, 2. to increase range of motion without causing aggravation of the underlying problem? Should the number of exercises per session be repeated once, twice, or ten times per day? Should resistive exercises be implemented, and if so how—isometrically, isotonically, isokinetically? How long should an isometric contraction be held and in what position? How many repetitions of an isotonic contraction should be performed and against how much resistance, and for how many times per day, per week, and for how many weeks? Should modalities (heat, cold) be prescribed in conjunction with exercise, before, during, after—if so, what modality and for how long—and why?

What bases are used to determine the indication for the use of one or more therapy modalities, the duration and frequency of their use, and the point at which one determines that the modalities are no longer of value in the patient's management?

OCCUPATIONAL THERAPY

The emphasis in many schools of occupational therapy is on psychosocial and eduational aspects of patient care rather than on physical disability management. Few occupational therapists have either specific knowledge about rheumatic diseases or have received supervised instruction from occupational therapists with that knowledge (4). The result is a hodgepodge of therapeutic assumptions and strategies that deal in generalities, but lack the sophistication needed for the evaluation of patient function, appropriate and precise training in joint protection, appropriate applications of splints and determination of their indications, and adaptations of functional activities to reinforce exercise therapy as well as apropriate body mechanics. The stress on the psychosocial aspects of occupational therapy training leads to problems of confusion in allied health professional role identification. Inevitable conflicts with psychology, social service, nursing, patient education, and physical therapy arise when occupational therapists and others attempt to establish their "turf" in the fringe areas of group activities, relaxation therapy, biofeedback and the like, and these conflicts become more intense and acute vis-á-vis psychological testing, counseling, and behavior modification programs.

PSYCHOLOGY-SOCIAL WORK

All of the previous mentioned sources of tension and confusion are exacerbated by the problems of splitting off psychological counseling from the psychiatrist on the one hand, and the social worker-psychiatric social worker and a variety of newly emerging lay and professional counselors (marriage counselors, death and dying counselors, and "holistic" health coordinators) on the other hand. The psychologist has a reasonable grasp on the domain of psychological testing, but can be in competition with a variety of other health professionals, and with the social worker in particular, in many of our rehabilitation settings for the privilege of counseling both individuals and groups.

The medical social workers tend to put some distance (usually as much as possible) between themselves and the traditional social problem solving aspects of patient care (e.g., meeting patient survival needs such as clothing, food, transportation, and shelter) for the more prestigious role of psychosocial counselor. Forays into patient education and even relaxation therapy by social workers are being reported as the social service profession attempts to "upgrade" its image and survive as a "cost effective" entity in the health care field. Conflict in institutions between the social worker and discharge planning nurse coordinators can be an additional source of confusion and inefficiency in the rehabilitation of the arthritis patient.

The nursing profession has emerged as a powerful resource in our health delivery system. A variety of specialists ranging from physician assistants to nurse's aides now adorn the nursing profession landscape. The idealized image promulgated by the nursing profession in this age of "person" liberation is no longer one of of a dedicated nurturing servant, but rather that of a sophisticated applied scientist-educator-administrator. The muscle exercised by the politicized nursing profession has provided it with real power in determining the allocation of resources in medical institutions. Today this professional nursing resource, already in short supply, is now moving into an ever expanding role development. Unfortunately, this can be at the expense of already highly trained and qualified existing health professionals and administrative specialists. Insistence that discharge planning and counseling be performed by a nurse and that patient education be taught and performed by nurses—regardless of qualifications of nonnursing professionals—has probably contributed in no small way to the dislocation of other allied health professionals, the distortion of their roles, and an aggravation of the nurse shortage.

There is no question about the appropriateness of the role of the specially trained rehabilitation nurse in a rehabilitation setting. The rehabilitation nursing staff is the key to the success of a comprehensive care program. The nursing staff is responsible for the round-the-clock monitoring and implementation of prescribed rehabilitation therapy programs. For these programs to be carried out effectively, the nursing staff cannot be fragmented in their responsibilities and expected to provide both acute general medical or surgical nursing care and comprehensive rehabilitation nursing care, because the pressing demands of the former preclude adequate attention to the latter. The priorities of rehabilitation nursing cannot be subservient to other needs, and ideally, arthritis rehabilitation care requires a segregated patient care unit.

PATIENT EDUCATOR

Health education has been everybody's business and nobody's business. The school or community health educator trained in education theory and practices as well as in elementary physiology and concepts of healthful living, sex education, and applied psychology has been called upon increasingly to develop specific programs in patient education. Today, many of our health care institutions and facilities and most of the categorical diseases or organ-oriented community health agencies (e.g., the Arthritis Foundation) have a patient education component. The responsibility of the health-patient educator to make himself highly knowledgeable about the diseases and disorders for which he assumes responsibility for education is implicit. The television channels, newspapers, and magazines are creating a constant infusion of arthritis related information for the public. If a patient goes to the library for better information about arthritis, he is likely to have to choose from a selection of books that are written predominantly by poorly informed lay authors and quacks. The health educator (or nurse patient educator) unless specially trained is often in no better position than the librarian when it comes to making a selection of what to teach about a specific disease, and he may contribute little that is helpful in arthritis patient education, no matter how skilled he may be in the application of educational theories.

VOCATIONAL COUNSELOR

The major concern of the vocational counselor is with job placement for the handicapped. Social, psychological counseling and specific knowledge and skills in job planning and training are requisites to the proper function of this health profession. The vocational counselor usually works out of a governmental organizational base and contracts to a varied extent with other health professionals for supplemental services. In this way the conflicts and overlaps of other health professionals may be minimized.

It should by now be obvious that the underlying theme of this discussion thus far is that there are far too few health professionals, including those who by title or other designation are considered to have specialized knowledge about the therapy of arthritis and related musculoskeletal disorders, who are truly competent to administer their therapies to the rheumatic disease patient no matter what the setting for that therapy may be (3–5). It is clear that research and training in rheumatological rehabilitation therapies from the level of the rheumatologist to and including all other physician and allied health professionals is deficient (4, 5). The priorities of our medical schools, our governmental institutions, and of the Arthritis Foundation have not included much more than lip service and token gestures to the various disciplines concerned with this aspect of arthritis care (with the possible single exception of the tremendous impetus given to joint replacement surgery) (4).

The lame hope that allied health professionals can do the bulk of their research independently of physicians belies the lack of background and training that the majority of these people has in research methodologies. It also ignores the obvious fact that most clinical research must rely on a physician for diagnosis and control of therapeutic variables (6). Incentives must, therefore, be created to involve interested and knowledgeable physicians in research in the various basic and applied aspects of rheumatological rehabilitation therapy so that coordination with qualified allied health professionals as coinvestigators can lead to a rational and cost-effective approach to rheumatological-rehabilitative therapies—appropriate to the setting in which they are administered.

Facilities—Where Do They Do It?

Just as a family practitioner cannot command the full array of integrated medical and surgical services for every arthritis sufferer, the small hospital in a community without the requisite specialized professionals must also make compromises. However, where the essential institutional and staff capabilities exist every effort should be made to address the issues of maximizing the effectiveness of comprehensive rehabilitative therapies. Even when resources are limited and the practitioner's office setting is equipped with a no-nonsense, no frills decor, many opportunities can be easily created to provide arthritis patients with the basic rehabilitative therapies. This section will attempt to delineate some of these opportunities, particularly as they apply to ambulatory care settings.

For the purpose of this discussion rehabilitative therapies include all of the aspects of patient management exclusive of conventional medical-pharmacological treatments and surgical procedures. Rehabilitation therapy for arthritis patients can be divided further into those *activities that enhance function and protect joints* against damage (activities of daily living (ADL) and functional adaptations), *modalities for pain relief* (including hydrotherapy), *exercises to maintain or restore mobility and strength* (including tank or pool therapy), and *counseling and environmental manipulations* designed to optimize coping for the arthritis sufferer—patient education, psychological, social, diet counseling, and vocational training.

In Table 1.1 the various therapies that can be adapted to the major categories of facilities for rheumatological health care are outlined. At each level of complexity of the facilities, the therapeutic options of the preceding level are retained and/or expanded to meet the additional capabilities for arthritis rehabilitation therapy of the larger and more complex facility and staff. Although the severely disabled arthritis patient, and those suffering from acute complications, severe systemic disease, or requiring surgical procedures, or those patients needing intensive multidisciplined services unavailable in their own communities may require acute in-hospital or convalescent care, *the vast majority of patients suffering from rheumatological disorders are preferably treated as outpatients.*

In order to implement the need to provide a practical facility for comprehensive care for patients suffering from arthritis and related disorders, the author designed and developed an ambulatory care facility (The Arthritis & Back Pain Center, Inc., A Medical Clinic). The Center's physical arrangements and staff are organized to meet most of the basic needs of comprehensive rheumatological care.

The Arthritis & Back Pain Center is specifically designed to provide two full-time rheumatologists with a competent multidisciplined supporting staff comprised of full-time, part-time and consulting health professionals, all of whom provide care for the patients at the Center. The basic staff configuration is outlined in Table 1.2. Figure 1.1 shows the facility floor plan and the location of therapy equipment and the arrangement of rehabilitative training and educational media and materials.

The configuration of any facility ideally reflects the architectural precept that form follows function. The Arthritis & Back Pain Center was designed after careful analysis of patient and staff traffic flow based on the assumption that on a fully scheduled day the two physicians would each see two consultations requiring an hour each and each would see in addition approximately twelve patients in 30-min follow-up visits. The distribution of diagnosis of the patients seen should, and does, reflect that customarily seen in rheumatological practice (7). The rehabilitative therapy needs including initial evaluations by physical and occupational therapists, therapeutic

TABLE 1.1. *Arthritis Rehabilitation Therapies in Various Settings*

Setting	Activities of Daily Living	Exercise Therapy	Modalities	Education
1-2 M.D. office	Orthopedic seating* in: waiting room, M.D. office, examining rooms, business office Adjustable height lab chair Portable raised toilet seat—restrooms Grab bars and rails Levers on door handles and on faucets Long handle: comb, shoehorn, dust pan Built-up handles: hairbrush, pen Loops on drawer pulls Lab refrigerator storage Step stool, footstool Parking lot—auto evaluation	Adjustable height therapy table (serves as exam table) Full length mirror Over door traction Over door pulley Belt/dental dam Beachball Adjustable cane, crutches	Cold pack Ice cups Moist heat pack (automatic) Paraffin Ultrasound Fluorimethane spray bottle	Pamphlets Basic patient education references Furniture and equipment catalogs Slides Models Audiotapes Therapy and consultant referral information Equipment resources files Bulletin board Posters
Group practice	Adjustable height chair and table (drafting type) in business office or lounge Shower/tub transfer seat, hose modifications, grab rails EKG room adjustable hospital bed Office storage lightweight objects high or low heavy bulky objects at counter height	Mat Walker, adjustable Wheelchair with adjustable foot rests, arm rests and brake extensions	Hot pack Diathermy Shower Tub with whirlpool Small extremity whirlpool	Blackboard Caramate Cine (motion pictures) Film strips Library
Rheumatology ambula-	O.T.—demonstration	Therapy office	Transcutaneous	Video-replay

tory care center	kitchen/office/shop (splinting and equipment adaptations) EKG—demonstration bedroom—dressing training area Bathroom—hydro, grooming training area O.T. desk; business office; M.D. office—work simulation areas Waiting room—low, middle, and raised garden beds lightweight tools with handle modified for joint and back protection instruction Car seat, back rests	Gym Raised mat area (group therapy) Open area—posture and exercise Mirrored walls Reciprocal pulleys Gait training areas (hall, stairs, parallel bars) Variable height split traction table Variety of canes, crutches, walkers Bicycle Restorator Treadmill Portable isokinetic exerciser	nerve stimulation Biofeedback	In-house miltipurpose consultation and counseling office for psychological, social, nutrition education Self-instructional program
Small community hospital	Bedroom dressing-transfer training area Light activity adjustable table with overhead suspension grid	Tilt table Multipurpose exercise table Gurney	Hubbard tank Hydraulic hoist	Nurse station Cafeteria—dining
University hospital referral center	Prevocational testing training area Orthotic department Furniture modification area Auto modification area Driver retraining Indoor-outdoor therapeutic gardening instruction area Home-community-school-work site visit capability Research laboratories	Multistation isokinetic exercise apparatus Adaptive recreation and exercise conditioning gym Outdoor physical training area	Therapeutic pool Power patient hoist	Dining-social recreation areas Classroom Closed circuit TV

* At least one tall, firm padded arm chair.

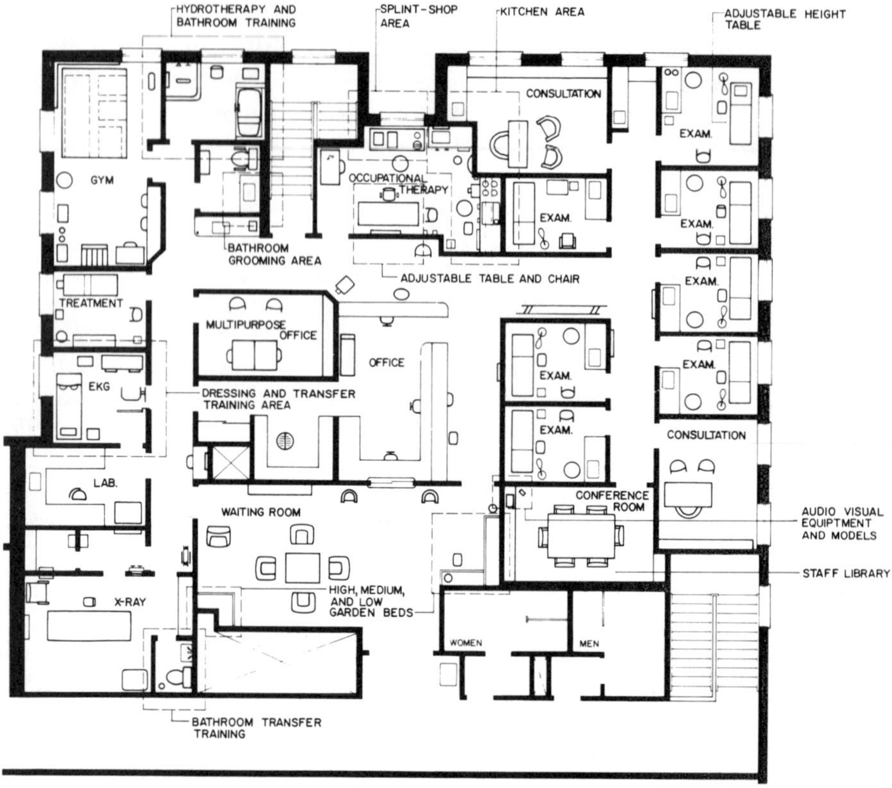

Fig. 1.1. Arthritis and Back Pain Center, Inc. floor plan.

therapy gymnasium area in the Center is a moderate sized room situated between the hydrotherapy-bathroom training area and a separate treatment-traction-modality room. The gymnasium contains a large elevated mat which is used for individual and group exercise therapy. The adjacent walls are mirrored for visual monitoring by the patients of their exercise and body mechanics. The variety of demonstration canes, crutches, walkers, corsets, and braces are stored in the gymnasium area. A wheelchair with multiple adjustments for arm and leg rests and brake handle extensions to facilitate its use by arthritis patients with limited ambulation abilities is kept in the nearby hall. The wheelchair is used to transport patients who are unable to walk from the parking area. The physical therapists' desks and files, hot and cold pack units, reciprocal pulleys, and essential exercise equipment are also situated in the gymnasium area.

Basic to the philosophy in the design of the Center is the provision for demonstrations of therapeutic options and regimens that can be adapted to the patient's home, work, or recreational locales. The two lavatories serve their customary functions for the Center, but each additionally provides a room in which a selection of raised toilet seats, toilet rails, grab bars, and

different faucet configurations can be tried. The bathrooms also contain a number of grooming assistive devices such as toothbrushes with built-up handles, long-handled combs, toothpaste tube squeezers, and one-handed nail clippers.

Hydrotherapy consists of a large standard bathtub with a commercial conversion to a multijet whirlpool. Tub transfer techniques are taught with the use of tub-attached grab rails and in-tub seating. Adjustable hoses and nozzles for in-tub showering for the seated or standing patient can also be demonstrated. A separate wall shower has two levels of faucet knobs to facilitate adjustment of water flow for patients who are showering when either seated or standing. There are two different types of shower heads which offer various combinations of jet and massaging pulsations so that patients can experience these options for possible home therapy use. Grab rails and low and high shower seats are used to teach safe transfer and showering methods.

One treatment room is equipped with an electric adjustable hospital bed so that patients can learn proper bed transfers and bed positioning. The decor of this room is that of a bedroom with the bedspread designed to cover the bed in order to minimize its hospital-like appearance. This bed serves as an auxiliary treatment table, rest area for patients (and staff) between treatments or after procedures, and as the electrocardiogram (EKG) station. An armoire in this room has a multilevel, adjustable clothes hanger, and is used to assist in the teaching of dressing skills. Various assistive devices such as reachers, long-handled shoehorns, prism spectacles (to allow patients with immobilized or rigid necks to read in bed), stocking and trouser donning assistive devices, and shoe removers are used in this room. The "bedroom" door is suspended on offset hinges designed to maximize clearance for wheelchair access, and it is also used to teach home cervical traction with an over-door traction suspension apparatus.

There are several important features in the waiting room that merit additional comment. The overall purpose of the waiting room, in addition to providing temporary seating for patients and their families and for its occasional use as a classroom, is to initiate awareness of good seating and body mechanics. The chairs provide various height configurations and arm and back supports. A custom car seat is placed against a decorative background mural depicting an automobile and is used to demonstrate a possible seating option for patients who cannot drive comfortably in standard car seats. Adjacent to the car seat area is a low garden bed, and on an opposing wall a middle level and a standing height level indoor garden are situated. The gardens not only fulfill a decorative purpose, but along with lightweight gardening tools, and tools carefully selected for their handle design or with adapted and built-up handles, serve as a demonstration area for hand joint protection and body mechanics screening and training. Different gradations of gravel in the low raking bed and in the middle level or seated gardening

bed can be used to grade the stresses and tolerances suitable for various patient problems. Reading and writing accessories for use in registering new patients or by patients and their families in the waiting room are designed for ease of use and to minimize joint stress.

The occupational therapy area features a small model kitchen in which the efficiencies of microwave cooking as well as the optimal use of a standard oven can be demonstrated. Knobs with large hand loops and grips designed to protect the small arthritic hand joints are used on the easily opened cupboard doors and drawers. A sturdy but easily pulled drawer has a butcher block work surface and is built into the kitchen counter area. When pulled out it can be used to facilitate wheelchair or seated kitchen activities. The counter surface has a flush line burner unit designed so that the lightweight, large handled pots and pans can be slid rather than lifted whenever possible. The overhead shelves are protruded to accommodate restricted shoulder mobility and to minimize reaching stress and strains that might be imposed on the neck, arm, or back (8). Storage of heavy articles at counter level and light or bulky objects below or above is also demonstrated. Footstools and various reachers, can openers, kitchen aides, easily opened storage containers, and hanging pots are also demonstrated in the therapy programs.

The occupational therapy area also has a workbench used for splint fabrication and equipment adaptation. The various hand tools have also been selected for ease of use by patients with upper extremity joint problems. The occupational therapist's desk and chair also serve as a work area demonstration facility. The telephone is equipped with a device attached to the desk that supports the speaker-receiver unit so that the patient does not have to hold a telephone in an arthritic hand or awkwardly cradle the telephone between the ear and the shoulder when suffering from a cervical disorder. All furniture and equipment items are catalogued and labeled so that the patients can, if indicated, readily order them from the providers. The occupational therapy area also serves as an informal conference room, a staff lunch room, and as the Center's minor repair and workshop.

In addition to the major treatment work areas, the Center utilizes one portion of a wide hall as a gait training area. There is a measured 50-foot walk, and there are parallel bars 10 feet in length that fold up to occupy minimal hall space when not in use. When opened the parallel bars are used in conjunction with a mirror placed at the end of the hall. A rear access staircase serves as a secluded area for stair climbing intruction. The parking lot adjacent to the building that houses the Center is also used to assess patients' car seating positions, back supports, and transfer techniques.

The business office is used to assess and teach body mechanics in a simulated work setting. The file drawer keys are placed in a rigid key holder designed to give greater leverage for patients with weak or painful hands. The laboratory has an adjustable height chair with the seat tilted slightly forward to facilitate working over a microscope or at similar tasks. In the physicians' offices the executive chairs and auxiliary seats serve as additional examples of well-designed seating, and the desk surface is angled to minimize neck stress, particularly for bifocal wearers with cervical disorders (8).

The staff library serves as a formal patient or staff conference area. Audiovisual equipment, including movie and slide projectors and screen, and video equipment for patient and staff education, are stored for viewing here. The Center has a video camera used for recording demonstrations of exercise treatment programs for staff as well as for patient education. The video camera is also used to help selected patients with problems learning exercise or body mechanics review themselves during a video replay. Anatomical models of the spine hands, shoulder, hip, knee, and foot are stored in the conference room when not in use for patient education in the treatment areas.

A multipurpose office serves as a consultation, small group counseling, psychological testing and privacy area for the consulting and regular staff. This provides the consulting staff with a formal location at the Center in which to see patients. Care is taken so that two consultants are not scheduled for the same time. The conference room and physicians' offices if not otherwise employed permit additional latitude in the scheduling of consultants and related activities. The patient and staff seating in the multipurpose office is also selected to demonstrate well-designed chairs.

Thus in a relatively compact facility most of the problems and activities that patients with rheumatological disorders might face in the course of a day or night can be assessed and solved under the supervision of a trained staff person. Ideally, every patient should be seen with his family and coworkers in his home or work situation, but the varieties of simulated situations provided at the Center—coupled with the various options for problem solving that can actually be tried on the premises—greatly minimizes the need for such site visits. In Table 1.1 the desired expansion of the facilities to meet the capabilities provided by a small community hospital and a regional arthritis referral center are outlined. The details of the organization and equipment requirements of these facilities can be found elsewhere (9–13). More important is the indication in Table 1.1 of rehabilitation therapy opportunities that can be readily instituted in the office of a generalist or a small group practice. The specific areas for demonstration of proper seating (physicians' offices, business office, laboratory, waiting room, patient examining rooms); bathroom transfer training (elevated toilet seat, grab bars, faucet levers, dressing and grooming aids); household adaptations (footstools, reachers, drawer knobs, storage arrangements); basic home gym equipment (elastic belt, beachball, adjustable cane); and automobile seating assessment (parking lot) applicable to almost any physician's office are listed (8, 14–16). Many of the features delineated in the foregoing discussion can be readily adapted to a variety of medical settings to help create an effective patient education awareness and training milieu.

Evaluation of Function—How Do They Know If They Did It?

If one is to design a facility to provide optimal rheumatological therapy, it is incumbent on the provider to determine if the patient's ability to function improves as a consequence of the treatment (measurement of outcome) and if and how the various components of therapy impacted on that outcome (measurement of process). Smits (17) has candidly added to these purposes for evaluation: the "vindication" of an approach, "salesmanship" for a particular treatment facility, and "security" for the health care provider that his programs can somehow be justified.

In a recent critical analysis Stewart et al. (18) defined good health in terms of functioning as "the performance of our capacity to perform activities that are normal for individuals in good health. Early attempts at classifying functional disability for the arthritic patient have focused on very gross descriptions of overall function (19, 20) (see Table 1.3). These criteria have provided useful thumbnail-sketch categorizations of gross levels of disability, but they lack the sensitivity and specificity to capture meaningful but less inclusive changes in function that may come about as a consequence of therapy or other changes in the status of a disease (21, 22).

At the opposite extreme are the activity of daily living (ADL) evaluations that are almost all-inclusive in their inventories of the various tasks that we all face in getting through each day. They can include literally everything from shoeshining to shampooing and golfing (divot digging) to ditch digging (23). For selected patients this kind of inventory may be essential to problem solving and rehabilitation therapy, but it is clearly impractical as a tool to

TABLE 1.3. *Functional Criteria*

American Rheumatism Association (U.S.A.)

1. Performs all usual activities without handicaps.
2. Performs adequately for normal activities despite discomfort occasionally in one or more joints.
3. Limited to little or no activities or usual occupation or self-care.
4. Largely or wholly incapacitated, bed-ridden, or confined to wheelchair, little or no self-care (19).

Joint Committee (Great Britain)

- Grade 1. Fully employed or employable in the usual work and able to undertake normal physical recreation.
- Grade 2. Doing light or part-time work and only limited physical recreation. For housewives, all except the heaviest housework.
- Grade 3. Not employed and unemployable. No physical recreations. Housewives, only light housework and limited shopping.
- Grade 4. Confined to house or wheelchair, but able to look after oneself and essentials of life. Hospital patients confined to bed.
- Grade 5. Completely bedridden (20).

Adapted from R. L. Swezey, *Arthritis: Rational Therapy and Rehabilitation*, W. B. Saunders, Philadelphia, 1978. Reprinted with permission of the publisher.

measure repetitively patients' progress in therapy. Gersten et al. (24) correlated joint mobility, strength, and a lengthy list of ADL activities and demonstrated the considerable overlap in these various measurements and the numerous redundancies in the ADL measurements per se.

An abbreviated self-administered inventory of patient activities (exclusive of psychosocial factors) has twelve categories of functional activity chosen to identify major and common functional deficits. This inventory has been successfully utilized in several arthritis clinics to determine needs for rehabilitation therapies (see Table 1.4) (25).

Two self-administered inventories designed to measure function in arthritis patients have been carefully studied from the standpoint of reliability and reproducibility of measures (22, 26). Both of these indices meet the additional requisites that they are easily administered and require little time to complete, as well as to score. The index described by Lee et al. (22), asks seventeen questions and requires but 2 min to complete. The method of Convery et al. (26) has 16 major categories of inquiry and a maximum of 64 possible questions (four in each category) which conceivably could require answering by a patient essentially totally disabled. Both of these methods have been found to provide highly reproducible scores when tested by various physicians, allied health professionals, and lay interviewers, and the method of Convery et al. was validated when used by two different institutions as well as by a telephone interview (22, 26). Both of these methods correlate well with the American Rheumatism Association (ARA) functional classification (1–4) and additionally provide more specific descriptions of the nature of the disability (19). They also avoid the classic pitfall of the ARA criteria whereby a nonambulatory patient with good use of his upper extremities (ARA class 4) is scaled below a more severely limited patient who is still able to walk short distances (ARA class 3) and vice versa (8, 19, 26).

The search for a practical and reproducible measure of function owes a great debt to the pioneering work of Barthel (27) and the adaptations for computer analysis of Barthel's criteria to an *objectively* scored Functional Status Measurement for use in a variety of disabling conditions studied by Granger and Greer (28). Convery et al. (26) adapted their arthritis functional assessment from the format put forth by Granger and Greer (28). The work of Granger et al. and a number of other authors, most notably Donaldson et al., Katz et al., Mahoney et al., Schoening and Iverson, and Scranton et al., raises the important question of whether or not objective data are preferable to a subjective inquiry as an instrument in the assessment of function (26, 28–33). The measurement of function is really an attempt to determine what behavior one can expect of or observe in a given patient. It seems ideal to quantify by objective tests a patient's actual ability to perform his essential functions (21). As a practical matter in any test situation one must arbitrarily select specific "representative" tasks and then develop a scoring system for

TABLE 1.4.
Rheumatic Disease Self-Assessment of Function

Dear Patient,
In order to help us learn whether you will need therapy in addition to the medicine prescribed for you, please fill out this form.
DIAGNOSIS
USUAL VOCATION (housewife, carpenter, etc.):
IF NOT EMPLOYED, retired?
Don't know
EMPLOYED?
YES
NO
on disability?
Please check (√) the best answer for you.

HOW MUCH PAIN and/or DIFFICULTY (stiffness, weakness, loss of balance) DO YOU HAVE WITH THE FOLLOWING ACTIVITIES?	AMOUNT			FREQUENCY	
	None	Some	Much	Sometimes	Usually
1. EATING:					
Cutting meat, drinking from a cup, etc.					
2. DRESSING:					
Arms and upper part of body					
Legs and lower part of body					
Fastening buttons, zippers, or snaps					
3. GENERAL HAND ACTIVITIES:					
Using key, writing, dialing phone					
Opening jars, drawers, or doors					
4. LIFTING:					
Holding objects					
Bending to pick up objects					
5. PERSONAL HYGIENE:					
Brushing teeth, combing hair, shaving					
Toileting after-care (wiping, washing, etc.)					
6. MOBILITY:					
Getting on and/or off toilet					
Getting into and/or out of chair					
bed					
car					
tub					
shower					
Walking inside home					
Walking outside home					
Walking up and/or down stairs					
7. HOME ACTIVITIES:					
Gardening					
Housekeeping					
Cooking					
Laundry					
8. ANY OTHER ACTIVITIES?					

9. How TIRED ARE YOU after an average day's activity?
Slightly Moderately Extremely Not at all
10. Do you perform any HOME EXERCISE PROGRAM? Yes No
If YES, was it prescribed by a doctor or therapist? Yes No
11. Check any of the following which you presently use:
Splints Canes or crutches Wheelchair Other aids None
12. What is your usual means of TRANSPORTATION? Drive self
Driven by family or friend Public transportation (taxi, bus, or van)

Table 2.4 is adapted from R.L. Swezey, *Arthritis: Rational Therapy and Rehabilitation* (Philadelphia: W.B. Saunders, 1978). Reprinted with permission of the publisher.

each task that can be scaled so that differences between scores for individual test subsets (e.g., subset under ambulation: 1. unable, 2. with great difficulty, 3. normal) and between various subsets are accurately reflected. There are two additional considerations that arise in attempting to quantify changes in function. One is that a limitation of function (such as stair climbing in an arthritic patient with cardiovascular disease) may actually reflect a usual (nonarthritic) level of function (34). Another is that the patient may perform at a high level in a test situation or in an institution environment and yet in his own home setting require assistance at the same task because of fatigue, variable pain, or psychosocial factors that reward dependency (35).

At this time one must concede that the Functional Status Measurement of Granger and Greer (28) represents the most sophisticated and comprehensive *objective method* to document the functional status of a patient with a physical disability. Their method includes criteria relating to the central nervous system and bowel and bladder functions that seldom apply to the arthritis patients, and hence the justification for the modifications used by Convery et al. (26) in their subjective test for arthritis patients.

Eberl et al. (36) have validated in a rheumatoid arthritis patient population an objective "functional" test that consists of 24 performance tests measuring mobility and strength in a variety of exercises or simple tasks (e.g., arising from a chair, or placing both hands behind the neck). Their test can be performed in 14 min, and serves as a useful indicator of arthritic disease activity, although it does not per se measure function (36). Jebsen et al. (37) validated a functional test for mobility, but it is primarily applicable to the more severely involved patients seen in a rehabilitation center because of its emphasis on wheelchair activities.

Although it is obvious that function implies more than an ability to perform and indeed should reflect what a patient actually does in his home, work, recreation, and interpersonal relationships, it is clear that many functional scales do not deal adequately with psychosocial issues. A surgical procedure performed on a hand may be judged a failure on the basis of tests of mobility, strength, dexterity, and activities of daily living, yet improved cosmesis may give a patient the self-confidence to reach out into a variety of social situations which previously he or she may have felt too self-conscious to attempt.

A comprehensive analysis of psychosocial testing is beyond the scope of this chapter, but it is important to note the contributions of Katz et al., Smythe, Sarno et al., Smits, Zung, Scorzelli et al., and Halstead for their studies and discussions of this area (2, 17, 30, 38–43). The Functional Life Scale of Sarno et al. (39) and the Vocational Diagnosis of Crewe et al. (40) are well-designed tests, but are slanted toward patients with impaired central nervous system function. Anderson et al. (44) have tried to scale psychosocial function into various levels, but their criteria lack sufficient semantic precision to eliminate the considerable overlap in judgment required to describe categories of social functioning (44). Smits' questionnaire (17) is quite inclusive regarding psychosocial functioning, and yet is not excessively exhaustive, and it has been validated in a variety of severe disability groups including rheumatoid arthritis. The ARA Uniform Database for Rheumatic Disease has expanded the original Steinbrocker classification to include indices of sexual function, vocation, and compliance (see Table 1.3) (45). Although the ARA functional data are limited, and when compared to the exhaustive laboratory measures that are tabulated in the same database appear almost inconsequential, they do represent a serious attempt to document the relationships of psychosocial function to other aspects of arthritis disease behavior (45).

Clearly one is tempted to select criteria that are not contaminated by subjectivity for studying the various components of a therapeutic process per se, as well as the effect of processes on outcome. Nonetheless, the practical administrative considerations required to carry out the various tasks of obtaining, recording, and analyzing desired functional data, coupled with the documented congruence of physician and patients' assessments of function, strongly bias support for the use of a well-designed, self-administered questionnaire (46). The inherent costs of observer time, "bookkeeping," motivation and consistency of observers over time, and bias of observers all tend to militate against the widespread use of multifactorial objective measures of function. Regardless of whether the data are collected from interview, objective measures, or a self-administered questionnaire format; the volume of data collected, the precision of the tools employed (both mechanical and written or verbal questionnaire), the complexity of the format for data retrieval and scoring will all impact on the accuracy of the examiner and the examinee. To the extent that any task is tedious, threatening, or otherwise difficult (exclusive of a test situation that stimulates the examinee by its inherent challenge), the likelihood increases that errors due to carelessness, guesswork, or failure to complete or record will occur.

In preparation for a study that was carefully designed to assess the impact of various health insurance plans on the behavior of health care consumers and providers, a group of investigators at the Rand Corporation analyzed a variety of methods of assessing health and function (47). This comprehensive study delineated six categories for assessing function. 1. Self-care activities: feeding, bathing, dressing, and going to the toilet. 2. Mobility: getting around indoors, outdoors, or in the community. 3. Physical activities: running, walking, using stairs, lifting, and moving one's body in a variety of ways. 4. Role activities: activities typical for an individual of a specified age and social role (work, school, or housework). 5. Household activities: housekeeping duties (major role activity for some and minor role activity for others). 6. Leisure activities: hobbies, clubs, church, sports, etc. (48). Each of these measures of function had to meet the five following tests for selection. 1. Measures must be comprehensive with respect to the major categories of functioning about which there is conceptual agreement. 2. Questionnaire batteries should represent state-of-the-art measurement strategies. 3. Measures in each category should contribute unique information about some aspect of functioning. 4. Measures should not be excessively confounded by other health status components (e.g., mental and social) or with nonhealth influences. 5. Measures should be both sensitive to the effects of medical care and applicable to general populations (a primarily healthy population) (49).

These authors have addressed themselves to the tasks of not only analyzing but field testing the various measures of function and performance as criteria for health. Using rigid criteria in which the statistical power of each measurement was established and, insofar as possible, validated as to its reliability, content validity (were the items representative of function and were all important areas of function accounted for), and construct validity (the high degree of association of measures of functional limitations and physical abilities or exercise capacities measures) was the basis for their partial synthesis reflected in the currently proposed format (see Table 1.5) (50). The specific questions used by the Rand group and the statistical

TABLE 1.5. *Hypothesized Item Groupings, Revised Physical Abilities Items (50) (Enrollment Medical History Questionnaire, Adults, Seattle, Fitchburg, Charleston)*

Hypothesized Item Grouping	Item No.	Abbreviated Item Content*
Basic abilities	12	Use bathroom without help
	11	Eat without help
	10	Dress yourself
	9	Walk to table for meals
	8	Walk around inside house
Moderate abilities	7	Walk a block or more
	6	Walk uphill or upstairs
	5	If wanted to, could run short distances
	4	Do light work around house like dusting or washing dishes
	3	Do moderate work at home like moving chair or table, pushing vacuum cleaner
Strenuous abilities	2	If wanted to, could participate in active sport such as swimming, tennis, basketball, volleyball, rowing boat
	1	Do hard activities at home, heavy work like scrubbing floors, lifting or moving heavy furniture

Reproduced with permission from the Rand Corp. from Stewart, A. L., Ware, J. E., Jr., Brook, R., And Davis-Avery, A., *Conceptualization and Measurement of Health for Adults in the Health Insurance Study*: *Volume II*, *Physical Health in Terms of Functioning* (July 1978).

* Three response choices are offered for each item: yes; yes, but slowly; and no. If a respondent endorses items 1 or 2, the remaining items in the battery are skipped.

justifications for their selection are described in the monograph which serves as the basis for much of this discussion (51).

Further field testing by this group is proposed to determine the validity of aggregation of categories into one of individual functioning, one of role or productive functioning, and one of leisure. The reliability of their scales used to measure function in a healthy nonaged population is about 0.90 (52). Applying these same measurement criteria to a population of patients suffering from some form of rheumatological disorder requires additional study, but one could argue that there would be less skewing of the distribution of each variable measured by the greater prevalence of functional disabilities in the patient group. The Rand group summarize their recommendations for further research on measures of physical health in terms of functioning in the 19 points listed below (53). It remains for those of us interested in the treatment of rheumatological disorders to address ourselves to these issues and in particular to validate these criteria in a population of patients with disorders of joint function.

1. The most appropriate way to score the leisure activities category needs to be determined.

2. The optimal scoring method for aggregating disability days items in a single index needs to be determined. This will provide the Health Insurance Industry with a measure of acute limitations. The functional limitations and physical abilities measures, as scored, assess primarily chronic limitations.

3. The addition of items pertaining to more strenuous activities will probably improve the variability of score distributions; whether this will improve the power of these measures with respect to testing hypotheses regarding the effects of medical care remains to be determined.

4. Reliability of measures of physical health in terms of functioning should be tested in socioeconomically disadvantaged populations to determine that it is adequate.

5. Further study is needed to determine whether aggregation across categories into summary indicators results in a significant loss of information.

6. Further study is needed to determine which categories of functioning can most appropriately be aggregated.

7. The nature of the positive association between socioeconomic status and limitations in functioning should be explored.

8. Whether there are differences in the meaning of physical health in terms of functioning across socioeconomic groups remains to be tested.

9. The nature of associations between measures of functioning and variables not traditionally included in the definition of health needs to be explored.

10. The extent to which response bias influences measures of physical health in terms of functioning should be tested.

11. The extent to which measures of physical health in terms of role

functioning and leisure activities overlap conceptually with measures of social health should be investigated.

12. Differences in the validity of items structured in terms of capacity or performance and whether (and which type of) experimental hypotheses are sensitive to these differences should be explored.

13. The validity of measures of functioning under varying conditions should be evaluated (e.g., in a disabled population).

14. Longitudinal studies such as those of predictive validity or of long-term effects of limitations in functioning would be useful.

15. The sensitivity and specificity of measures of functioning should be studied.

16. Whether value preference weights are necessary to achieve valid scores on physical health measures should be studied.

17. Whether functioning can be altered by changing any variable related to personal medical care needs to be determined.

18. Whether acute limitations are affected by use of medical care services in a different manner than chronic limitations in functioning needs to be investigated.

19. Further study is needed to determine how cost of administration can be reduced. Studies such as whether use of skip patterns in administering questionnaire items or whether reducing the number of items results in a loss of information would be useful (53).

Although it is clear that a practical global instrument to measure function is essential and that the previously described self-administered questionnaire approach appears highly likely to achieve that end, the need for specific evaluative instruments to measure specific kinds of function is also apparent. The most important areas of disability for many arthritis patients are those that impair manual dexterity, and therefore the analysis of hand function will be discussed as a separate topic.

HAND EVALUATION: MEASURES OF FUNCTION, DEXTERITY, AND PERFORMANCE

Selection of the various criteria for assessment of hand function and performance requires that the following tests for useful measure be met: 1. reliability—the tests should be standardized on a normal and rheumatoid arthritis population; 2. content validity—the test should represent the best consensus of reported studies for a specific function, which should be simple and economical and readily quantifiable, e.g., by a timed test; 3. construct validity—the associations between measures of function (buttoning) and measures of physical performance (such as strength and joint mobility) should be assessed and need further determination. The association among measures of function should be sufficiently discriminatory such that each test will measure a unique function specifically, e.g., tip pinch, palmar or pulp pinch, lateral pinch, and wrist mobility; 4. scaling—the test should be structured such that a test scale can be constructed. A timed test lends itself to this criterion because normative data on timed tests have been established and scales could readily be derived by bracketing a range of percent, e.g., 90–100% of "normal" equals 0, 75–90% equals 1, etc.

Based on the criteria above, the preferred method for measurement of overall hand performance include: for *power grip, the sphygmomanometer* because of its widespread usage, availability, prior standardization, and normative data; for measuring *pulp and lateral pinch, the standard pinch dynamometer* for similar reasons; for measuring *range of motion, the measurement of the fingernail tip to palm* in millimeters because it has had almost as widespread use as the cumbersome finger goniometry method and has been standardized, and is less subject to error; for *hand evaluation and gross appearance, standardized black and white photography* using full size prints on a mat finish including three views is suggested: 1. a posterior-anterior with the fingers actively extended and abducted to demonstrate ulnar deviation, 2. a lateral view in 15° of pronation with the fingers actively extended to demonstrate swan neck and boutonniere deformities.

A review of the various commonly used tests to measure hand function per se (see Tables 1.6–1.8) indicates that when the criteria that the test of choice should be simple and inexpensive, readily quantified (and therefore timed) and have had wide usage, previous standardization and validation are met; the following tests of function suggest themselves as being most suitable: 1. coin pickup, 2. peg or nail placement, 3. safety pinning, 4. buttoning, 5. simulated food cutting, 6. shoelace tying, and 7. writing. When the tests are further analyzed from the standpoint of minimizing redundancy and maximizing specificity, three tests seem to meet these more rigid standards. The unilateral coin pickup with coin placement into the ipsilateral hand will measure tip and pulp pinch, *and wrist supination*; peg or nail placement will also measure these pinch functions in a modified form and may indeed be redundant; safety pinning measures the above pinch functions *and strong lateral* pinch. Safety pinning additionally has the advantage that it can be performed either unilaterally or bilaterally. It would appear that none of the additional tests listed in Table 1.8 would add measurably to function except for pouring and moving various shaped objects. These latter functions may be actually a better measure of strength, however strength would be accounted for in the grip strength measurement with the sphygmomanometer (see Table 1.6).

In all matters where criteria for and methods of measurement are perforce arbitrary, those prescribed for specific projects or different perspectives may dictate alternative approaches. The use of motion pictures, three dimensional photography, radiographic measures, tests of sensory function, and many other criteria may need to be measured to evaluate adequately the outcome of specific medical or surgical treatments. Nonetheless, every

TABLE 1.6. *Hand Evaluation: Measures of Physical Performance*

Method	Reference
Strength	
Dynamometer—power grip	54, 57
*Sphygmomanometer**—power grip	59, 60, 62
Dynamometer—pinch (pulp/lateral)	54, 60†
*Sphygmomanometer**—pinch (pulp/lateral)	59, 62
Range of motion	
Goniometer	59, 60
Tip-palm (mm)§	60, 62
Grasp-Cylinder	58‖, 60
Grasp-Sphere	60
Grasp-Block	57, 58
Estimated	55

* *Preferred method* because of wide-spread usage and availability or standardized procedures and normative data (54, 59, 62).
† Electronic dynamometer.
§ Cylinder grasp measured indirectly in object placement test.
‖ *Preferred method* standardized (62) and used almost as widely as the more cumbersome finger goniometry.

TABLE 1.7. *Hand Evaluation: Measures of Function and Dexterity*

Method	References	Functions*					
		Tip Pinch	Pulp Pinch	Lateral Pinch	Wrist Action	Power Grip	Uni/Bilateral
Coin pick-up†	56_{st} 57_{st} 61_{st} 62_{st}	+	+	±	+		Uni
Peg or nail placement†	54_{st} 57_{st} 61_{st}	+	+		±		Uni
Safety pinning†	56_{st} 59_{st} 62_{st}	+	+	++			Uni/Bi
Buttoning	56_{st} 57_{st} 59_{st} 62_{st}	+	+	+			Uni/Bi
Food (simulated) cutting	56_{st} 59_{s} 62_{st}			++	+		Uni
Shoelace tying	56_{st} 59_{st} 62_{st}	+	+	+			Bi
Pouring	57_{st} 58_{t} 62_{st}			+	+	+	Uni
Writing	57_{st} 58_{s} 59_{st} 61_{st}		+	+			Uni
Zippering	56_{st} 59_{st}		+	+	+		Uni
Moving various objects	56_{s} 61_{st}	+	+	+	+	+	Uni/Bi

* Key: s, test has been standardized; t, test is timed; st, test is timed and has been standardized; +, mild strength required; ++, moderate strength required; ±, minimal supplementary function; Uni, unilateral testing; Bi, bilateral testing.
† Preferred method.

TABLE 1.8. *Hand Evaluation: Gross Appearance*

Method	References
Photography*	60
Tracing	62
Visual assessment	55, 59

* *Preferred method,* although not directly standardized it has been indirectly validated by visual assessment criteria (59) and widespread usage of photography to illustrate physical abnormalities. Suggested views are: 1. Posterior anterior with fingers actively extended and abducted to demonstrate ulnar deviation. 2. Lateral (15° pronation) with fingers actively flexed fully to demonstrate metacarpophalangeal joint subluxation. 3. Lateral (15° pronation) with fingers actively extended to demonstrate swan neck and boutonniere deformities. Full size black and white photographs on matte finish are recommended to minimize variations of color or glare.

measurement should be validated whenever possible so as to meet the criteria as described in the preceding discussion.

REFERENCES

1. Leviton, G. L. Professional-client relations in a rehabilitation setting, In *Rehabilitation Psychology*, edited by W. S. Neff. American Psychological Assoc., Inc., Washington, D.C., 1971, p. 215.
2. Halstead, L. S. Team care in chronic illness. A critical review of the literature of the past twenty-five years. *Arch. Phys. Med. Rehabil., 57:* 507, 1976.
3. Swezey, R. L. *Arthritis: Rational Therapy and Rehabilitation.* W.B. Saunders Co., Philadelphia, 1978, p. 5.
4. National Attack on Arthritis. *Congressional Record,* Volume 120, No. 155 (Part II). October 11, 1974, S-19129, pp. 1–10.
5. National Commission on Arthritis and Related Musculoskeletal Diseases. Arthritis: out of the maze. In *The Arthritis Plan Report to the Congress of the United States,* Volume I. United States Department of Health, Education and Welfare, Washington, D.C., April 1976, p. 79.
6. National Commission of Arthritis and Related Musculoskeletal Diseases. Arthritis: out of the maze. In *The Arthritis Plan Report to the Congress of the United States,* Volume I. United States Department of Health, Education and Welfare, Washington, D.C., April 1976, p. 101.
7. The American Rheumatism Association Committee on Rheumatological Practice. A description of rheumatology practice. *Arth. Rheum., 20:* 1278, 1977.
8. Diffrient, N., Tilley, A. R., Bardagjy, J. D., and Dreyfuss, H. *Humanscale 1/2/3.* The MIT Press, Cambridge, 1974.
9. Swezey, R. L. *Arthritis: Rational Therapy and Rehabilitation.* W.B. Saunders Co., Philadelphia, 1978, p. 8.
10. Erickson, E. R., and Pedersen, E. Design criteria for a rehabilitation unit. *Hospital, 39:* 53, 1965.
11. Boyle, R. W. The Therapeutic Gymnasium. In *Therapeutic Exercise,* edited by S. Licht. Elizabeth Licht, New Haven, 1961, p. 257.
12. Stewart, J. B. Exercises in Water. In *Therapeutic Exercise,* Ed. 2. edited by S. Licht. William & Wilkins Co., Baltimore, Waverly Press, 1965, p. 285.
13. Ehrlich, G. E. *Total Management of the Arthritic Patient.* J.B. Lippincott Co., Philadelphia, 1973, p. 209.

14. May, E. E., Waggoner, N. R., and Hotte, E. B. *Independent Living for the Handicapped and the Elderly.* Houghton Mifflin, Boston, 1974, pp. 153–174.
15. May, E. E., Waggoner, N. R., and Hotte, E. B. *Independent Living for the Handicapped and the Elderly.* Houghton Mifflin, Boston, 1974, p. 32.
16. Lucas, M. The place of physiotherapy in the management of lumbar disc lesions. *Physiotherapy, 50:* 189, 1964.
17. Smits, S. J. *A Model for Conducting Followup Studies in Medical Rehabilitation Settings.* RR&TC Monograph No. 4. University of Alabama, Birmingham, 1973, p. 4.
18. Stewart, A. L., Ware, J. E., Jr., Brook, R., and Davis-Avery, A. *Conceptualization and Measurement of Health for Adults in the Health Insurance Study*: Volume II, *Physical Health in Terms of Functioning.* Rand Corp., Santa Monica, Calif., July 1978, p. 1.
19. Steinbrocker, O., Traeger, C. H., and Batterman, R. C. Therapeutic criteria in rheumatoid arthritis. *J.A.M.A., 140:* 659, 1949.
20. The Joint Committee of the Medical Research Council and Nuffield Foundation on Clinical Trials of Cortisone, A.C.T.H., and Other Therapeutic Measures in Chronic Rheumatic Diseases. A comparison of cortisone and aspirin in the treatment of early cases of rheumatoid arthritis. *Br. Med. J., 1:* 1223, 1954.
21. Swezey, R. L. *Arthritis: Rational Therapy and Rehabilitation.* W.B. Saunders Co., Philadelphia, 1978, p. 18.
22. Lee, P., Jasani, M. K., Dick, W. C., and Buchanan, W. W. Evaluation of a functional index in rheumatoid arthritis. *Scand. J. Rheum., 2:* 21–77, 1973.
23. Robinson, H. S., and Bashall, D. A. Functional Assessment. In *Total Management of the Arthritic Patient.* edited by G. E. Ehrlich. J.B. Lippincott Co., Philadelphia, 1971, p. 219.
24. Gersten, J. W., Ager, C., Anderson, K., and Cenkovich, F. Relation of muscle strength and range of motion to activities of daily living. *Arch. Phys. Med. Rehabil., 51:* 137, 1970.
25. Swezey, R. L. *Arthritis: Rational Therapy and Rehabilitation.* W.B. Saunders Co., Philadelphia, 1978, p. 19.
26. Convery, F. R., Minteer, M. A., Amiel, D., and Connett, K. L. Polyarticular disability: A functional assessment. *Arch. Phys. Med. Rehabil., 58:* 494, 1977.
27. Mahoney, F. I., and Barthel, D. W. Functional evaluation: The Barthel Index. *Md. State Med. J., 14:* 61–65, 1965.
28. Granger, C. V., and Greer, D. S. Functional status measurement and medical rehabilitation outcomes. *Arch. Phys. Med. Rehabil., 57:* 103, 1976.
29. Donaldson, S. W., Wagner, C. C., and Gresham, G. E. Unified ADL evaluation form. *Arch. Phys. Med. Rehabil., 54:* 175, 1973.
30. Katz, S., Downs, T. D., Cash, H. R., and Grotz, R. C. Progress in development of the Index of ADL. *Gerontologist, 10:* 20, 1970.
31. Mahoney, F. I., Wood, O. H., and Barthel, D. W. Rehabilitation of chronically ill patients: Influence of complications on final goal. *S. Med. J., 51:* 605, 1958.
32. Schoening, H. A., and Iverson, I. A. Numerical scoring of self-care status: study of Kenny self-care evaluation. *Arch. Phys. Med. Rehabil., 49:* 221, 1968.
33. Scranton, J. M., Fogel, L., and Erdman, W. C., II. Evaluation of functional levels of patients during and following rehabilitation. *Arch. Phys. Med. Rehabil., 51:* 1, 1970.
34. Stewart, A. L., Ware, J. E., Jr., Brook, R., and Davis-Avery, A. *Conceptualization and Measurement of Health for Adults in the Health Insurance Study.* Volume II, *Physical Health in Terms of Functioning.* Rand Corp., Santa Monica, California, July 1978, p. 46.
35. Kelman, H. R., and Wilner, A. Problems in measurement and evaluation of rehabilitation. *Arch. Phys. Med. Rehabil., 43:* 172–181, 1962.
36. Eberl, D. R., Fasching, V., Rahlfs, V., Schleyer, I., and Wolf, R. Repeatability and

objectivity of various measurements in rheumatoid arthritis. *Arthritis Rheum,, 19:* 1278, 1976.

37. Jebsen, R. H., Treischmann, R. B., Mikulic, M. A., Hartley, R. B., McMillan, J. A., and Snook, M. E. Measurement of time in a standardized test of patient mobility. *Arch. Phys. Med. Rehabil., 51:* 170, 1970.
38. Smythe, H. A. Assessment of joint disease. Toronto, January 1975, p. 10. Unpublished data.
39. Sarno, J. E., Sarno, M. T., and Levita, F. The functional life scale. *Arch. Phys. Med. Rehabil., 54:* 214, 1973.
40. Crewe, N. M., Athelstan, G. T., and Meadows, G. K. Vocational diagnosis through assessment of functional limitations. *Arch. Phys. Med. Rehabil., 56:* 513, 1975.
41. Zung, W. W. K. A self rating depression scale. *Arch. Gen. Psychiat., 12:* 63, 1965.
42. Scorzelli, J. F., Goldthwait, J. C., and Myers, J. S. Rehabilitation and the arthritic client. A report on a seminar held June 11, 1976, Robert Breck Brigham Hospital, Boston, Mass. Northeastern University Rehabilitation Counselling Program, October 1976.
43. Smits, S. J. Variables related to success in a medical rehabilitation setting. *Arch. Phys. Med. Rehabil., 55:* 449, 1974.
44. Anderson, T., McClure, W., Athelstan, G., Anderson, E., Crewe, N., Arndts, L. G., Ferguson, M. B., Baldridge, M., Gullickson, G., Jr., and Kottke, F. J. *Evaluating Quality of Rehabilitation Using Outcome Assessment.* University of Minnesota monograph (undated).
45. Hess, E. V. A uniform database for rheumatic diseases. *Arthritis Rheum., 19:* 645, 1976.
46. Stewart, A. L., Ware, J. E., Jr., Brook, R., and Davis-Avery, A. *Conceptualization and Measurement of Health for Adults in the Health Insurance Study.* Rand Corp., Santa Monica, California, July 1978, p. 75.
47. Stewart, A. L., Ware, J. E., Jr., Brook, R., and Davis-Avery, A. *Conceptualization and Measurement of Health for Adults in the Health Insurance Study.* Volume II, *Physical Health in Terms of Functioning.* Rand Corp., Santa Monica, California, July 1978, p. 5.
48. Stewart, A. L., Ware, J. E., Jr., Brook, R., and Davis-Avery, A. *Conceptualization and Measurement of Health for Adults in the Health Insurance Study.* Volume II, *Physical Health in Terms of Functioning.* Rand Corp., Santa Monica, California, July 1978, p. v.
49. Stewart, A. L., Ware, J. E., Jr., Brook, R., and Davis-Avery, A. *Conceptualization and Measurement of Health for Adults in the Health Insurance Study.* Volume II, *Physical Health in Terms of Functioning.* Rand Corp., Santa Monica, California, July 1978, p. 81.
50. Stewart, A. L., Ware, J. E., Jr., Brook, R., and Davis-Avery, A. *Conceptualization and Measurement of Health for Adults in the Health Insurance Study.* Volume II, *Physical Health in Terms of Functioning.* Rand Corp., Santa Monica, California, July 1978, p. 190.
51. Stewart, A. L., Ware, J. E., Jr., Brook, R., and Davis-Avery, A. *Conceptualization and Measurement of Health for Adults in the Health Insurance Study.* Volume II, *Physical Health in Terms of Functioning.* Rand Corp., Santa Monica, California, July 1978, p. 170.
52. Stewart, A. L., Ware, J. E., Jr., Brook, R., and Davis-Avery, A. *Conceptualization and Measurement of Health for Adults in the Health Insurance Study.* Volume II, *Physical Health in Terms of Functioning.* Rand Corp., Santa Monica, California, July 1978, p. 139.
53. Stewart, A. L., Ware, J. E., Jr., Brook, R., and Davis-Avery, A. *Conceptualization and Measurement of Health for Adults in the Health Insurance Study.* Volume II, *Physical Health in Terms of Functioning.* Rand Corp., Santa Monica, California, July

1978, p. 140.

54. Kellor, M., Kondrasuk, R., Iversen, I., Frost, J., Silberberg, N., and Hoglund, M. Technical manual hand strength and dexterity norms. 1. Sister Kenny Institute Publ. No. 721. 2. *Am. J. Occup. Ther., 25:* 77, 1971.
55. Treuhaft, P. S., Lewis, M. R., and McCarthy, D. J. A rapid method for evaluating the structure and function of the rheumatoid hand. *Arthritis Rheum., 14:* 75, 1971.
56. Potvin, A. R., et al. Simulated activities of daily living examination. *Arch. Phys. Med. Rehab., 53:* 476, 1972.
57. Smith, H. Smith hand function evaluation. *Am. J. Occup. Ther., 27:* 244, 1973.
58. Carroll, D. A quantitative test of upper extremity function. *J. Chronic Dis., 18:* 479, 1965.
59. Carthum, C. J., Clawson, D. K., and Decker, J. L. Functional assessment of the rheumatoid hand. *Am. J. Occup. Ther., 23:* 122, 1969.
60. Swanson, A. H., Mays, J. D., and Yamauchi, Y. A rheumatoid arthritis evaluation record for the upper extremity. *Surg. Clin. N. Am., 48:* 1003, 1968.
61. Jebsen, R. H., et al. An objective and standardized test of hand function. *Arch. Phys. Med. Rehabil., 50:* 311, 1969.
62. Robinson, H. S., et al. Functional results of excisional arthroplasty for the rheumatoid hand. *Can. Med. J., 108:* 1495, 1978.

2

The Physiatrist in Arthritis Management

JOHN A. DOWNEY

Rheumatoid arthritis is a chronic disease of unknown etiology, the course of which is manifested by exacerbation and remission. The disease affects patients of all ages; however, there are very important differences in the conservative management of adults and children. The problems include those caused by the active growth of children as well as the tendency in the very young to develop difficult, early, if not fixed, joint contractures.

Until the etiology of the disease is found and an effective cure is developed, the central goal of all who care for rheumatoid patients is the maintenance of function which allows the patients to continue in their necessary or desired activities with as little limitation or modification as possible.

It is ideal when the specialist in Rehabilitation Medicine, the physiatrist, works in close association with a team of physicians trained in the diagnosis of both adult and juvenile rheumatoid arthritis. If not, then the physiatrist must take the responsibility of ensuring an accurate diagnosis before beginning his evaluation and therapy. With a specialized group of physicians it is usually the practice of the internist or pediatrician to prescribe and administer the medications; however, the physiatrist must not only be knowledgeable regarding the medications and their effects but must also be able to adapt the physical program to the optimum time of effect of the medicine, or to arrange medication time to fit the patient's daily schedule or needs. For example, with a patient having much early morning stiffness it is helpful to either take long-acting aspirin or take the aspirin ½ to 1 hr prior to arising, or both.

Maintenance of Function

To use the musculoskeletal system one must have joints which will move, muscles which can move them, and then the skill or dexterity for the act. Patients with rheumatoid arthritis have pain and inflammation of joints, often with deformity or contractures, weakness and inflammation of muscles due to disuse, myositis, and vasculitis (1–7). To manage adequately all aspects requires attention to each component contributing to the disability, as well as a strong supportive role by the rehabilitation physician and staff.

First, it is important to recognize that when dealing with a chronic disease, effective management as well as expediency and logistics require that the program should be home-based, materials used should be simple and inexpensive, and it should be flexible as to timing so that it will not unnecessarily interfere with the patient's life. Thus, the staff working with the physiatrist must be carefully instructed and trained in the special and peculiar problems of rheumatoid arthritis which include the fact that their role is to follow the physician's directions, act primarily as teachers of the desired program rather than therapist, per se, in the sense of "doing" for the patient. The therapist, after the initial period of instruction which will take three to six sessions, must be available to answer the patient's questions and at all times be ready and able to observe and bring changes in the patient's condition to the physician's attention. Acting as "eyes and ears" for the responsible physician is an essential and invaluable aspect of a comprehensive program, for without it and the cooperation of the therapist it is better not to have the therapist involved but to have the physician instruct the patient directly. Books or written programs of preprescribed exercises are less desirable than a program tailored to the problems and the specific needs of the patient. If no physician trained in prescribing such a program is available, then booklets available through the national and local arthritis agencies are the best and safest aids in patient care to avoid the ever increasing number of unproven or ineffective devices and/or programs being merchandized.

Management of Pain

The use of full dose antiinflammatory analgesic medications is the first line of treatment. These can and often must be supplemented by physical agents, the most common being the use of heat, although in rare situations, usually acute inflammation, cold may be useful. Other modalities, such as liniments, can be used if they are cheap and, as with the use of thermotherapy, make the patient feel better and thus able to move his joints, use his muscles, and perform activities.

The form of heat used should be simple and available at home. Frequently, hot baths, showers, or soaks are the easiest. Baths especially allow the patient to use the buoyancy of the water to begin active range of motion exercises. The criterion for use of any modality is whether or not it reduces pain. The patient should be allowed to experiment but should be warned against expensive devices and even the use of hospital or office treatment facilities and modalities. In general, deep heat devices (diathermy, microwave, ultrasound, etc.) cause greater pain, possibly by increasing deep tissue temperature (8), thus blood flow (9, 10) and congestion; a less likely explanation is that it works by increasing activity of destructive tissue enzymes (11).

Patients should be told that the purpose of the physical modality is to temporarily decrease pain to allow them to move their joints or to proceed to the next step.

Maintaining or Regaining Range of Motion

It is my opinion that passive motion or stretching of joints by anyone, therapist or otherwise, is contraindicated and frequently harmful. Patients respond to stretching with pain and fear. They resist both consciously and unconsciously, often using muscles that lead to increased contracture and after the procedure place the joints in a position exaggerating the deformity.

Exercise to increase range of motion is best done when the pain and stiffness are minimized by medication, analgesic physical modalities (heat, liniments, etc.) and time of day. The patient should be instructed as to what is the normal range and how it is obtained. For example, to elevate the shoulder, the patient must externally rotate the arm and be shown the bodily position whereby the motion can be obtained with the least stress such as lying down to eliminate gravity or during a bath using water for its buoyancy.

Patients should be instructed to perform a ritual during which all joints of the body are put through a full, normal range of motion each day including areas not currently inflamed. This will give them a sense of what is normal and an early indication of inflammation. In all instances and certainly with acute inflammation, resistive exercises or weight lifting should be avoided.

In those areas where there is restriction of motion, patients can be instructed to give themselves resistance using the other hand or part of the body; however, the resistance must be in the direction that motion is desired. If there is a flexion contracture of the elbow, the patient should be taught to extend the elbow and resist the extension with his other hand. In this way he has full control of the motion and will move into the pain zone. He will, if anything, be strengthening the elbow extensors and will automatically induce inhibition of the antagonist—the elbow flexors. This principle of resistance can be extended to most joints and in children may be given by a trusted family member as long as the patients know they will not be tricked by an unexpected release of the resistance.

Maintenance of optimal joint position and prevention of contractures by positioning and splinting will be dealt with later.

Muscle Strength

Patients with rheumatoid arthritis suffer a loss of muscle bulk, strength, and stamina around inflamed joints as well as elsewhere throughout the body. The primary cause of the atrophy and weakness is disuse because of the pain and limitation, but may also be the vasculitis and myositis that are parts of the systemic manifestation of the disease.

When pain and inflammation are present in a joint, active resistive exercises such as weight lifting will often cause an exacerbation of the inflammation, more pain, and less activity. Some of this is due to direct strain on the joints as they are given resistance through the full range of motion. However, increased joint temperature (12) and blood flow may also be factors.

In normal patients muscle strength, bulk, and stamina can be increased by isometric exercise even with surprisingly few repetitions (13, 14) and it has been shown that this can be induced in patients with rheumatoid arthritis (15–19). Therefore, even in early, relatively acute, situations patients can be instructed in isometric exercises with particular emphasis on those muscles around the inflamed joints as well as the antigravity muscles (especially the abdominals, gluteals, and quadriceps) when ambulation is anticipated. At the beginning as few as 1–2 repetitions of the isometrics should be prescribed and only as symptoms allow should they be increased to 10–15 per day.

In children with controlled disease activity who have little or no pain, it is usually not necessary to do other than allow and encourage normal life activities. In adults it may be necessary later (and only when the disease is inactive in all parameters) to progress to regular isometric resistive exercises, but even then only with caution and close supervision.

The development of dexterity in any task can only come from maximum repetitions of the desired activity but with as low or little resistance as possible. The numbers of repetitions will depend on the patient's clinical response and on the activity; more if it is a fine activity such as typing, less if it involves greater resistance such as operating a manual drill press.

Rest

There is controversy regarding the place of rest in the management of many illnesses and no less with rheumatoid arthritis (12, 20). Bed rest, even in normal persons, causes demineralization of bone, loss of muscle protein, cardiovascular deconditioning, and other effects discovered in studies preparatory for the effects of weightlessness in space (21). All of these occur in patients, with the added concern of developing complications of joint stiffness or contractures. However, it is a common, if not universal, experience that bed rest and reduction of stress and strain of painful joints reduce inflammation. Controlled trials with small numbers of patients on bed rest for several weeks with or without casting of severely inflamed joints have shown less inflammation and, in due course, no restriction of motion after reconditioning. Such a program, however, is highly expensive both in hospital cost and loss of function. It is more generally accepted that periodic, daily rest to avoid fatigue and to reduce joint strain, often supplemented by splinting joints (especially the wrist, knees, and ankles in optimum position, i.e., opposite of usual contracted position) allows rest and avoids trauma of motion even in bed is most efficacious. Regular adjustment of splints may even permit their use to correct deformity resulting from spasm and inflammation. Use of splints instead of casts at night and at rest periods also allows the limbs to be freed for the daily range of motion exercises generally, though not universally, advised (22, 23).

There is no doubt that children with juvenile rheumatoid arthritis should not be placed in casts, for they develop early and often intractable contractures. Active motion is always indicated. In fact, we advise and even mandate that the children not be allowed to miss school. We do not restrict their physical activity in any way, being willing to accept possible joint damage as preferable to the psychological crippling effect of enforced chronic invalidism.

I recommend and use resting splints for both children and adults, making them of the cheapest and simplest material (often plaster of Paris), regularly and frequently adjusting or renewing them until contractures are overcome and well past the time that inflammation has disappeared. Braces are rarely, if ever, used although small dynamic splints to support the wrists may be helpful during activity, if they enhance function.

It was stated that the goal of management was to return the patient to function at the normal capacity levels. The evaluation of ability to perform "activities of daily living" (ADL) is often requested from therapists, both occupational and physical. Too often patients return with gadgets to aid in their dressing or some other activity. This is undesirable. An adequate ADL evaluation determines the following.

1. What are the patient's needs to lead a normal life?
2. What of all these tasks or activities can the patient not do?
3. Why can the tasks not be performed? Is it due to stiffness, pain, loss of motion, or weakness?
4. Insofar as possible, therapy should be directed at correcting item 3.
5. Only when it is evident that the limitation cannot be quickly overcome are aids given with the object of being able to do the task in the unmodified way.
6. Finally, and only after all else has failed, are steps taken to modify tasks so that they can be done. A patient who can only function in a modified environment is truly disabled and restricted. It is better than not functioning, but it is certainly not ideal.

In certain patients the steps can be overlapped and devices can be used temporarily while physical goals are sought and then discarded. In other situations use of simple aids, such as knee cages or canes, can be continued on a long-term basis when they enhance performance and do not cause undue encumbrances.

In summary, physiatrists either independently or in conjunction with physical and/or occupational therapists who have been specially instructed in the principles and practice of rheumatology and who will work in close collaboration with the physiatrist can develop an individualized program for the rheumatoid patient which will minimize disability and enhance function (24). Most of the progress consists of patient education for self-care. The earlier in the course of the disease that this can be initiated, the better. The effectiveness of the progress depends on the compliance of the patient and much remains to be learned concerning how to present such programs (25).

REFERENCES

1. Tiselius, P. Studies on muscle weakness in rheumatoid arthritis. *Acta Rheum. Scand.*, (*Suppl.* 14 P) *14:* 75, 1969.
2. Tiselius, P. Studies on factors influencing quadriceps strength in rheumatic knee joints. *Acta Rheum. Scand.*, (*Suppl.* 14 P) *14:* 87, 1969.
3. Haslock, D. I., Wright, V., and Harriman, D. G. F. Neuromuscular disorders in rheumatoid arthritis. *Quart. J. Med.*, *39:* 335, 1970.
4. Lovgren, O. The Muscles in Rheumatoid Arthritis—New Findings and their Implications. In *Chronic Forms of Polyarthritis*, edited by F. J. Wagenhauser. Huber, Bern, 1976.
5. Edstrom, L., and Nordemar, R. Differential changes in Type I and Type II muscle fibres in rheumatoid arthritis. *Scand. J. Rheum.*, *3:* 155, 1974.
6. Magora, A., Wolf, E., and Gonen, B. Electrodiagnostic investigation of the neuromuscular lesions in rheumatoid arthritis. *Acta Rheum. Scand.*, *16:* 280, 1970.
7. Oka, M., Rekonen, A., and Elomaa, I. Muscle blood flow in rheumatoid arthritis. *Acta Rheum. Scand.*, *17:* 203, 1971.
8. Hollander, J. L., and Horvath, S. M. The influence of physical therapy procedures on the intra-articular temperature of normal and arthritis subjects. *Am. J. Med. Sci.*, *218:* 543, 1949.
9. Bonney, G. L. W., Hughes, R. A., and Janus, O. Blood flow through the normal human knee segment. *Clin. Sci.*, *11:* 167, 1951.
10. Harris, R., and Millard, J. G. Clearance of radioactive sodium from the knee. *Clin. Sci.*, *15:* 9, 1956.
11. Harris, E. D., and Krane, S. M. Collagenases. *N. Engl. J. Med.*, *291:* 557, 605, 652, 1978.
12. Smith, R. D., and Polley, H. F. Rest therapy for rheumatoid arthritis. *Mayo Clin. Proc.*, *53:* 141, 1978.
13. Hettinger, T., and Muller, E. A. Muskelleistung und Muskeltraining. *Arbeitphysiologie*, *15:* 11, 1953.
14. Rose, D. L., Radzyminski, D. F., and Beatty, R. R. Effect of brief maximal exercise on the strength of the quadriceps femoris. *Arch. Phys. Med. Rehabil.*, *38:* 157, 1957.
15. Liberson, W. T., and Asa, M. M. Further studies of brief isometric exercises. *Arch. Phys. Med. Rehabil.*, *40:* 330, 1959.
16. Machover, S., and Sapecky, A. M. Effect of isometric exercise on the quadriceps muscle in patients with rheumatoid arthritis. *Arch. Phys. Med. Rehabil.*, *47:* 737, 1966.
17. Ekblom, B., Lovgren, O., Alderin, M., Fridstrom, M., and Satterstrom, G. Physical performance in patients with rheumatoid arthritis. *Scand. J. Rheum.*, *3:* 121, 1974.
18. Ekblom, B., Lovgren, O., Alderin, M., Fridstrom, M. and Satterstrom, G. Effect of short-term physical training on patients with rheumatoid arthritis I. *Scand. J. Rheum.*, *4:* 80, 1975.
19. Ekblom, B., Lovgren, O., Alderin, M., Fridstrom, M. and Satterstrom, G. Effect of short-term physical training on patients with rheumatoid arthritis. *Scand. J. Rheum.*, *4:* 87, 1975.
20. Ferguson, R. H. Rheumatoid arthritis and rest. *Mayo Clin. Proc.*, *53:* 195, 1978.
21. Mills, J. A., Puials, R. S., Ropes, N. W., Short, C. L., and Sutcliffe, J. Value of bed rest in patients with rheumatoid arthritis. *N. Engl. J. Med.*, *284:* 453, 1971.

22. GAULT, S. J., AND SPYKER, J. M. Beneficial effect of immobilization of joints in rheumatoid and related arthritis: a splint study using sequential analysis. *Arth. Rheum., 12:* 34, 1969.
23. PARTRIDGE, R. E. H., AND DUTHIE, J. J. R. Controlled trial of the effects of complete immobilization of the joint in rheumatoid arthritis. *Ann. Rheum. Dis., 22:* 91, 1963.
24. KATZ, S., VIGNOS, P. J., MOSKOWITZ, R. W., THOMPSON, H. M., AND SVEC, K. H. Comprehensive out-patient care in rheumatoid arthritis. *J.A.M.A., 206:* 1249, 1968.
25. KARTEN, I., LEE, M., AND MCEWEN, C. Five year study of rehabilitation. *Arch. Phys. Med. Rehabil., 54:* 120, 1973.

3

Drug Therapy and the Rehabilitation Process: A Necessary Interaction

SANFORD H. ROTH

The rehabilitative management of the various rheumatic diseases provided by this text offers a well planned, organized, and systematic approach to the variety of problems characteristic of the arthritic and rheumatic disorders. From the most localized, simple mechanical joint problem to the most characteristic systemic disorder, rheumatoid arthritis (RA), some form of medical treatment will be and must be the center-point of an effective program. Whether a single intraarticular corticosteroid injection or a complex multiple drug regimen involving antiinflammatory/analgesic agents, and possible remittive or immunomodulating agents as well, is at issue, the key to planning and success of such a mangement program will in no small measure depend upon the clinical skill requisite to developing the appropriate medication regimen for the particular rheumatic disorder.

RA—a Model for Management

The acute inflammation which characterizes the early phase of RA (Fig. 3.1) evokes elaboration of direct simple mediators, such as the prostaglandins and the biogenic amines. In the absence of incitement of complex humoral and cellular immune mechanisms, salicylates, and nonsteroidal antiinflammatory drugs (NSAIDs) are often dramatically effective. These agents alone may quickly relieve pain, swelling, stiffness, and soreness through timely suppression of the acute inflammatory response.

By contrast the more complex stages of RA characterized by the later established disease (Fig. 3.2) are probably unresponsive to such limited measures alone. Here the acute inflammatory process superimposes intermittently on the underlying progressive, destructive granulomatous process which characterizes this stage. In this instance the salicylate and nonsteroi-

RX:

Antiinflammatory agents
Salicylates
NSAIDs
Steroids

General Medical Program
Home Instruction
PT/OT

Fig. 3.1. Early phase of RA.

RX:

Antiinflammatory agents
Remission-Inducing Drugs (SAARDs)
Rehabilitative Procedures

Fig. 3.2. Progressive phase of RA.

dal medications still effectively relieve acute episodes but are relatively powerless to suppress the chronic relentless granulomatous phase of the disease. Remission-inducing drugs (SAARDs, for slow-acting antirheumatic drugs) are required for this latter purpose.

In the late phase of inflammatory joint disease, as indicated in Figure 3.3, not only are acute inflammatory events superimposed on some degree of granulomatous progressive process (which by now may be "burning out") but secondary degenerative mechanical problems have evolved in the case of involved joints now damaged by RA. In this phase salicylates and nonsteroidal agents are not only effective in dealing with the acute inflammatory events but also relieve some of the fibrositic symptoms and pain associated with the secondary mechanical joint damage and its superimproved inflammation. SAARD may not be as appropriate in this stage unless the underlying granulomatous process has relentlessly persisted.

Thus, in order to envision management of the rheumatic diseases we must look upon them not only in relation to their individual peculiar presentations but also as to stage of activity. Drug therapy aims not merely for analgesia but also for antiinflammatory action. In some cases the potent suppressive action of SAARDs may, at times, approach remittive reversal in severe progressive stages of RA.

Efforts at rehabilitation in RA must, therefore, include successful drug therapy directed at uncontrolled pain, swelling, and systemic illness in order to achieve the exemplary goals detailed in this text.

The use of such drugs in the rheumatic diseases differs from usual therapy of pain or soreness in that it is oriented toward long periods of treatment for a chronic process. Thus short-term use of analgesics is often of less impor-

RX:

Antiinflammatory agents
Remission-Inducing Drugs (SAARDs)
Analgesics p.r.n.
Rehabilitative Procedures
Orthopedic Reconstructive Procedure

Fig. 3.3. Late phase of RA.

tance than long-term use of salicylates or NSAIDs which offer long-term analgesia as a secondary benefit of their acute antiflammatory activity.

Goals of Therapy in the Rheumatic Diseases

1. Long-term suppression of the inflammatory process with secondary relief of associated symptoms of stiffness, soreness and the pain of inflammation (this complex is often referred to as the "fibrositic process").
2. When necessary, induction of suppression of the chronic phase of the disease through a remission inducing drug (SAARD).
3. Maintenance of general health and well being, including measures directed towards general medical management and control of nutrition (i.e., therapy of anemia, prevention of obesity, correction of osteoporosis, etc.)
4. Attention to psychosocial needs, including individual and family counseling, direction and correction of environmental stress factors (vocational counseling, family social services, etc.), and medical attention to common problems or reactive depression and anxiety.
5. Appropriate rehabilitative programs directed towards basic instruction in home therapy, activities of daily living, joint protection procedures, etc.
6. Orthopaedic intervention and reconstruction in selected cases.

Basic to the achievement of such goals is control of the underlying inflammatory disease process, which to varying degrees contributes to all of the rheumatic disorders, including osteoarthritis. Use of antiinflammatory drug therapy is basic to the achievement of the fundamental goals set forth above. Without some degree of success in medical management of the rheumatic disease process the broad program directed toward maintenance of optimum medical, psychosocial, and rehabilitative goals is compromised. Conversely, attention limited to simply a pill or medication to treat such a long-term and complex disorder as RA is likely to fail without the broader attention to the general basic program of goals outlined.

Thus in this chapter we logically speak of an *interaction* between an appropriate antirheumatic drug regimen and ongoing basic attention to the personal, social, and environmental needs which combine to form the composite requirements for a well-balanced program necessary to the management of rheumatic disorders.

A Guide to Drug Selection

Patient education and understanding are the key to the achievement of a successful and effective drug therapy program in the rheumatic disorders. The following principles are suggested as guides to better understanding of the proper choice of agents for treating the particular rheumatic condition as well as to supplemental drugs that may be chosen to treat nonrheumatic complications incidental to the overall medical management program.

The patient seeks analgesia but must understand that he must not rely upon analgesics alone. That is to say, simple pain relief, though desirable on a short-term basis, is unsatisfactory without attention to suppression of inflammatory and disease activity as well as maintenance and protection of function and general health. Thus analgesic agents, particularly narcotics, are undesirable except in very limited and short-term circumstances. The patient must be able to rest at night and must be protected from severe or excruciating pain. If this can only be achieved with the use of narcotics it indicates a failure of the overall general management program.

The patient must come to understand that maximum symptomatic benefit can best be achieved through careful selection of the least toxic agent or agents which offer nonsteroidal antiinflammatory disease control. Traditionally, salicylate therapy, especially aspirin, has been given pride of place. More recently, NSAIDs have offered safe alternatives to aspirin with lower risk and equal antiinflammatory analgesic benefits. In such cases a selection of agent or agents will depend upon individualization based upon patient response and tolerance of drug or drugs without unpleasant side effects.

More potent medications including remittive drugs, or in special circumstances corticosteroids, will be limited to more important rheumatic disease activity and may well require experienced consultative opinion because of higher risks and toxicity complicating such difficult decisions.

Nonrheumatic drug therapy all too often must be considered in the overall management program. First, because drugs for treatment of unrelated nonrheumatic medical complications such as hypoglycemic agents, anticoagulants, diuretics, cardiovascular agents, etc. may importantly interact with antiinflammatory drugs with potentially serious toxicity unless appropriate adjustments in drug selection and therapeutic dosage schedules are allowed for. As an example, NSAIDs and salicylates avidly bind to serum albumin displacing such drugs as anticoagulants or hypoglycemic agents resulting in a magnified effect from the latter agents at a particular dosage. Some antiinflammatory agents, notably pyrazalones such a phenylbutazone, induce microsomal liver enzymes affecting the metabolism and half-life of other drugs, such as the barbiturates. Thus both the patient and physician must not only be alert to nonrheumatic drugs the patient brings to his new antiinflammatory regimen but conversely concern about superimposition of such drugs at a later stage upon a previously established regimen. Second, drugs used to treat the complications of the rheumatic disease process become an all too common part of the long-term medical program of the arthritic patient (Table 3.1). At the forefront are such drugs as antacids, anticholinergics and, more recently, cimetidine to treat the all-too-common upper gastrointestinal disorders. In the presence of previous or ongoing acid peptic disease, such treatment measures may not only be desirable but may be required on a long-term prophylactic basis because of the high recurrence rate of such complications in the rheumatic diseases. Other examples from Table 3.1, including antidepressants and diuretics, suggest the potential for more complicated drug regimens than may always be desirable in the long run. The clinical therapist must always balance the need for treating an additional problem with the concern for drug interactions and overall patient compliance problems in a multiple drug regimen. As compliance is inversely proportional to the number of drugs, the number of tablets or capsules, and the number of doses, a problem of "polypharmacy" readily emerges.

Nature of the Rheumatic Disorder

Usually, rheumatoid arthritis is used to illustrate inflammatory joint disease and osteoarthritis localized disease without important systemic inflammatory components. Paradoxically, both diseases respond to salicylates and NSAIDs.

However, rheumatoid disease and its variants often require higher dosages than osteoarthritis and more often require a combination of agents including at times low-dose corticosteroids and/or SAARDs, whereas these systemic agents are inappropriate in osteoarthritis. Nonarticular fibrositic disorders, especially polymyalgia rheumatica and collagen vascular disorders such as systemic lupus erythematosus and polyarteritis, are very corticosteroid sensitive. However, because of the multiple complications complicating long-term corticosteroid therapy these agents are usually limited to lower dosages except in the face of life-threatening complications. Heroic use of cytotoxic and immunomodulating experimental drugs is presently the province of specialists under controlled, protocol-monitoring, conditions.

TABLE 3.1. *Treatment of Rheumatic Disease Complications*

I. Gastrointestinal (primarily acid peptic disease)
   - Antacids
   - Anticholinergics
   - Cimetidine

II. Cardiovascular (fluid retention, hypertension, congestive failure)
   - Diuretics

III. Reactive depression
   - Antidepressants

Adapted from S. H. Roth, *New Directions in Arthritis Therapy*, Publishing Sciences Group, Littleton, Massachusetts, 1980. Reprinted with permission of the publisher.

Recent appreciation of the role of crystal-induced inflammatory joint disease has expanded in understanding of metabolic arthritis, from the classic gout induced by monosodium urate crystals, and featuring altered uric acid metabolism to pseudogout, a calcium pyrophosphate dihydrate crystal-induced disorder often seen in combination with various osteoarthritic and other apparently unrelated medical disease states (1) (e.g., hypothyrodism, hemochromatosis). A transient synovitis is also induced by the microcrystals formed after injection of some corticosteroids into joints, leading to the misconception that such intraarticular injections can cause arthritis (2).

The infectious forms of arthritis include septic states responsive to specific antibiotics (determined by culturing joint fluid) combined at times with orthopedic incision and drainage. Arthritis associated with venereal disease, such as gonorrhea, is now the leading infective arthritis, tends to respond to early attention and appropriate antibiotics. The reactive arthritis seen with various viral states, such as rubeola and serum B hepatitis tends to be more self-limited; thus, primary attention needs to be directed toward systemic supportive measures rather than toward drug therapy.

Rheumatic fever is on the wane in civilized nations. Its early diagnosis is still important, because it yields to antibiotics, salicylates, and supportive therapy, as a rule when these are started early in the course. Less common causes of arthritis, serum sickness and drug-diathesis states such as systemic lupus and hypersensitivity angiitis, often require massive intervention with corticosteroids, and careful appropriate follow-up alert to complications.

Rheumatic Diseases Induced by Drugs

A secondary form of systemic lupus erythematosus probably tops the list of the rheumatic disorders which are most likely to be induced by a variety of drugs. First of all, such patients are historically more sensitive to many drugs, including penicillin, sulfa, and iodides (3), and have stronger allergic background. Isoniazide, used to treat tuberculosis, hydralazine, used to treat hypertension, procainamide given for management of arrhythmias, and various anticonvulsants, such as hydantoin phenytoin, and mesantoin can induce lupus-like states with production of lupus erythematosus cells and induction of antinuclear antibody titers (4). Although such autoimmune activity appears to be self-limited, cases have been reported which evolve into chronic systemic lupus erythematosus, suggesting such agents may have "uncovered" or stimulated actual basic underlying disease (5). At times gold therapy, and more recently d-penicillamine, have been associated with such a diathesis (6).

Diazide diuretics and pyrazinamide can elevate serum uric acid, so can small doses (under 3 g a day) of aspirin, doses likely to be taken by patients self-medicating. In some predisposed patients, this can precipitate an acute gouty synovitis. Secondary hyperuricemia resulting from cytotoxic drug therapy is seen in leukemia and psoriasis when increased breakdown of nucleoprotein occurs.

Of much concern is the osteoporosis seen particularly in postmenopausal women who have rheumatoid arthritis and are beging treated with corticosteroids. For here we see the combination of multiple catabolic factors from the disease, the hormonal state, and the steroid effect combining to produce a potentially relentless condition. This requires graduated tapering of corticosteroids, taking care to avoid exacerbation of the rheumatoid disease. It will not prove easy to treat this condition, often discovered because of severe sudden pain produced by compression fractures, usually of one of more vertebrae, that are it consequence. Calcium and fluoride supplementation in combination with intermittent vitamin D, anabolic hormones, and temporary bracing and rehabilitative measures are usually indicated for a considerable time, together with attempts at corticosteroid withdrawal. Pain relief can be achieved, but reossification may be more difficult to achieve. Salicylates and NSAIDs can give additional symptomatic aid.

Aseptic necrosis is a consequence of both systemic and intraarticular corticosteroid therapy, as is secondary septic arthritis.

Serum sickness and hypersensity drug vasculitic reactions are associated with a more benign, self-limited rheumatic disorder. The long list of ubiquitous therapeutic culprits so often part of such problems obfuscate easy determination of the offending agent in the case of a mixed drug regimen. This requires a careful process of elimination.

Choice of Therapy

ANALGESICS

Surely pain is the calling card of the arthritic/rheumatic processes. Yet pain relief alone, devoid of any antiinflammatory or antirheumatic properties, is not a desirable long range or even short-term goal. For that reason, above all others, primary reliance or analgesic medication, whether nonnarcotic or narcotic, in the absence of a supervening antiinflammatory or antirheumatic drug regimen is usually unacceptable. Exceptions may be simple mechanical osteoarthritic disorders involving the spine or weight bearing joints when surgery is contemplated in the not-too-distant future or involvement not characterized by a propensity to recurrence. Yet even here, localized tissue inflammatory activity can most often be demonstrated suggesting the advantages of the mixed antiinflammatory analgesic approach.

However, the addition of an analgesic agent to allow relief from pain for a night's sleep or reduction of agony when the patient's medical condition will not allow adequate other antirheumatic therapeutic measures, as in the case of acute bleeding ulcer, may require implication of a rule of therapeusis, "relieve pain".

As indicated in Table 3.2, paraaminophenol derivatives (acetaminophen, phenacetin), narcotics (codeine, oxycodeine, morphine, and others), narcotic-like agents (propoxyphene, ethoheptazine) are present examples of analgesics commonly in use.

Certainly all of the above agents are used not only alone but often in combination with aspirin and caffeine. Whether these combinations are justified is open to legitimate inquiry and controversy. Nevertheless, the fact remains that it is simpler for the physician to order acetaminophen in combination with codeine as a refillable prescription drug over the phone rather than plain codeine, which requires a written prescription, although enhanced efficacy is doubtful and cost is certainly higher in the case of the combination. This argument can be carried through the whole range of combination medications described here. Suffice it to note that the physician should avoid addictive narcotic medications except for extreme cases or limited use, especially in the face of the chronic pain conditions he must treat. At the same time, a judgment must balance adequate analgesia with the immediate needs of the clinical situation.

Substantial pain relief from most oral analgesics will not be achieved until approximately 45 min have passed, but the habituating potential or parenteral agents, which work faster, make them poor alternatives except in the most acute situations. Rectal suppositories containing such medication are generally not well accepted in the United States despite their more rapid absorption and onset of efficacy and low incidence of gastrointestinal upset. However, while such suppositions enjoy considerable popularity in Europe, they have not really been available in the United States and few attempts have been launched to assess acceptance or popularity of this mode of treatment.

Moertel (8) has probably one of the best discussions of the advantages of

TABLE 3.2. *Analgesics of Oral Use*

Paraaminophenol derivatives
Acetaminophen
Phenacetin
Narcotics
Codeine
Oxycodeine
Morphine
(Others)
Narcotic-like agents
Propoxyphene
Ethoheptazine
Pentazocine
Others

Adapted from S. H. Roth, *New Directions in Arthritis Therapy*, Publishing Sciences Group, Littleton, Massachusetts, 1980. Reprinted with permission of the publisher.

various analgesics, both alone and in combination, and of common undesirable side effects associated with their use. Of particular significance is the consistent analgesic efficacy of placebo in about one-fifth of patients in various double blinded situations. The proper place of the analgesic agent is not usurped by such data, but temporary placebo response must be kept in mind in evaluating the clinical situation. Both the patient and the therapist interact to meet some needs through placebo response.

Newer analgesic agents, some perhaps soon to be introduced to the American market and already available elsewhere, include anthranilic acid derivatives such as mefenamic acid, and more recently floctafenine, which probably are especially appropriate because they do have mild antiinflammatory efficacy as well. Indeed the most potent of the anthranilic acid series in this regard is meclofenamic acid which has been used extensively in rheumatoid arthritis and variant diseases as an NSAID (9). This series is flawed by a propensity toward bowel irritation and colitis which, however, is reversible[10]. In those patients not susceptible to this disorder the drugs of this series have minimal upper gastrointestinal toxicity and no apparent addictive potential (11). Table 3.3 offers common dosages of analgesics and their side effects.

SALICYLATES

Consistently the most effective analgesic and the most commonly used, averaging billions of dosage units daily, is aspirin in all of its forms. Yet, paradoxically, it is aspirin that has stimulated the enormous recent resurgency of antirheumatic nonsteroidal investigative drug research. For despite the consistent unchallenged antiinflammatory efficacy of this ancient derivative of salix, willow bark, noted in the ancient writing of Hippocrates, Pliny, and Galen, the difficulties in side effects of its often not well monitored use in therapeutic dosages has aroused interest in less toxic, more simply

TABLE 3.3. *Analgesics*

Drugs	Efficacy*	Dose	Side Effects
Aspirin	++	1–2 g/day	Primarily upper gastrointestinal, tinnitus, blood coagulation (see Table 3.4)
Acetaminophen	+	1–1.5 g q 3–6 h	Hepatic necrosis (overdosage)
Codeine	++	15–60 mg q 4 hr	Primarily constipation, nausea, vomiting, dizziness, sedation
Dihydrocodeine	++	60 mg q 4 hr	Same as for codeine
Propoxyphene	++	65 mg q 4 hr	Nausea, vomiting, dizziness
Pentazocine	++	50–75 mg q 4 hr	Nausea, vomiting, dizziness, hallucinations

* ++, highly efficacious; +, moderately efficacious.

Adapted from S. H. Roth, *New Directions in Arthritis Therapy*, Publishing Sciences Group, Littleton, Massachusetts, 1980. Reprinted with permission of the publisher.

administered, nonsteroidal alternatives (to be discussed next). Thus we seem to be passing beyond the hallowed "Age of Aspirin" to newer interest in alternative NSAIDs as well as to a resurgence of interest in nonacetylated cation salicylates, which also offer lower toxicity, and simpler dosage forms for easier compliance.

Although acetyl salicylate (ASA) may confer unique analgesic potency, newer clinical investigative efforts suggest that the nonacetylated cation salicylates may be equally potent antirheumatic agents for chronic administration (12). Thus although the acetyl radical transiently confers additional "fast, fast pain relief", the probably more meaningful therapeutic salicylate level confers the sustained antiinflammatory benefit desirable in long-term rheumatic disease control. Of the various salicylates listed in Figure 3.4, choline magnesium trisalicylate (CMTS) described in Figure 3.5, has probably been the most widely tested of these newer salicylates against traditional aspirin therapy, NSAID therapy, and in combination with various other antirheumatic agents including corticosteroids and gold therapy. CMTS has the advantage of simple two or three times a day dosage. It achieves a desirable therapeutic salicylate level at between four to six tablets (of 0.5 g each) daily with minimal upper gastrointestinal toxicity and fecal blood loss compared to clinical experience with therapeutic dosage of ASA (13) (4.0 g daily or more).

As Table 3.4 indicates, the most serious and most common side effects associated with therapeutic ASA sustained therapy are those affecting the upper gastrointestinal tract, the blood clotting mechanism, and the severe hypersensitivity reactions fortunately less common. Teratogenic acid and renal toxic effects and altered liver function also occur. These reactions are peculiar to ASA. The cation salicylates, though also likely to cause tinnitus and acid-base imbalance problems at high doses, infrequently are flawed by the major problems characteristically induced by acetylated salicylates, like aspirin (15).

Furthermore, the less expensive varieties of aspirin store poorly and decompose to salycilic acid, useful for corns and calluses but corrosive to the mucosal lining, when in contact with glass, as in the storage bottle. When inadequately dissolved in the stomach, ASA may come to nestle in its own private erosive pocket. This acid peptic pock mark not infrequently punctuates the chronic peptic disease of the rheumatoid patient and may erode into a blood vessel, provoking serious hemorrhage.

Nonacetylated salicylates, as is also the case for some of the newer benign propionic acid NSAIDs, seem to be bereft of such serious acid peptic potential. In contrast to ASA they do not potentiate back diffusion of hydrogen ions through the vulnerable mucosal barrier, which could lead to erosions, inflammation of the lining, loss of mucosal barrier, and even bleeding.

Although salicylates seem to be successful antiinflammatory agents for

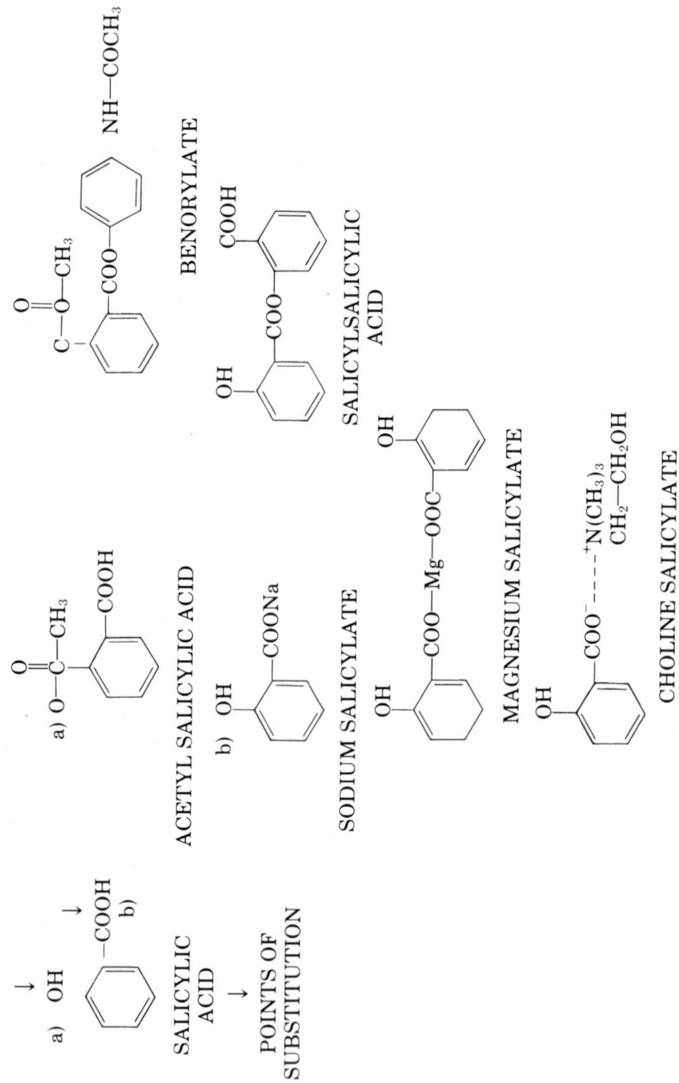

Fig. 3.4. Salicylic acid derivatives.

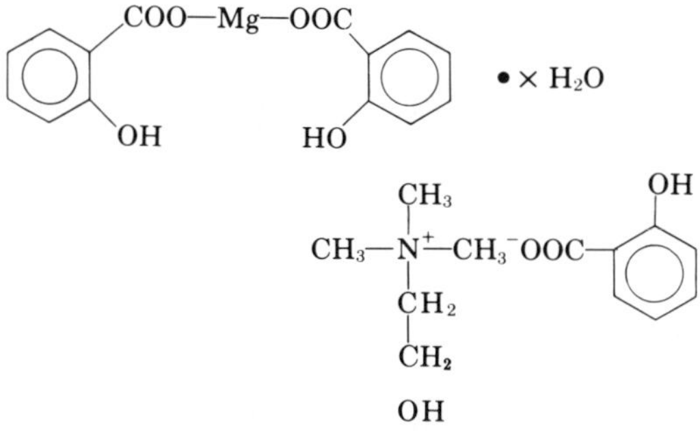

TRILISATE (CMTS)

Fig. 3.5. Trilisate (CMTS).

TABLE 3.4. *Salicylates: Adverse Effects*

1. Gastrointestinal, upper	AC*
2. Central nervous system	
3. Hepatic	
4. Renal	
5. Blood clotting	AC*
6. Hypersensitivity	AC*
7. Pregnancy	
8. Anemia	AC*

* Acetyl group aspirin.

Adapted from S. H. Roth, *New Directions in Arthritis Therapy*, Publishing Sciences Group, Littleton, Massachusetts, 1980. Reprinted with permission of the publisher.

the gamut of rheumatoid and osteoarthritic problems, they are not quite so simple to administer in order to achieve optimal effect. Desired therapeutic salicylate levels are not easily achieved. Some patients may absorb their salicylates poorly while others, because of a peculiar conjugation excretion mechanism, may suddenly achieve unusually high levels, with undesirable side effects. This, especially in the very young or very old, includes potentially dangerous metabolic acid-base imbalance. Tinnitus is common, unpleasant, and though usually readily reversible, may frighten the unsuspecting patient who fears for his hearing. Another unrecognized complication of high salicylate levels is central nervous system depressant effects including at times severe obtunding of affect leading to the impression in the elderly of senility. This is rapidly reversible upon discontinuance of salicylate. Of all medications, salicylates are the prime example of a group of drugs whose pharmacodynamics a physician must well understand in order to use properly.

To achieve and maintain ideal therapeutic levels the patient cannot simply be told to buy any over the counter ASA preparation and "learn to live with his arthritis". Rather he must be directed toward a salicylate that he will tolerate well, that he ideally can take in a simple manner to insure long-term compliance, and finally, at appropriate intervals his serum salicylate level must be monitored appropriately to determine that maximum efficacy is attainable. Under such circumstances the patient as well as the physician may often be well rewarded by sustained efficacy with safety from this form of initial therapy for the treatment of inflammatory joint disease or osteoarthritis.

Table 3.5 lists the most common salicylates by equivalent dosage schedules and side effects.

NONSTEROIDAL ANTIINFLAMMATORY DRUGS (NSAIDS)

Up to one hundred new nonsteroidal, nonsalicylate, organic acid derivatives for antiinflammatory analgesic therapy have been and are being developed. The general characteristics common to the NSAIDs are listed in Table 3.6.

Rather than consider the whole potpourri of current clinical investigative trial and failure, as well as some atypical though not necessarily promising structural exceptions to the organic acid rule, we will concentrate on those groups of drugs immediately available or about to appear in the medical marketplace.

Propionic Acid Series

The propionic acid series (Fig. 3.6) is really the prototype of the present nonsteroidal crop of drugs of lower toxicity with acceptable antiinflammatory efficacy.

Ibuprofen is the forerunner of this series. Its predecessor, ibufenac, was far more potent but as is so often the case in antirheumatic drug therapy—the more potent agent also tends to produce more and more severe toxicity. The hepatotoxicity seen with ibufenac has not recurred to mar the ibuprofen experience. After a decade of attempts to find an optimal therapeutic dosage

TABLE 3.5. *Salicylate equivalents**

Name of Medication	No. of Tablets	Tablet (mg)	Salicylate Content (mg)	Content of Other (mg)
ASA	1	325 (5 grains)	244	81.3–acetyl
	2	650 (10 grains)	487	162–acetyl
Liquid Arthropan salicylate	1 tsp	870	496	374–choline
Mobidin salicylate	1	600	447	65–magnesium

* Thus when a physician prescribes ASA for patients with RA at either 3 tabs. q.i.d. or 4 tabs. t.i.d., the total mg dose of aspirin is 3.9 mg. However, the total mg dose as *salicylate* is only 2.925 mg. Since one teaspoonful of Arthropan Liquid or one tablet of Mobidin is equivalent in salicylate content to 2 ASA tablets, appropriate conversions would be required when prescribing these medications.

Adapted from S. H. Roth, *New Directions in Arthritis Therapy*, Publishing Sciences Group, Littleton, Massachusetts, 1980. Reprinted with permission of the publisher.

TABLE 3.6. *Antiinflammatory Drugs*

I. Pharmacological Properties
   A. In general, all well and rapidly absorbed from the upper gastrointestinal tract.
   B. All, in general, tightly bind to plasma albumin competing for sites with other drugs.
   C. All prostaglandin synthetase inhibitors (sulindac exception in that it's biometabolite sulphide performs this active function).

II. NSAID Activity
   A. All fast acting with symptomatic benefit within days although full antiinflammatory effect may not be evident for weeks.
   B. Upper gastrointestinal side effects are uniformly most common. Side effects especially peculiar to some groups:
      1. Pyrroles–fluid retention
      2. Indoles–central nervous system effects
      3. Fenamates–diarrhea

III. Choice of NSAID
   A. Propionic acid derivatives, lowest incidence of long-term side effects and alternative first choice to salicylates.
   B. Appropriate trial of any of less toxic NSAIDs individualized to a particular patient response within first 2 weeks.
   C. More potent but toxic NSAIDs such as indomethacin and phenylbutazone. Keep in mind drugs for more resistant inflammatory problems.
   D. Combination therapy with background steroids, gold and other remission-inducing drugs acceptable.
   E. Combination with salicylates and multiple NSAIDs still under investigation.

Adapted from S. H. Roth, *New Directions in Arthritis Therapy*, Publishing Sciences Group, Littleton, Massachusetts, 1980. Reprinted with permission of the publisher.

range, ibuprofen has evolved to the present 1200–2400 mg dosage range to achieve its optimum analgesic/antiinflammatory potency.

Partly because of a short, 2-hr half-life, at least a four times daily dosage is required. However, the drug is well absorbed, even with food and meals, and achieves a rapid serum concentration in 1–2 hr after a single 400 mg dose.

Although drug interactions occur with hypoglycemic agents and corticosteroids, displacing them from albumin binding sites, ibuprofen has been given safely in combination with warfarin without undue anticoagulation interference. Nevertheless, it should be appropriately monitored. It produces little upper gastrointestinal toxicity, as documented by endoscopy studies, and this may be of importance for the all too common problem of arthritis with preexisting upper gastrointestinal disease. It has been used in combination with essentially all forms of other background antirheumatic drug therapy. Aspirin seems to increase excretion of the drug and lower its serum level.

Huskisson et al. (16) suggested, on the basis of his studies, that various

ALCLOFENAC (Mervan, Warner-Lambert; Prinalgin, Berk)

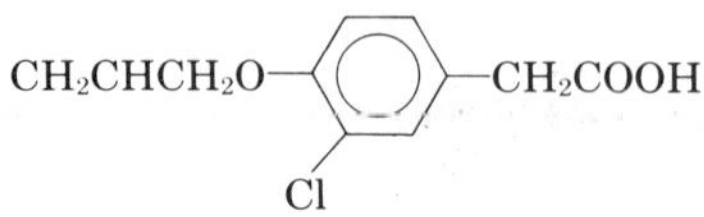

4-ALLYLOXY-3-CHLOROPHENYLACETIC ACID

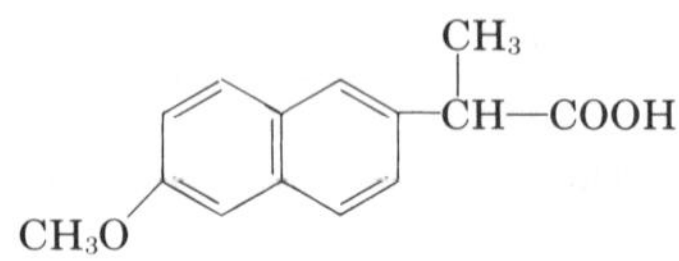

NAPROXEN (Syntex)

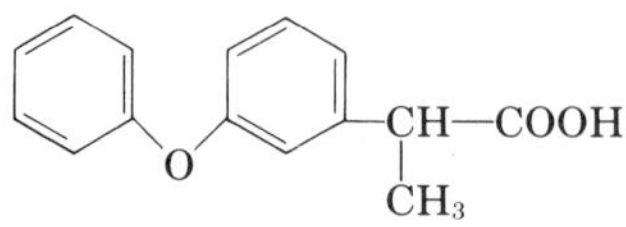

FENOPROFEN (Dista)

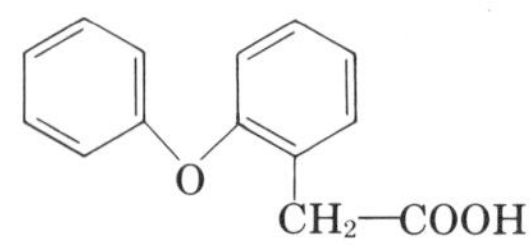

FENCLOFENAC (Reckitt-Norwich)

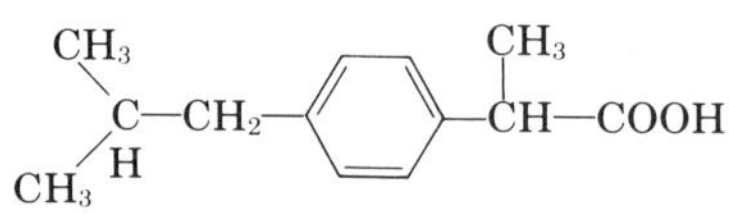

IBUPROFEN (Boots-Upjohn)

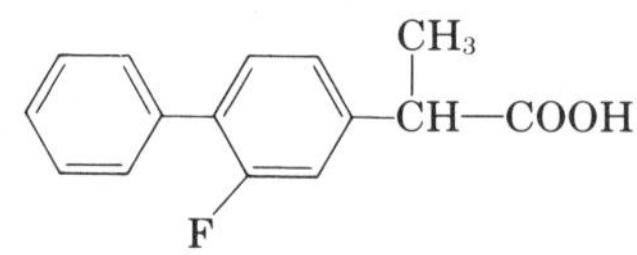

FLURBIPROFEN (Boots)

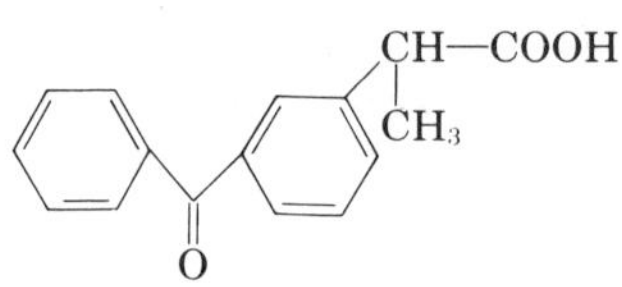

KETOPROFEN (Ives-Rhone)

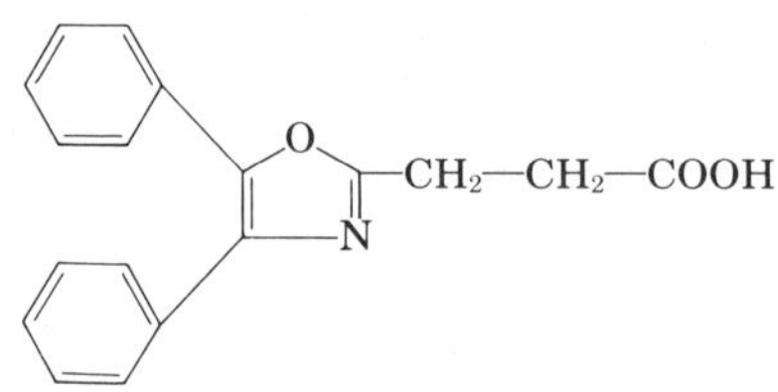

OXAPROZIN (Wyeth)

Fig. 3.6. Arylalkanoic acids (Propionic acid series).

RA patients, when tried on a cross-over regimen of ibuprofen, ketoprofen, fenoprofen calcium, and naproxen, generally tended to respond to one agent better than to the others and to tolerate others less well. His study has since been repeated under different dosage circumstances by Fries and his co-workers (17), and both tend to point to subsets of patients who respond best to one particular agent but not always as well as to others. Generally, in both Huskisson's and Fries' experience naproxen was the preferred agent, with the maximum efficacy and lowest toxicity. However, there may be chemical groupings that help one population more than another (18).

Naproxen has a 13-hr half-life, allowing a simple twice daily dosage for the recommended 500–750 mg total daily dose. However, with sustained use it has been determined that once daily dosage at 500 mg may offer simple maintenance advantage (19). Especially of interest, naproxen is the only NSAID to date with published evidence of enhanced clinical efficacy in combination with salicylate (20). Thus in our experience, a twice daily salicylate, such as CMTS, can be given to a patient together with naproxen to achieve a simple dosage regimen with enhanced compliance for greater efficacy when one or the other agents alone proves less than optimally effective at therapeutic dosage. This also appears to sidestep the additive upper gastrointestinal toxicity of ASA.

Of further interest, a databank analysis of comparable subsets of RA patients on ASA with background therapy versus naproxen with background therapy suggests that naproxen may have greater efficacy in patients under nonstudy conditions (21) (Fig. 3.7). These patients remained on a particular drug only when they appeared to benefit from that agent in contrast to usual imposed protocol requirements to complete a controlled study. This demonstrates the "real world" comparison of the subset of RA patients that does best with naproxen compared to usual ASA response in RA.

Naproxen has a wider therapeutic to toxicity ratio than many of the NSAIDs, allowing higher than recommended dosages without untoward side effects, and accelerated renal clearance above 750 mg. This may explain why 500 mg twice daily is often well tolerated when warranted by the clinical situation, again confirmed by the same databank experience (22).

Other propionic acid agents include fenoprofen calcium, given 300–600 mg three to four times daily, and ketoprofen, 150–300 mg three times daily, to provide alternatives with similar properties and pharmacological profiles.

We would agree with Huskisson that patients not responding optimally to one of this group after an appropriate trial of weeks could be switched safely to another for comparison purposes. Table 3.7 lists equivalent dosage schedules and comparisons of side effects for NSAIDs.

Indole Series

This series, which began a decade ago with indomethacin, has now spawned the indene, sulindac, and the pyrrole, tolmetin sodium (Fig. 3.8).

Indomethacin is well recognized as a standard in therapy for rheumatoid variant diseases, especially ankylosing spondylitis (23). In that disorder, especially, it is well tolerated even in higher dosage, up to 150–200 mg daily. Unfortunately, central nervous system side effects may flaw use of this agent (because of its serotonin-like chemical structure), as do fairly frequent upper gastrointestinal intolerance problems (24).

Its successor from the same manufacturer, sulindac, has a longer half-life of 16 hr, which allows twice daily dosage. In early studies it is reputed to have less side effects (25) and little gastrointestinal erosive potential. The full dosage of 200 mg twice daily might induce side effects similar to those of indomethacin in large doses, but are that uncommon. One hundred fifty milligrams twice daily may be less efficacious than optimal indomethacin doses, especially for treatment of negative spondyloarthropathies and osteoarthritis of the hip (26).

Tolmetin sodium has a short half-life but relatively long action, and therefore becomes a reasonable alternative to the previous two agents.

RA, DX PHOENIX ARTHRITIS CENTER
Date: MAR 21, 1979 COMPUTER PROGNOSTIC ANALYSIS
325 patients have been selected with the following criteria: See Subset Library Listing for criteria defining Subset 2 Diagnosis: RA

PRE-TREATMENT COMPARABILITY

Descriptor	Aspirin		Naprosyn	
		+		+
Age (mean years)	52.46		53.45	
Sex: percent Female	71.01		64.37	
Arthritis (% of patients)	100.00		100.00	
Symmetry of Arthritis (% of patients)	88.41		88.51	
PIP Involved (% of patients)	62.32		58.62	
Wrists Involved (% of patients)	81.16		71.26	
Knees Involved (% of patients)	66.67		52.87	
Subcutaneous Nodules (% of patients)	23.19		14.94	
Dry eyes (% of patients)	5.80		3.45	
Hematocrit (mean)	38.23		38.76	
White blood count (mean)	8.28	*	7.03	
Grip strength (mean)	60.00	*	83.40	
FANA (mean)	64.00	*	33.33	
Latex Fixation (mean)	219.53		236.92	*

THERAPY

Drug	Pts.	Mean Dose	Associated Therapy	Subsequent Therapy
Aspirin	69	7.6 tabs/day	Nap(19)Indo(10)*	Plaq(9)Gold(4)Indo(3)
Naprosyn	87	877 mgm/day	ASA(19)Gold(12)*	Pred(2)ASA(9)Plaq(5)*

Other Therapy (43):
Ibuprofen (15), Nalfon (9), Phenylbut (6), Penamine (6), Methotrexate (5), Azathioprine (1)

OUTCOME

Per cent of patients experiencing each event.

End Event	Months									
ASPIRIN GROUP	1	2	4	6	8	10	12	14	16	18
Death (cumulative %)	0	0	0	0	0	0	0	0	0	0
Arthritis, exacerbated (%)	3	5	5	14	25	25	47	47	47	47
Arthritis, remission (%)	0	0	0	0	0	0	0	0	0	0
MCP joint improvement (%)	10	12	18	37	37	37	37	69	69	69
Prednisone, increased (%)	0	0	0	0	0	0	0	0	0	0
Neuropathy, observed (%)	3	3	3	3	3	3	3	3	3	3
Patients followed (number)	69	23	13	9	6	4	3	3	1	0
NAPROSYN GROUP	1	2	4	6	8	10	12	14	16	18
Death (cumulative %)	0	0	0	0	0	0	0	0	0	0
Arthritis, exacerbated (%)	3	3	3	3	3	3	3	3	3	3
Arthritis, remission (%)	1	1	5	12	12	12	12	12	12	12
MCP joint improvement (%)	23	26	31	47	47	47	47	73	73	73
Prednisone, increased (%)	0	0	0	0	0	0	0	0	0	0
Neuropathy, observed (%)	3	3	3	3	3	3	3	3	3	3
Patients followed (number)	87	28	18	10	6	5	5	5	4	2

Fig. 3.7. Computer prognostic analysis.

TABLE 3.7. *Nonsteroidal Antiinflammatory Agents*

Drugs	Efficacy	Antiinflammatory	Dose	Side Effects
Aspirin	++	+++	3.6 g or more	Primarily upper gastrointestinal, tinnitus blood coagulation (see Table 4)
Indomethacin	++	++++	25–200 mg (1–4 times divided dosage daily)	Upper gastrointestinal, central nervous system; muzzy headed, headaches, disorientation, personality changes, visual disturbance
Phenylbutazone	+++	++++	100–400 mg (2–3 times divided dosage daily)	Primarily gastrointestinal, fluid retention skin reactions, stomatitis, hematuria
Oxyphenbutazone	++	++++	100–400 mg (2–3 times divided dosage daily)	Same as for phenylbutazone
Ibuprofen	++	++	900–3600 mg (3–4 divided doses daily)	Infrequent gastrointestinal
Ketoprofen	++	+++	150–300 mg (3–4 divided doses daily)	Similar to ibuprofen
Fenoprofen calcium	++	+++	900–3000 mg (3–4 divided doses daily)	Same as ibuprofen
Naproxen	++	+++	500–750 mg (2–3 divided doses daily)	Same as ibuprofen
Sulindac	++	+++	300–400 mg (2 divided daily doses)	Similar to indomethacin but less frequent
Tolmetin sodium	++	++++	1200–3000 mg (2–3 divided doses daily)	Similiar to indomethacin but fewer CNS reactions
Sodium meclofenomate	++	+++	200–400 mg (3–4 divided doses daily)	Gastrointestinal, skin

Adapted from S. H. Roth, *New Directions in Arthritis Therapy*, Publishing Sciences Group, Littleton, Massachusetts, 1980. Reprinted with permission of the publisher.

Maximum efficacy is achievable by 200 mg capsules taken three to four times daily. Central nervous system toxicity is seen less often than with indomethacin, and gastric tolerance appears equivalent to the propionic acid series (27). Some patients unresponsive to drugs cited earlier may prove to be responsive to tolmetin sodium.

Tolmetin sodium also has the best substantiated early experience as an NSAID in the treatment of juvenile rheumatoid arthritis (28). Juvenile rheumatoid disease consistently responds to therapeutic dosage of salicylates. Yet, owing to oto-toxicity, hepato-toxicity, acute salicylism, and upper gastrointestinal toxicity on full dosage of ASA, unfortunately all too frequent, NSAIDs have logically evolved as alternatives to more toxic forms of therapy, including corticosteroids and aspirin in the juveniles.

Others

The pyrazolone group continues to be effectively represented by phenylbutazone and oxyphenbutazone as very potent nonsteroidal agents for short-term acute antiinflammatory use. However, because of potential bone marrow and renal toxicity, as well as major upper gastrointestinal toxicity, they have been increasingly replaced by previously discussed NSAIDs for long-term chronic rheumatic disease therapy. Short-term use is reserved for the acute inflammatory syndromes involving the axial skeleton and centri-

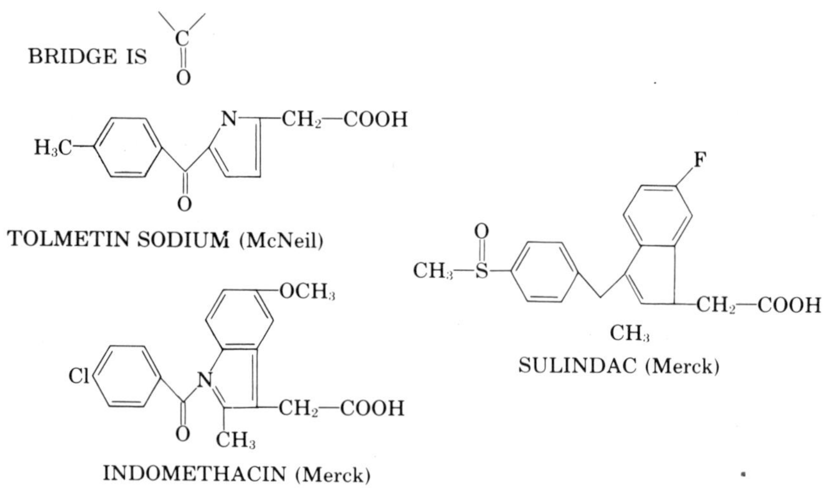

Fig. 3.8.

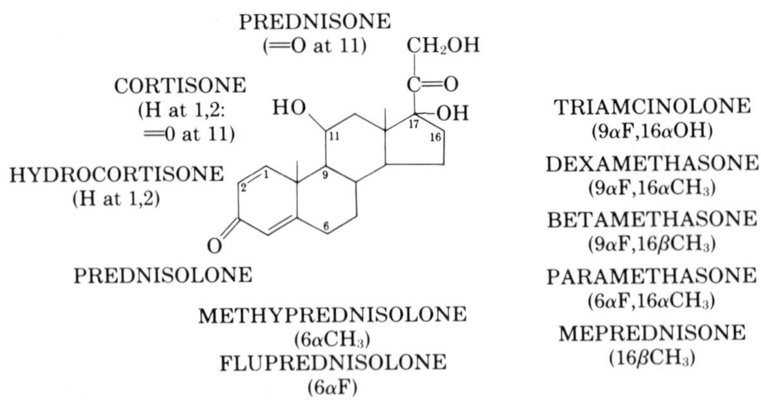

Fig. 3.9.

petal joints. If desired efficacy is not apparent within 36 hr, it is safe to assume that alternative agents are indicated. Three hundred to 400 mg daily, divided into three or four doses, are usually appropriate for such inflammatory syndromes, but somewhat higher doses, up to 800 mg daily, may be used in acute gouty arthritis for very short intervals (not to exceed 2, maximally 3 days). Usually the dosage is rapidly tapered downward because of the toxicity of this group, and repeated laboratory monitoring is required.

Other agents, such as meclofenamate sodium, alclofenac, and diclofenac, have appeared in many foreign marketplaces, but they are not yet available in the United States at the time of this writing. They are being tested and may yet appear for prescription use. They are flawed by rare but serious side effects—serious diarrhea for meclofenamate and vasculitis and severe skin rash problems with alclofenac, perhaps also diclofenac (29, 30).

Corticosteroids

No drug brought more excitement or hope to the treatment of inflammatory joint disease than that seen with the introduction of corticosteroids by Hench and coworkers in 1947, which was greeted by a Nobel Prize. This story by now is well known, as are the many side effects and unwanted effects of corticosteroids listed in Table 3.8. Hormonal toxicity is dosage dependent, age and sex dependent, and characterized by wide individual variation.

Corticosteroids almost always effectively relieve the symptomatic inflammatory fibrositic stiffness, fatigability, and discomfort of inflammatory joint disease. Even in small dosages they can dramatically alter the functional impairment that accompanies such rheumatic disease states. For this reason, they are not infrequently used in practice. A review of a national rheumatic disease databank produced data from a number of university and community arthritis centers that confirmed that up to one-third of patients with rheumatoid arthritis are taking corticosteroids, usually in lower physiological dosages (31). The drugs were not necessarily started by these centers, but discontinuation is difficult. Molecular modifications of the basic steroid molecule, as indicated in Figure 3.9, represent the transformation of the original cortisone through prednisone and analogues. Once the mineral corticoid side effect was stripped from cortisone, little change in antiinflammatory activity or toxicity was noted on a relative dosage strength basis.

Table 3.9 represents relative prednisone dosage equivalents of the steroid analogues. The physiological dosage is considered to be an amount not exceeding the endogenous production of 7.5 mg or from 5 mg and below for postmenopausal females.

Even lower dosages produce increased susceptibility to infection as part of their action. Chemical alteration of carbohydrate metabolism and fluid retention are also part of the basic action of these hormones. Easy bruising

TABLE 3.8. *Corticosteroid Side Effects*

I.	Cosmetic
	Acne
	Ecchymosis, petechiae
	Moon face
	Fatty deposition
	Hirsutism
	Striae
II.	Hormonal
	Carbohydrate intolerance
	Hyperlipidema
	Electrolyte intolerance
	Hypertension
	Heart failure
	Menopausal symptoms
	Menstrual disorders
III.	End Organ
	Gastrointestinal ulcers
	Glaucoma
	Steroid myopathy
	Arteritis
	Osteoporosis
	Pancreatitis
IV.	Psychological
	Agitation
	Euphoria
	Restlessness
	Stimulation
	Psychotic state
	Manic-depression
V.	Systemic
	Edema
	Infections
	Thromboembolism

Adapted from S. H. Roth, *New Directions in Arthritis Therapy*, Publishing Sciences Group, Littleton, Massachusetts, 1980. Reprinted with permission of the publisher.

and osteoporosis in the postmenopausal women are all too common problems. Particular analogues, such as dexamethasone, have a marked stimulant effect, overcoming fatigue, but enhancing obesity through stimulation of the appetite center; thyroid and pituitary suppression may develop. The halogenated corticosteroid analogues have the greatest propensity for steroid myopathy.

In the face of stress related to surgery, trauma, or infection, mineralcorticoids may be required to prevent collapse from relative adrenal insufficiency.

The attraction of corticosteroids in the face of disability and suffering can be enormous until the clinician considers the increasingly wide array of

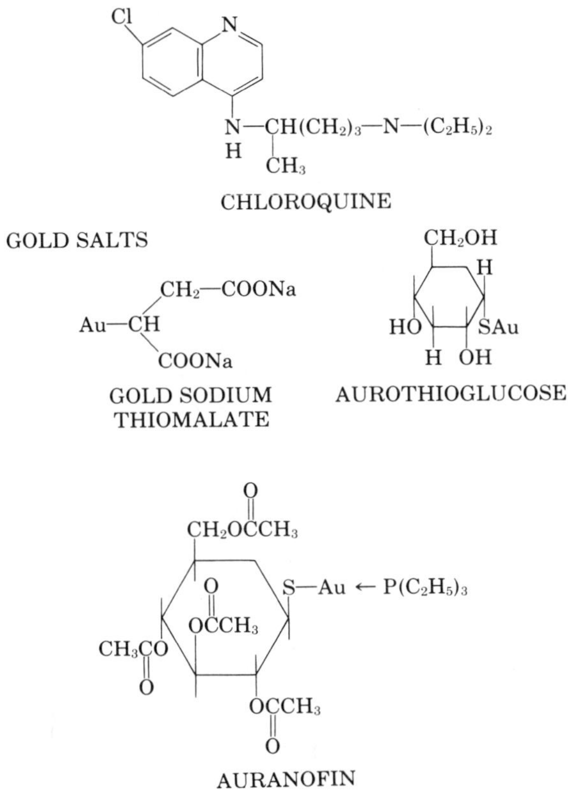

Fig. 3.10. Gold compounds and antimalarials.

nonsteroidal alternatives now available. Weighed against the almost addictive potential of corticosteroids in rheumatoid diseases the substitution, whenever possible, of nonsteroid alternatives appears justified.

By contrast, adrenal corticotrophic hormones (ACTH) can be dramatically effective in acute inflammatory events such as gouty arthritis or the severe exacerbation of rheumatoid disease. It is best suited for inpatient use and short-term therapy. A suggested dosage regimen is outlined in Table 3.10.

Intraarticular corticosteroids offer consistent and sometimes dramatic benefit in resistant proliferative synovitis whenever sepsis can be safely ruled out. Secondary aseptic necrosis or accelerated wear in weight bearing joints can occur in cases where the procedure is repeated with undue frequency.

Remission-Inducing Drugs (SAARDs)

Gold salts and antimalarial medications (Fig. 3.10) (in the form of chloroquine and hydroxychloroquin) are time-honored SAARDs. Only the latter

TABLE 3.9. *Comparison of Steroid Equivalent Dosages*

Name	Structure of Synthetic Analog	Equivalent Dose (mg)
Cortisone		25.0
Prednisone	δ-1-cortisone	5.0
Prednisolone	δ-1-cortisol	5.0
Triamcinolone	9-α-fluoro-16-α-hydroxy-prednisolone	4.0
Dexamethasone	9-α-fluoro-16-α-methyl-prednisolone	0.75
Methylprednisolone	6-α-methyl-prednisolone	4.0
Fluprednisolone	6-α-fluoro-prednisolone	1.5
Betamethasone	9-α-fluoro-16-β-methyl-prednisolone	0.6
Paramethasone	6-α-fluoro-16-α-methyl-prednisolone 21-acetate	2.0
Meprednisone	16-β-methylprednisone	4.0

Adapted from S. H. Roth, *New Directions in Arthritis Therapy*, Publishing Sciences Group, Littleton, Massachusetts, 1980. Reprinted with permission of the publisher.

TABLE 3.10. *ACTH Dosage Schedule in Rheumatoid Arthritis*

Dose (units)	Frequency	Clinical State	Duration
30–120	q	Severe flare	×1
40	q.d.	Active rheumatoid arthritis	×3–5
20	q	Active maintenance	×3–4
20	q.o.d.	Maintenance	prn
10	q.d. to q.o.d.	Taper off	prn

Adapted from S. H. Roth, *New Directions in Arthritis Therapy*, Publishing Sciences Group, Littleton, Massachusetts, 1980. Reprinted with permission of the publisher.

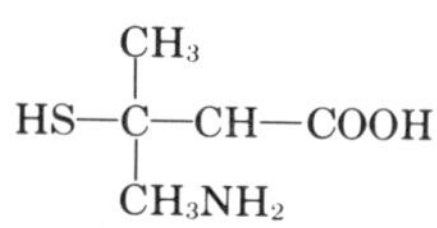

PENICILLAMINE

Fig. 3.11. Penicillamine.

is used in systemic lupus erythematosus and certain collagen-vascular diseases. They are not usually used in the rheumatoid variant disease nor have they any place in degenerative arthritis or metabolic arthritis.

More recently, d-penicillamine has been approved for use in rheumatoid arthritis. Its side effects are similar to those produced by gold therapy but this chelating agent appears to have immunomodulating effects that are especially desirable when vasculitis is superimposed upon RA. Nevertheless, experience with this agent is far more limited than with gold therapy and it remains at this point a potent backup drug for patients resistant to more conventional therapy, including chrysotherapy (Fig. 3.11).

All these agents are slow to produce effects (3–4 months) and suppress the underlying granulomatous, destructive disease process when effective. A newer gold compound, auranofin, given orally, may act with greater alacrity (4–6 weeks); it is currently being tested and, at the time of this writing, is strictly experimental. This newer agent seems to have immunoregulatory potential in addition to usual effects on basic sulfhydral and lysosomal mechanisms common to traditional gold therapy. Further experience will be necessary to document whether auranofin has less serious, especially renal, toxicity than traditional gold therapy.

Other immunomodulating drugs such as cyclophosphamide, chlorambucil, azathioprine, methotrexate, and, more recently, levamisole are reserved for the most severe recalcitrant cases of rheumatoid disease or limited to clinical investigators under rigidly monitored protocol conditions. Nevertheless, they do point to new directions in medical therapy of previously untreatable disease. Other compounds of different chemical structure, with different times, are in the trial stages.

Summary

The foregoing series of drugs summarizes the groups of agents at the command of the physician treating rheumatic disorders. Prescription based on experience can achieve relief from pain and suppression of rheumatic activity in even the most advanced cases, with enhanced systemic well-being and the increased mobility necessary to the individualized rehabilitation program.

The program must be closely individualized to the particular problem at hand. For example the osteoarthritic patient may require only simple local attention to a problem induced by a symptomatic weight-bearing joint. In the short run, intraarticular corticosteroids may be adequate for a start whereas long range plans might include a moderate dose of NSAID.

By contrast, systemic inflammatory rheumatic disorders will involve ever more sophisticated combined treatment programs. No one program will generally work over sustained periods of time without intermittent reevaluation and adjustment to the changing needs of the patient. Without such careful attention long-term management goals may be lost. Moreover, during postoperative periods, little alteration in the program, even needed corticosteroid decrements, should be undertaken as adverse effects upon compliance with a physical and occupational therapy program might result.

Less common forms of arthritis, including metabolic arthropathy, infectious arthritis, the arthritis associated with hematological and neoplastic diseases, and various collagen diseases, all require more specific detailed medication discussions than appropriate here. Suffice it to add that the peculiar agents required by these disorders for medical control are just as necessary to the success of any rehabilitation attempt planned.

Similarly, appropriate therapeutic response to such common rheumatic disease complications as anemia, reactive depression, osteoporosis, and especially gastrointestinal dysfunction demands acute intervention as well as long-term prophylactic measures. The attentiveness and preparedness of the physician are equally demanded for the umbrella of good general medical care that must cover the requirements of a successful rehabilitation program.

In planning treatment it must be appreciated that patient compliance with the physician's instructions is not only related to *hope* of the patient for important help controlling disease and relief of discomfort, but is inversely related to such factors as concern for toxicity of the medication, number of tablets, frequency of dosage and finally, cost of medication itself. However, cost considerations must be tempered by overall successful impact of the particular therapeutic regimen on the success of the demanding rehabilitation goals. Certainly inefficacious therapy or undesirable toxicity have a built-in cost beyond the price of an individual tablet, no matter how inexpensive!

In summary then, it is clear that a balanced general medical program with appropriate antiarthritic agents is an intimate part of the immediate and long-range planning for both treatment and rehabilitation of the arthritic patient. To achieve these goals requires close physician-patient rapport and cooperation with an experienced, expert team of health professionals that closely communicate continuous interest and expert experience. It is through such effective interaction that appropriately determined drug therapy will allow for maximal rehabilitative direction of the patient toward successful management.

REFERENCES

1. McCarty, D. J., Jr. Pseudogout: Articular Chondrocalcinosis. In *Arthritis,* Ed. 9., edited by J. L. Hollander and D. J. McCarty, Jr. Lea and Febiger, Philadelphia, 1979.
2. Hollander, J. L. Intra-Synovial Corticosteroid Therapy. In *Arthritis,* Ed. 9., edited by J. L. Hollander and D. J. McCarty, Jr. Lea and Febiger, Philadelphia, 1979.
3. Hart, F. D. Drug induced arthritis. *Curr. Med. Res. Opinion, 2:* 505, 1974.
4. Blomgren, S. E. Drug-induced lupus erythematosus. *Semin. Hematol., 10:* 345, 1973.
5. Alacaron-Segovia, D. Drug-induced lupus syndromes. *Mayo Clinic. Proc., 44:* 664, 1969.
6. Hill, H. F. H. Treatment of rheumatoid arthritis with penicillamine. *Semin. Arthritis Rheum., 6:* 361, 1977.
7. Fessel, W. J. Hyperuricemia in health and disease. *Semin. Arthritis Rheum., 1:* 275, 1972.
8. Moertel, C. J. Relief of pain with oral medication. Symposium on analgesics. *Aust. N.Z. J. Med.,* (Suppl. 1) *6:* 1, 1976.
9. Dresner, J. A. Multicenter studies with sodium meclofenamate in the United States and Canada. *Curr. Therap. Res.,* (Suppl.) *23:* S90, 1978.
10. Preston, S. N. Safety of sodium meclofenamate. *Curr. Therap. Res.,* (Suppl.) *23:* S107, 1978.
11. Roth, S. H. Meclofenamate sodium long term open label experience. Presented at the American Society of Clinical Rheumatology, New Orleans, November, 1978.
12. Roth, S. H. Salicylate therapy: challenge and change. Presented at the UCLA Symposium on Pain, Los Angeles, May, 1977.
13. Multicenter Choline Magnesium Trisalicylate-ASA Study, Purdue Frederick Files.
14. Caravati, C. M., and Cosgrove, E. F. Salicylate toxicity—the probable mechanism of action. *Ann. Intern. Med., 24:* 638, 1946.
15. Roth, S. H. Salicylate therapy. *Florida Family Phys., 28:* 33, 1978.

16. HUSKISSON, E. C., WOOLF, D. L., BALME, H. W., SCOTT, J. AND FRANKLYN, S. Four new anti-inflammatory drugs: responses and variations. *Br. Med J., 1:* 1048, 1976.
17. WASNER, C., KRAINES, R. G., BRITTON, M. C. AND FRIES, J. F. A randomized double blind crossover trial of six nonsteroidal antiinflammatory agents in rheumatoid arthritis and ankylosing spondylitis. *Arthritis Rheum., 22:* 671, 1979.
18. HUSKISSON, E. C. Nonsteroidal antiinflammatory analgesics: basic clinical pharmacology and therapeutic use. *Drugs, 15:* 387, 1978.
19. ROBBINS, S. Personal communication, Syntex Files.
20. WILLKENS, R. F., AND SEGRE, E. J. Combination therapy with naproxen and aspirin in rheumatoid arthritis. *Arthritis Rheum., 19:* 677, 1975.
21. ROTH, S. H. Future trends in antiinflammatory drug therapy. Presented at the Annual Meeting of the American Society of Clinical Pharmacology and Therapeutics, Atlanta, March, 1978.
22. ROTH, S. H. ARAMIS: new insights into rheumatic diseases and management. Presented at the Kansas Veterans Administration, Kansas City, March, 1979.
23. CALABRO, J. J. Arthritis of the spine: early diagnosis and management of ankylosing spondylitis. *Med. Times, 105:* 80, 1977.
24. LOCKIE, M. D. Phenylbutazone, Indomethacin and Chloroquins in Therapy of Rheumatoid Arthritis. In *Arthritis*, Ed. 8., edited by J. L. Hollander and D. J. McCarty, Jr. Lea and Febiger, Philadelphia, 1972.
25. ROONEY, P., BUCHANAN, W., HAIGH, B. S. AND ROYLANCE P. J. A clinical assessment in general practice of sulindac. *Eur. J. Rheumatol. Inflamm., 1:* 66, 1978.
26. GRIBRAU, F. W. J., AND LISSONE, D. A. Experiences during double-blind study with MK-231 versus indomethacin in patients suffering from ankylosing spondylitis. *Dutch Med. J. (NTvG), 119:* 1135, 1975.
27. EHRLICH, G. E., AND ROTH, S. H. Rheumatoid arthritis: long term therapy with tolmetin sodium. *Orthop. Digest, 4:* 16, 1976.
28. LEVINSON, J. E., BAUM, J., BREWER, E., FINK, C. W., HANSON, V. AND SCHALLER, J. Comparison of tolmetin and aspirin in the treatment of juvenile rheumatoid arthritis. *J. Pediatr., 91:* 799, 1977.
29. PRESTON, S. N. Safety of sodium meclofenamate. *Curr. Therap. Res., 23:* S107, 1978.
30. HORT, J. F. Adverse reactions to alclofenac. *Curr. Med. Res. Opinion, 3:* 333, 1975.
31. ROTH, S. H. *New Directions in Arthritis Therapy.* Publishing Sciences Group, Littleton, Massachusetts, 1980.

4

The Rheumatic Disease Nurse Practitioner

COLLEEN CAVANAH MILLER

The nurse practitioner emerged in the mid-1960s as a new health professional trained to meet the public's primary health care needs. Today, there are scores of programs across the country preparing nurse practitioners in such speciality areas as pediatrics, adult health, women's health, geriatrics, mental health, family health, and the school-aged child. These health professionals practice in neighborhood health centers, hospital out-patient clinics and inpatient units, private medical offices, long-term care facilities, and schools.

Through didactic instruction and supervised clinical practice, nurse practitioner programs prepare registered nurses to obtain a complete health history, perform a comprehensive physical examination, identify health problems, assess laboratory data, and to develop and implement health care plans which include treatment goals, health education, referral to appropriate members of the health team, and evaluation of outcomes of care. Course outlines of nurse practitioner programs include normal and pathophysiology of the cardiovascular, musculoskeletal, respiratory, endocrine, neurological, and gastrointestinal systems, and eye, ear, nose, and throat; cultural implications for patient care; principles of teaching and learning; principles of management of chronic disease; and principles of management of episodic illness.

Medical supervision of nurse practitioners is often provided through the use of protocols written collaboratively. These protocols define areas of accountability of the nurse practitioner and the physician in planning and implementing the patient plan of care.

In the specialty of rheumatic disease, adult, family, and geriatric nurse practitioners identify their roles and responsibilities as including evaluation of new patients; ongoing management of the chronic disease; management of episodic illness; education of the patient and family, coworkers, and the community; and quality assurance.

Evaluation of New Patients

Often the nurse practitioner is the first health professional to assess the new patient. The responsibilities may include taking the health history, performing the physical examination, ordering appropriate laboratory tests and x-rays, establishing the data base and then referring the new patient to the physician to establish the diagnosis and to prescribe the treatment plan.

Most health care settings have developed special forms to record the history and physical examination. For a review of the components of the health history, the reader is referred to Reference 1.

A good checklist for inspection and palpation of the musculoskeletal system can be found in Reference 2.

Patient and family education for the new patient begins with an explanation of how a diagnosis is made and why an accurate diagnosis is essential.

Through words and behavior, the nurse practitioner can convey the attitude that "something can be done". The need for regular follow-up visits is emphasized. The nurse practitioner allows the patient and family time to ask questions, and offers support and understanding. These elements constitute the beginning of the nurse-patient relationship which may influence patient compliance with the prescribed medical regimen.

Ongoing Management

When the diagnosis of a specific rheumatic disease is confirmed, the physician may refer the patient to the nurse practitioner for follow-up. During subsequent visits, the nurse practitioner will perform the joint examination and screen laboratory data in order to evaluate the patient's response to the medical program. Changes in medication may be prescribed and laboratory tests ordered according to established protocols. An example of such a protocol is the following, which is offered as a model for the monitoring of patients receiving gold.

Gold Patients

		YES	NO	
SUB:	1.	____	____	Any changes in general health?
	2.	____	____	Any sudden changes in status of arthritis?
	3.	____	____	Any psychosocial changes influencing status? Explain.
	4.	____	____	Urticaria (hives) 24–48 hr after last gold shot?
	5.	____	____	Flushing 15–60 min after last gold shot?
	6.	____	____	Weakness, dizziness, or palpitations 15–60 min after last shot?
	7.	____	____	Any rash or pruritus (itching)?
	8.	____	____	Mouth or throat ulcers?
	9.	____	____	Recent diarrhea?

If Positive Response to 7, 8, 9, Withhold Gold. Treat Symptomatically.

		YES	NO	
	10.	____	____	Recent onset of visual changes? IF POSITIVE RESPONSE, REFER TO PHYSICIAN.
OBJ:	11.	____	____	Protein in urine____. IF OVER 1+, DO NOT GIVE GOLD. INSTRUCT PATIENT TO RETURN IN 2 WEEKS.
	12.	____	____	Change from normal in white blood count
	13.	____	____	Specific joint inflammation. Explain:

Plan: Symptomatic

1. Rash or pruritus	Synalar Cream 0.025% Sig: Apply b.i.d.
2. Mouth or throat ulcer	Folvite 5 mg, #50 Sig: One daily
3. Diarrhea	Lomotil #50 Sig: One tablet after each stool

Nurse Practitioner May Regulate Dosages as Follows:

1. Gold—increase or decrease time between injections, as indicated by side effects.
2. Indomethacin—increase to 200 mg/day. Decrease as indicated.
3. Ibuprofen—increase to 2000 mg/day. Decrease as indicated.
4. Aspirin—increase to tolerance (tinnitus)
5. Naproxen, fenoprofen calcium, tolmetin sodium, sulindac—increase or decrease as indicated.

X-rays and laboratory tests may be ordered by the nurse practitioner as indicated on a symptomatic basis.

Specific joint and system examination is to be done by the nurse practitioner every two months.

Patient to have office visit with nurse practitioner every third injection.

Review and audit to be done on regular basis, every sixth visit, jointly by physician and nurse practitioner.

Patients will be seen by physician as necessary at nurse practitioner's discretion. (Reproduced with permission from Mrs. Beverly Burton, R.N., A.N.P.)

Joint Aspiration and Injection

If the rheumatic disease patient has a limited number of painful, inflamed joints, the nurse practitioner may consult with the physician to determine if joint aspiration and local corticosteroid injection is indicated to relieve

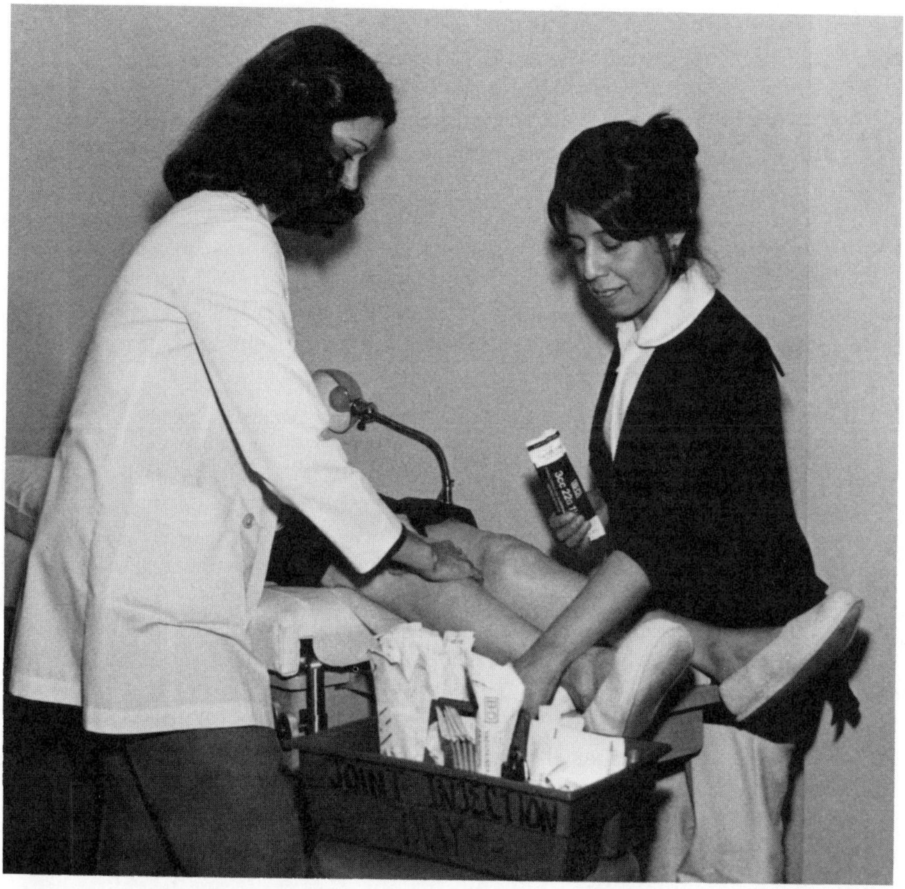

Fig. 4.1. If the rheumatic disease patient has a limited number of painful, inflamed joints, aspiration and injection may be indicated. (Colleen Miller, R.N. and Marie Ball, L.P.N. Patient is Mosstella Beaubien.)

symptoms temporarily. In addition, local therapy may preserve musculoskeletal function, prevent contractures, delay muscle atrophy, and prevent capsular and ligamentous laxity secondary to prolonged distension of joints containing effusions (3) (Fig. 4.1).

Intraarticular injection is contraindicated if infection or fracture of the joint is present, if the patient did not have a satisfactory response to a previous injection, if the patient has a systemic fungal infection, or if the joint to be injected is unstable.

Realizing the possibility of introducing infection into the joint capsule and the importance of obtaining a sterile specimen to culture, the nurse practitioner uses strict aseptic technique in preparing the injection site. The reason for the injection and the procedure which will be followed should be explained to the patient. Many patients do not appreciate the difference between oral corticosteroids and local corticosteroid injections.

The nurse practitioner will ask the patient if there is a history of allergy to local anesthetics. Any signs or symptoms of a reaction are to be reported as soon as practicable. Reactions may occur several minutes to several hours or days after injection.

Minor reactions from lidocaine may consist of any of the following: slight dizziness, pallor, diaphoresis, weakness, nausea, rarely fainting, and elevated pulse (4). Postinjection flare may occur a few hours after injection and may last up to 24 hr. Ice and analgesics will usually control the symptoms. For a detailed review of joint aspiration and injection technique, the reader is referred to Reference 4.

Signs of infection after a joint injection include an increase of pain, with or without swelling, occurring a few days to a week after injection. Immediate aspiration and culture should be performed.

The rheumatic disease nurse practitioner realizes the diagnostic value of the aspirated synovial fluid. The following are recorded: the gross appearance of the fluid including color, clarity, viscosity and occurrence and size of clots, and the quality of the mucin clot. Proper handling of the fluid is necessary to yield accurate laboratory results. Usually 15–20 ml of synovial fluid is sent to the laboratory for the following determinations: 2–5 ml in a sterile test tube containing heparin to be used for routine bacteriologic cultures; 2–5 ml prepared as above for cell count, differential, examination for crystals and cell inclusions; 2–5 ml in a test tube without anticoagulant for analysis of clot, hyaluronic acid, appearance (and possible protein, enzyme, and lipid studies) and examination of cells for inclusions and crystals; 3–5 ml in a tube containing potassium oxalate for sugar analysis and other determinations if clotting occurs in the above tube (5). For a comprehensive explanation of synovial fluid analysis, the reader is referred to Reference 5.

Hazards from multiple injections include accelerated destruction from overuse of a diseased joint, avascular necrosis (especially the hip and shoulder joints), osteoporosis, and delay in other more appropriate therapy such as surgery. Some practitioners follow the rule of thumb that if a joint requires more than three or four injections in a year, a surgical procedure may be indicated. An orthopedic surgeon should be consulted to evaluate the patient.

The topic of surgery produces anxiety in most people. Patients and their families usually need as many facts as possible to help them decide if and when to have surgery. Explaining the indication for the type of surgery, anticipated results, estimated length of stay in the hospital and cost will answer a few of the patient's questions and relieve some of his anxiety. Talking to other patients who have had the surgery and seeing models of the joint prosthesis can provide the patient with additional and very helpful information (Fig. 4.2).

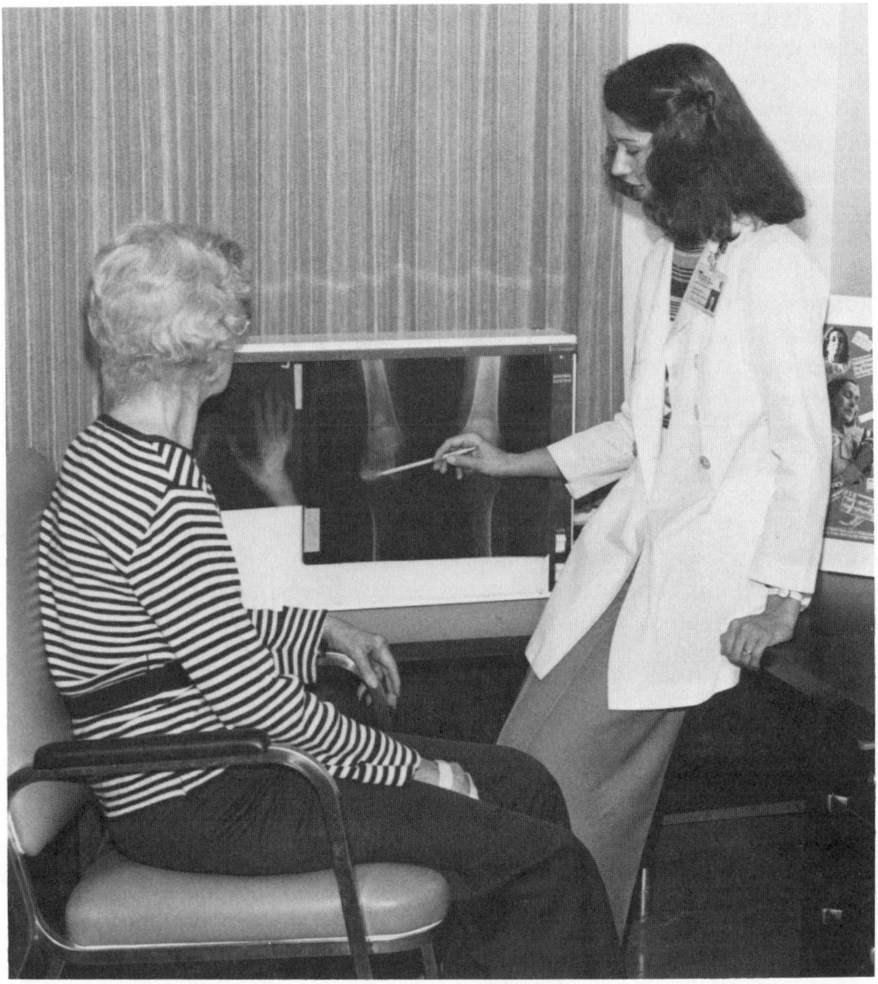

Fig. 4.2. Patient education includes an explanation of how a diagnosis is made. (Colleen Miller, R.N. and patient Mosstella Beaubien.)

Psychosocial Aspects

The rehabilitation of the rheumatic disease patient includes not only the medical management; the psychosocial aspects of chronic illness must also be considered as a province for the nurse practitioner. The patient and family are encouraged to discuss the frustrations caused by dealing with a rheumatic disease. The nurse practitioner then helps them understand that the remissions and exacerbations of some rheumatic diseases force the patient and family to continually readjust, and that an ill person at home imposes physical and psychological difficulties on the patient, family, and society. The patient or family may not want friends or employers to know that a diagnosis of some type of rheumatic disease has been made. A very real concern is the financial burden which may result from loss of earnings, the need to hire household help, and the cost of health care including medications, office visits, laboratory and x-ray charges, transportation, adaptive equipment, therapy, and hospitalizations. Adverse reactions can be discouraging to the patient. Add to this the sense of failure when medications do not produce the desired effect; the patient's feelings of helplessness, of being a burden to the family; physical deformities; pain, fatigue, the realization that there is no known cure, and the depression felt by many patients can be appreciated.

Besides listening to patients, understanding and accepting their feelings, the nurse practitioner may be instrumental in identifying a group of patients to form a self-help club. Many patients learn to deal effectively with changes caused by illness. Often patients who have "been there" can be extremely supportive to other rheumatic disease patients.

The nurse practitioner can also help by participating in public forums and other types of community education programs, such as speaking to industries, schools, citizen's groups, and professional organizations in order to educate them about current management of rheumatic diseases and to help change society's attitudes.

Patient Education

The nurse practitioner's role includes teaching informally as she sees each patient individually, performing an examination, preparing the patient for a procedure, interpreting laboratory results, and adjusting medications. In addition, many nurse practitioners have established formal, structured educational classes for rheumatic disease patients based on principles of learning and teaching (Fig. 4.3). These principles are summarized for the reader's review.

Principles of Learning

1. Perception is necessary for learning. 2. Conditioning is a process of learning. 3. Learning may occur through imitation. 4. The process of trial and error is a way of learning. 5. Problem solving is a method of learning. 6. The development of concepts is a part of the learning process. 7. An individual must be motivated to learn. 8. Physical and mental readiness are necessary for learning. 9. Effective learning requires active participation. 10. New learning must be based on previous knowledge and experience. 11. The emotional climate affects learning. 12. Repetition strengthens learning. 13. Reinforcement influences learning (6).

Principles of Teaching

1. Good nurse-learner rapport is important in teaching. 2. Teaching requires effective communication. 3. Knowledge of cultural patterns of

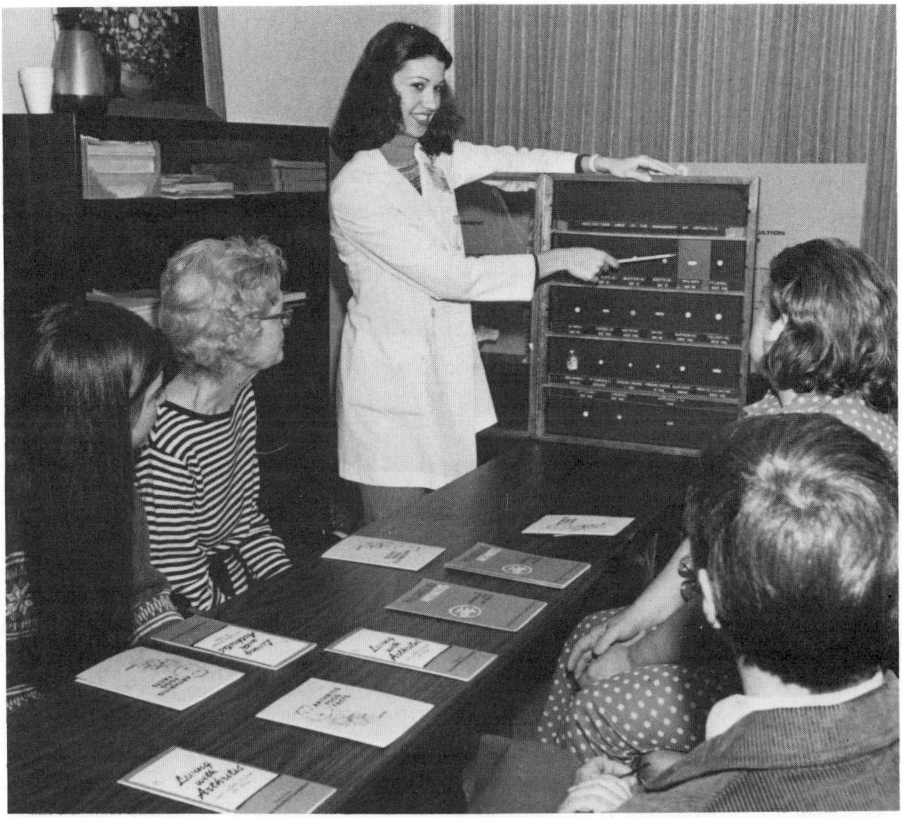

Fig. 4.3. Using a medication display made to facilitate discussion. The nurse practitioner teaches a group of rheumatic disease patients. (Colleen Miller, R.N., Mosstella Beaubien, Shann Taylor, Karen Vowells, and Jean Hoffman. All but Mosstella Beaubien are staff who posed as patients.)

ethnic groups to be taught is essential. 4. The teaching-learning process requires client-nurse cooperation. 5. Learning needs of clients and coworkers must be determined. 6. Objectives serves as guides in planning and evaluating teaching-learning experiences. 7. Planning time for teaching and learning requires special attention. 8. Control of the environment is an aspect of teaching. 9. Learning principles must be applied appropriately. 10. Evaluation is an integral part of teaching (7). For additional guidelines in patient teaching, the reader is referred to References 7 and 8.

Applying the general teaching and learning principles to rheumatic disease educational programs, the nurse practitioner first identifies the participants' special learning needs. Factors to be considered include their level of pain; disease history; relationship with the teacher and other participants; previous educational efforts; educational background; age; sex; social and cultural attitudes about illness; limitations, such as ability to ambulate, hearing or vision deficits, or a language barrier; and their receptivity to education. Learner's objectives and course content are based on the needs identified. Also to be considered are teaching resources available. The reader is referred to Reference 9. The purpose of this publication is to offer guidelines to design an educational program to meet the needs of your patient population and your health care setting. It contains an excellent bibliography of patient education materials.

In general, learners' goals for the rheumatic disease patient may include the following: at the end of the series of classes, the participant will be able to: 1. state the type of rheumatic disease; 2. state that there is no known cure at present; 3. state that the goals of the management program are to decrease pain and inflammation, to increase independent functioning, and to prevent deformity; 4. identify the patient's medications and list side effects of each; 5. demonstrate joint protection principles; 6. demonstrate range of motion exercises; 7. identify feelings caused by living with a chronic illness.

Typical classes conducted in a series may include such topics as joint anatomy and pathophysiology; control through medication, joint protection; exercise programs, proper use of heat and cold, balancing rest and activity, and proper follow-up care; proper nutrition; quackery; and living with arthritis.

Often other members of the multidisciplinary health team as well as lay volunteers, such as selected patients, may help plan and teach the classes (Fig. 4.4). Formats of the classes may be lecture, group discussion, demonstration or a mixture. It is helpful for the nurse practitioner to explain the objectives of each class and to summarize at the end. The date, time, place and topic of the next class are also announced. Handouts which the patients review between classes can strengthen learning.

To evaluate the classes, feedback from the participants is essential. Their comments will help the nurse practitioner and other teachers learn if content, speakers, length and location of the classes meets the needs of the participants and if the objectives were realistic.

In order to have an effective educational program, the comfort of the rheumatic disease patient must be considered. Evaluate the classroom for proper chairs, easy access, accessible bathroom, adequate ventilation, and good lighting. It is helpful to offer a "stand-up" break during the class so that the participants do not have to sit in one position more than twenty or thirty minutes. Active participation by the patients, such as doing the exercises or joint protection principles being demonstrated will not only facilitate learning, but will also give the participants an opportunity to change position.

Family should be encouraged to participate in the classes. Special "family nights" may be scheduled to offer the family the opportunity to hear up-to-

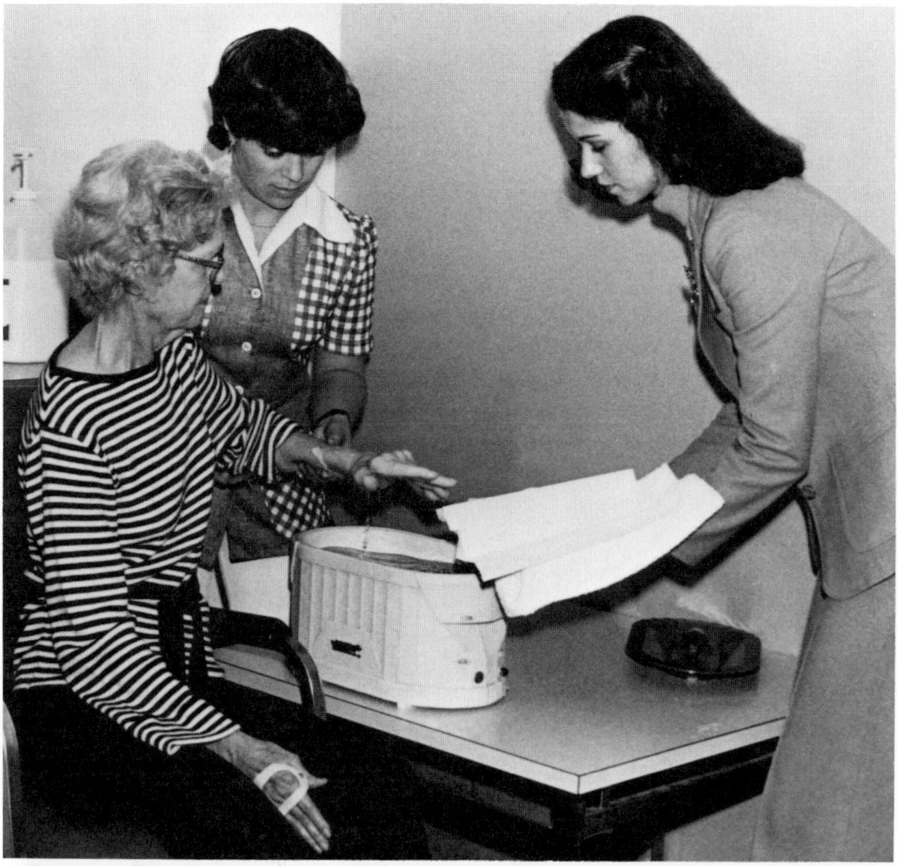

Fig. 4.4. One of the health professionals often asked to evaluate, educate, and treat the rheumatic disease patient is the physical therapist. (Colleen Miller, R.N., Jan Hanson, R.P.T., and Mosstella Beaubien.)

date information concerning rheumatic disease management and to have their questions answered.

While many books and films are available commercially for rheumatic disease patient teaching, the nurse practitioner may find that certain materials needed are unavailable. Individual nurse practitioners have made various teaching materials such as medication instruction cards, medication displays, slides, and tapes to supplement their programs. A bulletin board in the waiting room of the office or clinic or on a prominent wall on a hospital unit can display current information and announcements of future meetings and classes.

Referral to Other Health Professionals

Successful rehabilitation of the rheumatic disease patient requires the expertise of various health professionals (Fig. 4.5). Those professionals often

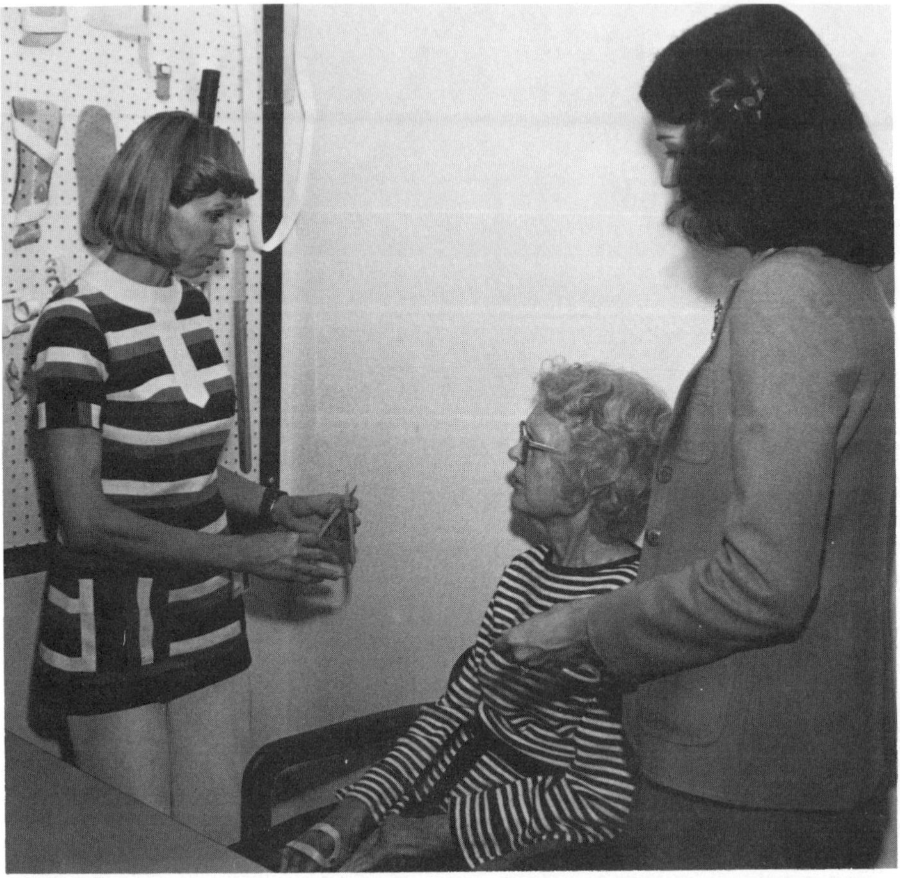

Fig. 4.5. Referral to other members of the rehabilitation team is the responsibility of the nurse practitioner. (Colleen Miller, R.N., Sherrill Musser, O.T.R., and Mosstella Beaubien.)

asked to evaluate, educate and treat the rheumatic disease patient include the physical therapist, the occupational therapist, the dietitian, and the social worker. Referral to appropriate members of the rehabilitation team, coordination of efforts and follow-up are major responsibilities of the nurse practitioner.

Management of Episodic Illness

The nurse practitioner may often manage episodic illness in rheumatic disease patients according to written protocols. The reader is referred to Reference 10. This reference offers initial guidelines to manage common patient problems. Included are protocols for eleven acute self-limiting illnesses such as nausea and vomiting, abdominal pain, and upper respiratory infection and for five chronic diseases. Each protocol gives an overview of the disease process, management goals, and worksheet. The worksheet guides the nurse practitioner to elicit and explain subjective and objective data in order to make an assessment and to establish the diagnostic, therapeutic, and patient education plan.

Professional Education

The nurse practitioner may have a clinical faculty appointment to schools of nursing and medicine, and may offer classroom instruction and clinical supervision to students and coworkers. Many nurse practitioners serve as preceptors for nurse practitioner students (Fig. 4.6). The nurse practitioner may also plan and present continuing education and "in-service" programs

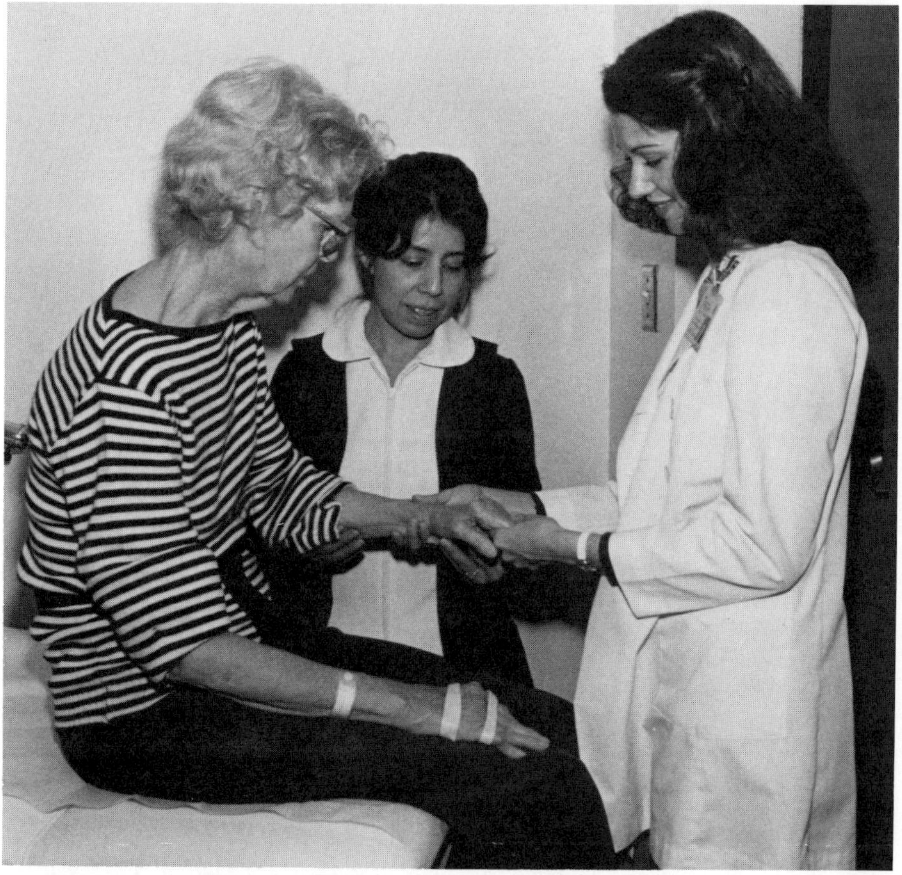

Fig. 4.6. Many nurse practitioners serve as preceptors for nurse practitioner students. (Colleen Miller, R.N., Marie Ball, L.P.N., and Mosstella Beaubien.)

to various hospital, office, long-term care, and home care health professionals.

Quality Assurance

Because of the nature of this expanded role, the nurse practitioner accepts responsibility for delivering quality care. Quality care to the patients is assured in the following ways.

1. Ongoing updating of knowledge and skills by attending continuing education seminars, teaching rounds, study hours, etc. (Fig. 4.7).

2. Facilitating patients' moving within the health care system. For example, when an out-patient nurse practitioner's patient is admitted to a hospital unit, the nurse practitioner may perform the admitting history and physical, write certain orders, and meet with the hospital nursing staff and other members of the health team to assure continuity of care, and actively plan and evaluate care, including discharge planning.

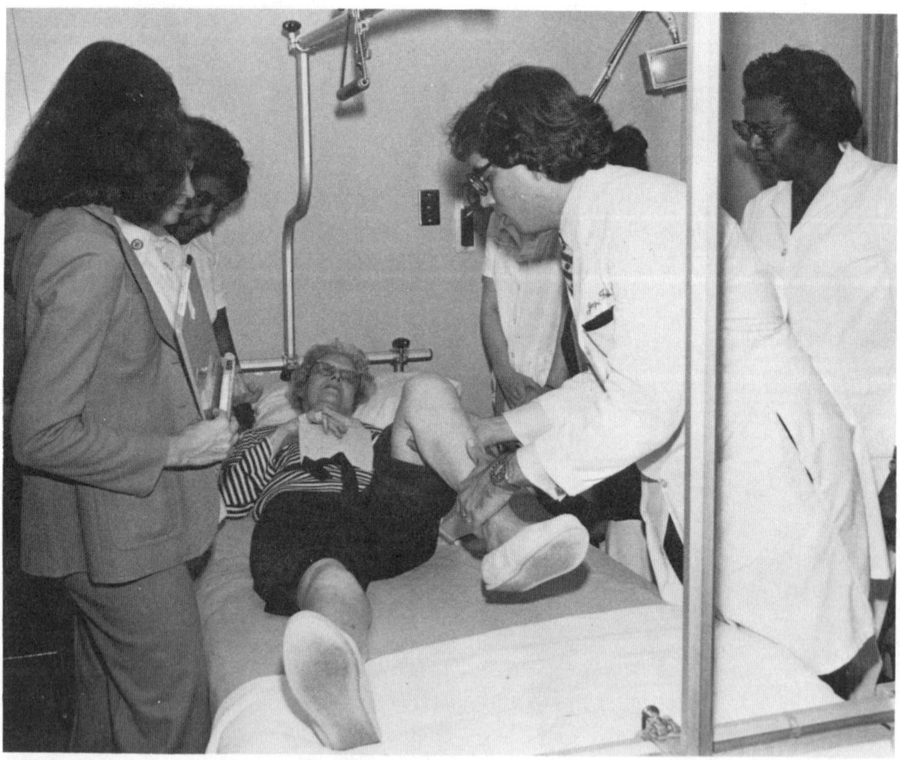

Fig. 4.7. The nurse practitioner updates her own knowledge and skills by attending teaching rounds. (Colleen Miller, R.N., Margaret Williams, Willie Mae Jones, R.N., Joseph Forstot, M.D., and Mosstella Beaubien).

3. Applying for certification when available, in addition to state R.N. licensure.
4. Participating in peer review audits of quality patient care.
5. Having access to medical consultation and supervision.
6. Being knowledgeable about community resources available which offer services to the rheumatic disease patient.

Summary

Through formal educational programs, registered nurses expand their traditional roles to become nurse practitioners.

In the specialty of rheumatic disease, nurse practitioners function collaboratively with physicians and other health professionals to assess the patient, establish a plan of care, and continually evaluate the results of care. The patient and family are actively involved in educational efforts which will help them understand and manage the illness, in order to achieve the highest level of functioning possible. This goal-directed teamwork is the process of rehabilitation.

REFERENCES

1. MAHONEY, E., ET AL. *How to Collect and Record a Health History*. J.B. Lippincott Co., Philadelphia, 1976.
2. BROWN, M. S., ET AL. *Student Manual of Physical Examination*. J.B. Lippincott Co., Philadelphia, 1977.
3. COHEN, S. Regional Corticosteroid Therapy. In *Rheumatic Diseases: Diagnosis and Management*, edited by W. Katz. J.B. Lippincott Co, Philadelphia, 1977, p. 910.
4. STEINBROCKER, O., AND NEUSTADT, D. *Aspiration and Injection Therapy in Arthritis and Musculoskeletal Disorders*. Harper and Row, Hagerstown, Maryland, 1972, p. 17.
5. COHEN, A. S. *Laboratory Diagnostic Procedures in the Rheumatic Disease*, Ed. 2. Little, Brown, and Co., Boston, 1975, p. 12.
6. POHL, M. *The Teaching Function of the Nursing Practitioner*, Ed. 3. Wm. C. Brown, Dubuque, 1978. p. 35.
7. POHL, M. *The Teaching Function of the Nursing Practitioner*, Ed. 3. Wm. C. Brown, Dubuque, 1978, pp. 53, 54.
8. REDMAN, B. *The Process of Patient Teaching in Nursing*. Ed. 3. C.V. Mosby Co., St. Louis, 1976.
9. Arthritis Foundation, Allied Health Professions Section. *Patient Education in Arthritis "How-To" Packet*. Atlanta, 1977.
10. HUDAK, C., ET AL. *Clinical Protocols: A Guide for Nurses and Physicians*. J.B. Lippincott Co., Philadelphia, 1976.

5

Nursing Care of the Hospitalized Patient with Rheumatic Disease

JANICE SMITH PIGG

It is important that nurses and nonnurses understand the contribution nursing can offer patients with rheumatic disease so that there can be proper utilization of nursing skills. This can be demonstrated in the inpatient unit where the nurse is the health professional with whom the patient has the most contact.

Certain needs of patients with rheumatic diseases can best be met within the controlled environment of the hospital (or similar care institution). Obviously, conditions that can best be corrected or improved by a surgical approach require professional nursing care (see Chapter 6). In addition, the chronicity of most of the rheumatic diseases mandates that the patient have the ability to make proper decisions regarding his way of living. The nurse can help the patient with an educational program as an integrated part of the treatment program. Such as a program incorporated into the daily schedule, physical care and environment requires close supervision and instruction by professional nurses. As the most constant care provider, the nurse is the logical coordinator of the patient's time. Because of this close association, the nurse can contribute practical information about the patient and his perceptions and reactions to other care providers. As the basis for all these activities, the nurse provides physical care for the patient as she assists him in regaining maximum independent status.

If nursing care is a major reason for hospitalization, the quality of that nursing care becomes increasingly important. What this nursing care consists of has been ill-defined and sometimes misunderstood by nurses as well as by nonnurses. Perhaps this is because of the sensible and sometimes basic nature of the nursing care. This leads to a lack of recognition of the nursing intervention. Nurses themselves often have not recognized or have undervalued their contribution.

It must be remembered that most nurses caring for people with arthritis will also be caring for patients with strokes, gallbladder disease, and pneumonia. Therefore, expectations of level of practice will be necessarily limited by the exigency of each individual situation. Just as there is currently increased emphasis being placed on upgrading the rheumatology knowledge and skills of the primary physician, so too, attention must be paid to upgrading the rheumatology knowledge and skills of the nurse generalist since the majority of patients will be cared for by the generalist rather than the rheumatology nurse specialist. This enables the rheumatology nurse specialist to be available to upgrade basic nursing rheumatology knowledge by research, publication, role-model practice, preceptorship, teaching, and staff development.

This chapter will examine the hospital nursing staff in regard to preparation, role, and environment in which the nurse practices. Nursing implications and interventions in regard to some of the common problems of patients with rheumatic diseases will be explored in three different ways: the task or function performed by the nurse, the skill used by the nurse, and the patient problem to be addressed.

The Nursing Staff

The caliber of the nursing staff determines the quality of the rheumatology nursing care. Formalized basic entry level preparation for nurses varies from the 2-year Associate degree, to the traditional diploma program of 3 years' preparation through the 4 or 5-year Baccalaureate programs. All can lead to the Registered Nurse. Too often these various levels of preparation are not taken into consideration in the expectations of how the nurse functions. Yet they reflect a difference in emphasis, exposure, and experience. Advanced degrees in nursing specialty areas are also available, although at this time the nurse interested in rheumatology would have to seek a master's program in medical/surgical nursing, rehabilitation, or possibly chronic disease nursing. With the exception of these advanced programs, the nurse will probably have had limited formal background in the rheumatic diseases. Only recently have instructors in some nursing schools given specific attention to rheumatic disease, and only in a few schools has arthritis become a model for chronic disease.

Beyond the formalized basic educational program, nurses have variable opportunities to learn about rheumatic diseases through continuing education programs as well as through experience in the care setting. Again, the quality of these learning experiences will reflect the expertise of the teachers and the individual nurse's ability to incorporate her learning into her nursing practice.

Often nurses do not realize the potential challenge of rheumatology nursing. Instead, they are apt to label people as having "arthritis" without being aware of the tremendous diversity of the over 100 rheumatic diseases.

They may only be aware of a few of the more commonly known rheumatic diseases such as osteoarthritis, rheumatoid arthritis, and gout. And the information taught may possibly be outdated. For example, the attitude toward a patient with systemic lupus erythematosus may reflect an earlier time when such patients were primarily seen with end stage kidney involvement. Or the earlier emphasis on diet in the treatment of gout will be known rather than the more recent control of the disease by medication.

Unfortunately, nursing, like other disciplines, sometimes reflects a mirror image of society's view of arthritis. Nurses, like the general public, are exposed to the media presentation of arthritis as an inevitable consequence of old age or as a minor affliction easily overcome by the touted product.

Fortunately the quality of nursing literature and instruction in schools of nursing is rapidly improving and being updated. Once a nurse is exposed to the dynamic and diversified care of this patient population, she recognizes how she can draw from her knowledge and experience in other areas and apply and adapt it to the needs of patients with arthritis and she will likely be challenged and enthused.

If one has the opportunity to employ a rheumatology nurse (be it specialist or generalist), there are certain qualities that may be particularly desirable to seek, despite the problems previously discussed. Currently, it is rather unlikely that a nurse with rheumatology education and experience will be found.

First consideration should be given to the desired outcome of the nursing activities in terms of patients status. If the purpose of the nursing care is to have an educated, independently-functioning patient, then nursing ability and interest in patient education should be sought. Content knowledge about rheumatology is more easily and quickly acquired than basic skills and experience. Ideally, of course, both would be found. Areas of preparation and experience that would be valuable vary according to the desired outcomes, but particularly skill and experience in rehabilitation and the psychosocial areas as well as patient education are helpful. Previous experience with other chronic diseases such as diabetes, hypertension, obesity, etc. would be very useful.

Orientation of new nurses and staff development of currently employed nurses requires careful attention if quality nursing care is to result. This will not happen without planning and organization. Although nonnursing personnel can certainly contribute valuable expertise to this process, only nurses can teach about nursing. When the physician gives a lecture, this should be supplemented by a nurse skilled in identifying the nursing implications and interventions. Nurses can then be held accountable for changes in their practice. Planning for either orientation or a staff development program can be overwhelming when confronted by the large amount of information to be transferred and the limited amount of routinely available time. Rather than the traditional approach by disease entities (teaching about rheumatoid arthritis, degenerative joint disease, etc.), focus is on specific patient problems (pain, stiffness, etc.) and their assessment and proper intervention such as is briefly done in the latter portion of this chapter. Medical education with its major focus on diagnosis and treatment rightfully is directed at specific diseases. Nursing, with its efforts directed at the patients' problems within the context of the person and his milieu, may be better approached in a different way.

The role or function of nursing in relationship to the patient with any one of the rheumatic diseases is more than simply carrying out physician orders. The broader aspect of comfort and caring makes nursing's contribution essential to the patient with rheumatic disease. Nursing's patient-problem oriented approach is more comprehensive than is usually assumed under the medical-model's traditional disease orientation. The nurse will be concerned (in addition to the arthritis) with nutrition, psychological adjustment, health habits, and general state of well-being. This adds confusion to the nurse's role and the expectations of her by the patient/family, other care providers, and most unfortunately, sometimes the nurse herself. While not under the same pressure as their medical counterparts to diagnose, nurses respond to the patient's need for help in dealing with problems such as pain, without having to pinpoint the exact cause. In the process of assessing the nature of the pain and evaluating the results of their intervention, they can furnish the physician with additional data that will assist him to carry out his specific responsibilities to the patient and family.

Nursing can give physical care, comfort, counseling, and guidance, and help the patient/family cope with the rheumatic disease. To do this, the nurse assumes responsibility for assessing, planning, coordination, intervention, and evalution of the patient's care and status. The role of the nurse is not carried out in a vacuum, but the nurse is not dependent upon other care providers to "nurse." Indeed, her functions are best carried out in an interdependent manner with other care providers. For example, the nurse helps reinforce to the patient what has been explained or taught to him by other health professionals. This carries the educational process nearer to completion. As the patient tells the nurse what was said, she is in a position to evaluate and validate his perceptions and clarify any misconceptions. The patient who aks if he will feel better right away when the nurse is administering the gold can then be helped to recall what the doctor said about the cumulative effect and the teaching be reinforced. The nurse is more likely to be present at opportune moments during self-care, making it possible to recognize problems and needs and interpret them to other members of the health care team.

The nurse serves as a liaison with other team members, for the patient's benefit, in order to insure a consistency and uniformity in plans and goals. This includes coordination related to patient needs rather than coordination of others' services. Recognition of the nurse's role as a coordinator focused on patient needs allows for nursing the patient, and not the various parts or persons of the care system. When nurses spend the majority of their time responding to the demands of all the various people who come and go seeing to the patient's needs, little time is left for the nurse to care for the patient.

As an example of coordination of patient needs: numerous tests are frequently ordered when a patient is admitted to an inpatient unit. The nurse who has assessed her patient well, recognizing physical and psychological factors as well as other pertinent variables (such as financial problems that may have a bearing on length of stay), and who has a good understanding of the physician's plans, may well decide to schedule the tests over 2 or 3 days so as not to overwhelm the patient physically or emotionally. Such an action requires nursing knowledge of the value and need for rest and pacing to be incorporated in the care plan of the rheumatology patient.

The traditional role of the nurse in providing physical care to the patient with arthritis is better understood and accepted. Staffing levels can have a definite effect on the level of physical care. It takes more time to allow functionally-limited patients to be independent in their self-care than for nurses to perform the same tasks for them. Physical care must always hold a high priority and not be sacrificed, but rather be incorporated into the plan of care that includes the provision of emotional support and patient/family education. The nurse, by her close and prolonged proximity to the patient, is able to monitor and report progress, not only in the traditional areas of vital functions, but in the patient's functional ability, emotional status, and problem solving ability. The nurse can provide an evaluation of the effectiveness with which the patient can carry out the treatment plan or assume responsibility for self care.

The nurse also plays a large role in teaching and counseling the patient and family, helping them to achieve a better understanding and improving their ability to cope with the arthritis. Her teaching function should be both formal (with a plan, documentation, and evaluation) and informal, to take best advantage of the many "teachable" moments that arise throughout the patient's stay. This can include teaching about a medication while giving it to a patient, or it may be answering a question or providing information to an anxious patient in the middle of the night.

Nurisng is particularly well suited to provide emotional support both by formal preparation and by the nature of the traditional nurturing role. This is often a time consuming, ongoing process. The need may be greatest when other care providers are not available.

Nurses have opportunity for in-depth knowledge of the patient and the potential problem areas. For example, the nurse who is aware of factors influencing the greater risk of noncompliance can take steps to counter this, such as providing anticipatory guidance by helping the patient develop ways to deal with side effects of medications.

Medical staff and administration (both nursing and hospital) play an influential part in the quality of nursing care of the patient with arthritis. It has been said that nurses are viewed by hospital administration as someone to manage and coordinate activities on the patient unit; and by physicians, as an additional pair of skilled hands. Granted, these are activities that can benefit the patient with arthritis. What nurses have to offer in addition, and how nurses see themselves, is sometimes blurred as they try to meet the expectations of patient, employer, and physician (not necessarily in that order of priority). To only manage and coordinate unit activities or provide another pair of skilled hands minimizes the problem solving, therapeutic, and personal care functions of the nurse.

Administration, in conjunction with rheumatology nursing input, determines those elements of the physical setting that can enhance or hinder the nursing care of patients with arthritis. Often those things that will improve the quality of care are directly proportional to the amount of flexibility the system will allow. Administration generally controls this flexibility. This would include provision for bedside self-administered medications and daily schedules for patients that place a high priority on elements of the therapeutic program such as rest or patient education.

The staffing quota of professional nurses will quite decidedly influence the level of nursing care. There is no pat formula or ratio of nurses to patients. This is better based on results expected and what it will take to achieve the desired outcome. Quality of care does not necessarily increase directly with increased numbers of nurses.

One way to improve quality of nursing care without necessarily increasing the number of nurses is to look at tasks performed by nurses and relieve them of those tasks not requiring their professional skill and judgment. If nurses are performing functions of other disciplines or departments, it may be decided that their time is more worthwhile spent in nursing. For example, if the nurse is responsible for the exercise routine on the weekend, what nursing activities are left undone to allow time for this additional duty? If she supervises the exercises on the weekend, why does she not also do this during the week? If nurses apply hot packs during the night, why should another department assume this function during the day? Nurses are guilty of assuming as theirs, that which no one else does, irrespective of the appropriateness.

Physicians also are in an excellent position to influence the quality of nursing care, not so much by the "completeness" of their orders but by their acceptance of the nurse as a partner who contributes unique skills and knowledge to the care of the patient. Physicians and nurses should make daily patient rounds together, and discuss, evaluate, and revise their joint plans of care. This joint caring for and treating the patient in a colleague fashion provides an excellent educational experience for both parties. The patient stands only to benefit rather than being confused by different goals, plans and priorities.

The Patient-Centered Environment in Which the Nurse Practices

The type of nursing unit will in a great part determine not only the way in which the nurse practices but also the quality (amount and type) of care the patient receives. If the arthritis patient is on a or general medical/surgical nursing unit, he will quite likely have to compete for nursing time with patients whose needs are perceived to be more acute or critical. Because of the slower pace mandated by many of the rheumatic diseases, there will be less opportunity for the patient to be independent. The nurse with many demands on her time will be more inclined to do for the patient rather than assist him to independence. The increased demand for rest, and its use as a treatment modality, is less likely to be met as the patient is forced into a care schedule dictated not by his needs but by the needs of a busy unit or the needs of other patients. Although less than ideal, this is the setting in which the majority of arthritis patients must be cared for.

The advantages in patient care and potential for high quality nursing care on a specialty unit are obvious. However, specialized or segregated rheumatology units are few in number. There are several options in the type of segregated unit. Among these are: medical rheumatology alone, medical rheumatology and orthopedics, medical rheumatology and rehabilitation, and comprehensive medical, orthopedics, and rehabilitation. The specialized unit lends itself more readily to meeting the needs of its specific patient population because indeed it exists for this purpose. This can include routines or schedules that differ from other nursing units. The tempo is slowed to provide an unhurried environment which allows the patient to function at his own pace with frequent rest periods to meet the demands of his disease process. Problems may be encountered with other departments such as physical medicine, X-ray, dietary, and laboratory, where there is apt to be a stronger orientation to the hospital system than to the patient's needs. With education of other care personnel to the special needs of persons with arthritis, changes and compromise can bring about more suitable ways of accomplishing the function. Satellite therapy units located on or near the rheumatology unit can eliminate transportation waits. They do away with the long line of patients sitting in wheelchairs along the wall in the corridor, waiting for therapy or waiting to return to their rooms—an all too familiar and undesirable sight. Arrangements can be made with radiology departments to take nonemergency rheumatology patients later in the afternoon when morning stiffness is not as much of a problem and at a time when it is less likely to interfere with vital therapy or educational programs. Similar agreements can be facilitated with other departments. The x-ray technologist who has a better understanding of persons with arthritis is less apt to rush the patient, try to straighten a contracted elbow or knee, or move him abruptly. This can lead to increased patient satisfaction and positive feelings about hospitalization.

Nursing, too, must not sacrifice the patient's needs to the demands of a traditional or ritualistic schedule. There is nothing that says patients must be bathed before 10 AM or be awakened at 6 AM to have temperatures taken. Warm showers or baths in the middle of the night can relieve pain and stiffness and promote sleep. These are effective interventions which do not require a physician's order. Patients who are capable of taking their own medications before admission, and who will be expected to do the same after discharge, should be allowed to do so during hospitalization. Patients who are not acutely ill or having specialized tests, can be permitted and encouraged to dress in comfortable casual clothes. This will enhance a more positive self-image in addition to providing an opportunity for others to observe problems in dressing.

Some components of the specialized unit may be able to be incorporated on the more general unit. Nursing care in either setting is still based upon the nursing process and its foundation of assessment, planning, intervention, and evaluation.

The physical environment in which the nurse practices can influence the care she gives. A decentralized environment places the equipment, linens, medications, patient records in the patient's room. This optimally places the nurse in greater proximity to the patient for longer periods of time. Most importantly, the environment should provide for meeting patient needs. This includes appropriate beds (firmness and height), chairs (with good back and arm support, the right depth of seat, and a height that allows for easy entry and exit), as well as safe and easy access for wheelchairs, walkers, and crutches and other assistive aids. The environment can be supportive of good mental health for both patients and care providers if it is cheerful and colorful.

The influence of the medical staff and nursing administration on the environment in which the nurse practices can considerably benefit the patient, family and nurse. Nursing administration can control the degree of patient/nurse interaction by decentralization and by the level of staffing. This will be dependent upon how the patient population and the nurse's role are viewed. Both require defining in order to be understood by all. The subtleties of rheumatic disease nursing are not widely understood.

The medical staff in influencing the placement of patients must recognize the amount of nursing care required is not always proportional to the amount of needed medical care. For instance, the stabilized postcardiovascular accident patient may require relatively little in the way of medical care, yet the amount of nursing time required for care of the same patient can be considerable. The organization of a unit from a medical (disease) orientation is different than when the organization is the patient-centered approach of nursing. Nursing must have a voice in the location of patients to optimize nursing care.

Nursing Implications and Interventions Related to Common Problems of Patients with Rheumatic Diseases

The patient with arthritis must be able to adapt to the demands of his disease on a day-to-day basis for an indefinite period of time. The physical care the nurse provides the hospitalized patient must consist of more than "doing" for the patient what he cannot do for himself. Interwoven into the nursing plan of care, the nurse teaches the patient/family unit skills to promote independence and self-management of the chronic disease in preparation for discharge to the home environment. The nurse is one of the care providers who helps the patient incorporate in his lifestyle the changes demanded by the disease.

The nursing care can be traditional physical care or providing more highly developed care skills such as patient education. Nursing care can also be in the form of options of nursing intervention for the identified patient problems, i.e., hot packs, warm showers, or analgesics. These are different but not necessarily uncomplementary to the focus of the medical model upon the disease. These nursing approaches of physical care, teaching, and support, are not necessarily an either/or matter. It may be any one or a combination of all these ways of bringing nursing to focus on the special needs of the person with arthritis.

When the approach is task oriented, certain adaptations can be made to make the function performed more specific to the patient with rheumatic disease.

BATHING

Bathing is a long established nursing ritual. Whenever possible, means other than the traditional bed bath should be used. Certain adaptations in regards to bathing need to be made for the patient with arthritis. While cleanliness is important, the warm moist environment of the bath or shower can provide relief of pain and/or stiffness and and an increased sense of well-being. So for these reasons, the time of the bath may need to be other than the accustomed after-breakfast time. The patient with the severe morning stiffness of rheumatoid arthritis or ankylosing spondylitis may benefit more from a tub bath or shower immediately upon awakening. In the same way, a patient awakening during the night in discomfort might also benefit from a warm bath or shower at that time.

The patient may need physical and/or mechanical assistance to use the tub or shower but that is preferable to the bed bath in providing comfort and self-esteem. Adaptations, such as grab-bars or tub-seats also must be made for the patient who cannot maneuver in and out of the bathtub. As an alternative, the patient may be limited to the shower, where a stool should be provided. A telephone-type spray nozzle that can be hand-held and directed may be useful.

The nurse teaches the patient the rationale for the use of warm water, selection of the proper mode (shower, tub) to be used at home, and safety factors. Patients should know that 15–20 min will probably give the maximum relief, and that to sit in a bathtub for longer may accomplish little more in the way of relief. Patients sometimes ask about the use of whirlpools at home. Generally, these are not as satisfactory for use in the tub at home as in the hospital department because of the smaller size and difficulty in keeping the water warm.

Bath time provides a time of quietness and an atmosphere conducive to patients sharing their thoughts and concerns with the nurse. It can be prime assessment and teaching time. It is also a time that lends itself well to increasing the patient's independency towards self care.

Water therapy in the form of Hubbard tubs and therapeutic pools can usually be found only in hospital settings. These can be even more effective than the bathtub or shower, but it must be remembered that seldom can they be duplicated in the patent's home environment. And even in the hospital, they are usually only available on a limited basis and at specific times. The patient may become dependent upon the tub or pool as the preferred treatment to the exclusion of other forms of treatment such as medication or exercises. When these modalities are used, the purpose for using them should be known so that the time of their use can be appropriate. If the patient is receiving the Hubbard tub for relief of morning stiffness but is not scheduled to receive it until 3 PM, little purpose is served. If several patients are receiving the Hubbard tub, the patient with the longest period of stiffness should be given priority in morning scheduling. This is a situation requiring coordination by the nurse.

The hospital is a good place for the patient to learn what will benefit him most and ways in which he can adapt his home environment to his needs.

NUTRITION

It is generally well understood that diet plays no direct role in either the cause or cure of arthritis, with the exception of gout wherein it can be a factor in control. (Nurses are usually aware of the role of diet in relationship to gout but they may not be as aware of the influence of the newer uricosuric drugs in lessening the previous dietary restrictions for these patients.)

Health professionals may have difficulty in dealing with the patient's susceptibility or conviction that altering his dietary pattern might effect a change in his disease state. This unproven area of treatment is widely disseminated by personal testimony and capitalized upon by entrepreneurs. It generally takes the form of adding or excluding certain foods from the diet. The nurse needs to be prepared to deal with both the questions and erroneous beliefs.

This is not easily done as little direct research has been done in the area of nutrition and diet in relationship to arthritis. The reasons for this omission include limited research dollars and the reluctance of competent investigators to spend time and energy to prove something is of no value. The public finds this difficult to understand.

The nurse is left with reinforcing to the patient and his family that there is no evidence to believe that diet influences arthritis. In recognizing the patient's need to have a feeling of control over his dietary means, the nurse should capitalize on the opportunity and teach the value of maintenance of optimal weight and a well-balanced, nutritious diet for anyone with chronic disease. Because of the proven value of reinforcement as a teaching method, the specifics of a well-balanced, nutritious diet should be spelled out in detail.

The nurse has a major role in assessment of the patient's nutritional status since adequate nutrition is an important general measure in the treatment program. The assessment can be by observation, questioning, or utilizing such tools as 72-hr diet recall. The assessment is aimed at discovering the underlying cause of the nutritional deficit (if present) or its relationship to a less obvious problem such as depression, fatigue or lack of mobility. A patient who cannot move around well may not be able to shop for food or even prepare it. Unless this information is directly sought, it may not be realized while the patient is hospitalized.

Obesity is usually readily assessed, although the length of time the patient has been overweight, his perception of this as a problem and its cause, and the presence of a similar problem in other members of the family, can have a bearing on the appropriate selections of options of intervention. Most attempts at dealing with this problem are doomed to a low rate of success because of the relatively short length of intervention time in the hospital environment. The patient should be instructed in a weight reduction diet plan and can be assessed of his understanding by demonstrating his ability in proper selection of foods while hospitalized. The nurse reinforces the instruction and supports the patient in this process of incorporating new eating habits. In addition, definitive plans need to be made in regard to proper and adequate follow-up and intervention after he has left the protective hospital environment. This needs to be on a regular and frequent basis. It can be provided by community agencies such as public health or visiting nurses, or the commercial self-help groups that have sprung up. If the latter are utilized, some communication is necessary to ascertain the group leader's understanding of the effect their usual program (such as exercise) may have on the patient's arthritis. Supervision can also be provided by dietitians or nurses from the hospital setting.

If anorexia, or undernourishment, seems to be the problem the nurse should work with the dietitian in seeing the food is presented in an attractive manner. Smaller and more frequent settings as well as attempting to meet the patient's preferences sometimes helps. Offering variety in the foods is another measure. Warm, steamy foods may increase the appetite. Socialization by means of communal dining at mealtime may help. Often the stimulation of eating with other patients and the diversion of conversation will make the patient less aware of the food as a chore to be consumed, and previously long-established habits of eating will prevail.

Dysphagia may be a problem as a result of polymyositis or systemic sclerosis. In this case the patient may benefit from small frequent feedings, softer consistency of food, and/or sitting while eating. Instruction should be given to eat/chew slowly and take frequent sips of liquid. If gastric reflux is troublesome, in addition to the above mentioned items, the patient should remain sitting for an hour or so after eating, and may benefit from having the head of the bed elevated.

Nurses should be aware that the temporomandibular joint may be involved and can present a mechanical problem in chewing. Proper intervention would be directed toward attention to the consistency of the food. Some conditions such as systemic sclerosis may limit the patient's ability to open the mouth. Again, the types of food presented can ease the problem.

Patients with impaired usage of their hands are likely to have problems in their ability to eat. Because of the insidious onset of this decreased hand function, the patient may not be aware of this problem because he has compensated in other ways. Adaptive equipment may be required. Appropriate tray set-ups with light-weight cups with wide handles, light-weight (plastic throw-away) silverware, and tossed salads substituted for lettuce wedges, will all increase the patient's ability to function independently and improve his dietary intake. Paper covers may need to be removed from butter, salad dressing, jelly, or other condiments. Milk cartons should be opened, both for ease in access as well as to protect joints. When possible, it is better for the patient's self-esteem to have these things done before taking the tray to him. Milk can be served in a glass instead of the usual carton container. Sometimes these arrangements can be made with a cooperative dietary department. The indirect benefits in patient morale and cooperativeness can be considerable and long reaching. If this attention to detail is not possible, certainly nursing and its ancillary personnel should provide the needed services such as cutting meat, buttering bread, etc. The manner in which this is done is very important. The patient should be taught to assume some responsibility in this by requesting the needed service if it is not offered. Fear that the nurse is "too busy" should not be accepted by the nurse, nor be used by the patient as an excuse. The nurse may wish to secure a referral to the occupational therapist for their additional expertise.

The nursing assessment of these items and the appropriate interventions do not generally require a physician's order. The patient should understand the rationale behind all these measures of intervention such as adaptive devices, patterns, and methods of eating, so they may be applied as appropriate in the home environment.

MEDICATION

Another traditional function of nurses is the administration of medicines. With consideration for the special needs of patients with arthritis, this area too can require special nursing knowledge and intervention.

After the physician has determined and prescribed the appropriate drugs, the nurse has the primary responsibility for the medication portion of the treatment regime. She must have knowledge and understanding of the actions of the various drugs used in treatment of the rheumatic diseases. She is responsible for their safe and accurate administration. Beyond this nursing role in pharmacologic therapy, the rheumatology nurse must have an appreciation for those things that are unique in the relationship of medicines and arthritis. These would include timing, adherence and education. The nurse must not only be able to understand and apply these considerations as a part of her nursing care, but she must also be able to help the patient/family understand them.

Most hospitals require that any medications a patient brings with him on admission be relinquished to the nurse as a part of the admission process. If orders are not secured for their replacement within a reasonable period of time, this can result in the patient's missing a dose and can have considerable impact on their physical well-being and the patient's impression of the health care institution and the care providers. The nurse should make every effort to avoid such an occurrence.

One of the common errors in the nursing care of patients with arthritis has to do with the timing of administration of medications. Hospitals frequently have routine times assigned for the administration (b.i.d., t.i.d., q.i.d., etc.) of drugs. These times are designed either for the convenience of the system or have become so routine that no one stops to ask why. This ritualization results in patients being awakened to take their medicine or not receiving them at the optimum time, such as immediately upon awakening, when it may best provide relief from stiffness. Often the physician's orders allows the nurse flexibility in determining the timing, in which case the nurse should exercise that option. The physician's input should be sought for more reasonable timing, individualized to that patient's needs or home schedule. The more the patient can link and identify his medication schedule to his daily routine at home, the more likely he is to comply.

If the patient is taking a variety of drugs at many different times, the nurse, in consultation with the physician, can seek to group the times as much as possible. This will be less disruptive of the patient's rest and will be more conducive to patient compliance after discharge.

Because nurses are aware of the gastric irritability of many of the antiinflammatory drugs, they often encourage patients to eat something or take milk with their medications. For many people this can be appropriate, especially those who are below optimal weight. However, if the patient is overweight, this is another factor that should be taken into consideration. Arthritis, by restricting mobility, often limits activity. That, plus food (additional calories) taken routinely with medicine over long periods of time, can result in increased weight and subsequent increased stress on joints already jeopardized by disease. In such cases, it is a better solution for the nurse to teach patients to take their medications with a full 8-oz glass of water. The nurse should also provide an adequate amount of water for the patient when passing medications. This amount provides sufficient solution for adequate dissolving and dilution of the drug to minimize irritation of the gastric mucosa.

People have a tendency to think more is better. Patients are people and must be carefully instructed to follow the physician's directions and not to increase the dosage to try to either speed up or improve the results. Conversely, there is also a strong tendency for patients with arthritis to take less medication because they are feeling better. This can be very detrimental in the case of a drug like aspirin where a certain amount must be taken to achieve an antiinflammatory effect instead of merely an analgesic effect.

Another noteworthy feature about drugs used in treating arthritis are the medications which have a cumulative effect with delayed results. Patients need to know not only what to expect in the way of a positive response to the medication, but when to expect it. This time span should not be vague, yet should be sufficiently general to allow for individual variations. Such information may keep the patient from prematurely discontinuing the drug because of lack of perceived results. It should be recognized that it is difficult for patients to take medication when they are symptom-free, such as is the case in gout. The realization of this should be shared with the patient. The patient needs a degree of monitoring and support to maintain the regimen. The nurse in the hospital setting that recognizes this need can arrange for follow-up monitoring by the office, clinic, or community health nurse.

Other patients may have difficulty maintaining the medication regimen and require the support services of the nurse as well as anticipatory guidance. For example, some patients (systemic lupus erythematosus, polymyalgia rheumatica, polymyositis) may be on high doses of corticosteroids. They need help in understanding the necessity of treatment and with dealing with the possible side effects. Particularly they must be counseled on adherence and be carefully instructed on the tapering program so abrupt discontinuance does not produce harmful results. They need guidance in their understanding of salt restriction in their diet. It may additionally be advisable for them to wear a Medic-Alert or some other type of medical information identification.

The same way medications are only a part of the treatment program, the distribution of them to patients is only a portion of the nurse's role. Patient education about medications is an important and shared responsibility with the physician. It is difficult for patients to accept that medicine can often control their disease but not cure it because it is contrary to previous experience or what they would like to believe.

The length of time that a patient has had his arthritis does not guarantee there is a good understanding or adherence to the prescribed program. The nurse must reassess compliance and the patient's feelings about his medicine. The large numbers of pills that a patient may need to take per day may create concern on the part of the patient and his family as to possible harmful effects. A question asking the patient what he is taking and comparing the answer to the record can be very revealing.

Because over-the-counter drugs are so easily obtained, their effect is often underestimated. And this is very important since aspirin plays such a major role in the treatment of many kinds of arthritis. The patient may not understand or appreciate the antiinflammatory action involved. To protect his stomach he may succumb to misleading advertising and substitute a product that has only analgesic effects.

Patients tend to blame untoward things that happen to them, if not on their arthritis, then on the medicine the doctor prescribed. Particularly this is so if it is a new drug. In anticipation of this reaction, they need information about side effects and what action should be taken if they should occur. This needs to be sufficiently specific so as to elicit the desired behavior.

Patients should be aware of the need to keep their physician informed of all medicines (prescribed and otherwise) and not assume the doctor will remember from one time to the next. This is part of a program to involve the patient, making him responsible for portions of his medication program.

Attention to small details may increase the patient's positive outlook towards his medication program. This includes a sensitivity to the patient/family's feelings about the medications and awareness of how they may reflect an underlying denial or fear. Anticipation and discussion with the patient of possible vulnerability to high pressured advertising may help the patient make better decisions at a later date. Knowledge of how to secure easy-open containers may prevent unneeded frustration and anger. Learning to secure new medications in small amounts until their effectiveness and long-term usage is assessed and purchase of heavy usage drugs in quantity will help conserve financial resources.

One must not overlook the family's role or influence when it comes to medications. They can aid or hinder compliance. If they are taught along with the patient, their involvement may be in the direction of positive support. However, the responsibility is ultimately the patient's, if we assume ours in providing adequate instructions and proper skills.

PHYSICAL COMFORT

The nurse plays a primary and traditional role in providing for the comfort of the patient while in the hospital and in teaching him comfort measures that can be used at home. One of the method used to promote comfort is positioning. Nurses should sensitize patients to their standing, sitting, and lying postures. Individualization is once again important.

Good body alignment is often in conflict with the position of comfort. The most comfortable position is usually one of flexion. That is why so many patients put pillows under their knees, which can quickly and easily lead to joint contractures. All patients need to be aware of this hazard, as such contractures are easier to prevent than to correct. If the contracture has already occurred, then the joint should be supported along its length, unless the force of gravity is being used to straighten it. Extension when sitting, standing, and lying is to be encouraged.

Pillows are often misused through incorrect placement under the head. It is almost axiomatic that all hospital beds are made up with two plump pillows which, if used, put the neck into a position of acute flexion. Pillows can be beneficial if they are used to support the cervical spine and ease the stress on neck muscles. There are pillows made especially for this purpose. Otherwise the patient is best taught the value of and helped to grow accustomed to using a single small flat pillow.

Bed cradles or foot boards to take the weight of the bedclothes from painful lower extremities are a necessity in gout and useful in other cases where ankles and feet are a problem. Patients can be instructed in using a cut-out cardboard box or straight chair to accomplish the same purpose at home. Unless specifically ordered, patients should be encouraged to get up to go to the bathroom and to sit in a proper chair. In addition to being taught the value of good postural habits, patients need to learn body mechanics and joint protection.

Splints are sometimes used to reposition or rest an affected joint. If the patient is having difficulty adjusting to wearing the splint, a gradually increasing program of off and on times should be instituted in the hospital. This can lead to better patient acceptance and follow-through at home. The nurse should carefully inspect the skin, so pressure areas caused by the splint can be treated and the splint modified promptly. The nurse can supervise and evaluate the patient/family's ability to take the splint off and on and check for pressure areas.

Comfort is a state of mind. The caring supportive nature of nursing may often be as helpful as the analgesic. In the hospital such intervention is possible if it is recognized, provided for, and expected to be a part of the function of the nursing staff.

The three previous areas (bathing, medication administration, and providing for physical comfort) are examples of how traditional nursing functions can become more than performed tasks or a caretaker-type of nursing service when adapted to the special needs of the patient with arthritis.

Another approach and one requiring greater depth in nursing care of the patient with arthritis is to use the application of special and sometimes unique skills that the nurse brings to the care of the patient. Two examples of these would be patient education and interpersonal relationship skills applied to developing coping/adaptation resources of the patient. While other care providers also practice these skills, only the nurse has the intensity of time and flexibility to provide them on the patient's time schedule.

PATIENT EDUCATION

Patient education incorporates more than just teaching. The goal is learning, leading to a change in behavior. To tell a patient what to do, provide facts or information is only a small part of the total educational process. The patient must be assisted to incorporate this data as a part of his belief system and apply it to his daily life. This "working through" is accomplished in a variety of ways in which the nurse can play a part. It is also the reason that the rheumatology nurse's knowledge and experience in patient education and principles of adult learning are so valuable. It is often the nurse to whom the patient ventilates his fears and concerns or tests his plans for change. She must be able to respond in such a way as to help him build his problem-solving abilities.

Since most forms of arthritis are basically chronic in nature, it is crucial that the patient learn self-management for that considerable period of time outside the hospital and between physician visits when there is no direct supervision by professional care providers. The hospital provides both a controlled environment for teaching the patient/family as well as an opportunity for more in-depth and concentrated learning experiences than are usually available in the ambulatory settings.

All care providers are involved either directly or indirectly in the process of teaching/learning and helping the patient/family live with the arthritis. Patient teaching is recognized as an independent function of nursing practice. The nurse does not need a direct order from the physician to instruct the patient. The nurse and the physician teach in a wider variety of areas than do most other disciplines. Usually the physician teaches more theoretical information while the nurse pays greater attention to practical details.

The physician bases most of his teaching on the diagnosis, explanation of the disease process, the treatment program, and the prognosis. Within the hospital setting, the nurse should be present during this process so she is aware of what has been said and can communicate (preferably by written documentation) the information the patient has received to the other care providers. The nurse who has heard or knows what the doctor has told the patient is then in a position to listen to the patient's perception of what the doctor told him, evaluate his understanding, clarify misconceptions or refer him to an appropriate resource. As the patient with a new diagnosis or new information is going through the process of incorporation, the nurse can also broaden his informational background as he indicates the need for more knowledge. The specificity of her information is dependent upon the patient's perceived need for more information and her familiarity with his individual case.

The nurse's role deals not only with what is commonly thought of as patient teaching or information specifically about arthritis but she is also concerned with setting the climate for learning.

The nurse should be aware that the patient often perceives himself as improved by hospitalization when he is less irritated by the admitting procedure, by his room environment, as well as when he receives information about his illness. Her teaching in these areas can then be beneficial as she explains and helps him deal with hospitalization. This is particularly important in the care of the patient with arthritis who often has extended contact with the care system and is the most apt to be dissatisfied.

The nurse is often in position to identify the fatigue or pain that interferes with the patient's ability to learn. Her intervention can contribute to the learning process.

The nurse's role in patient education may include assisting the patient in learning how to be an active responsible participant in his therapeutic program. The patient can be helped to incorporate new skills and attitudes into his life style and be directed toward assuming responsibility for his (the patient's) part in the program.

Involved in the nursing process of patient education is assessment of the patient's status of what he needs to know to safely and effectively manage his rheumatic disease and what his deficiencies are in this body of knowledge. One can then match assessment with behavior. If the patient can identify his medications, tell about their actions, etc., but doesn't take them, the problem may not be one of lack of knowledge, but one of fear of side effects, influence of family or friends, or inability to incorporate the medication schedule in his daily life. One must also know his perception of his problem, not only what he knows but what his goals are. Understanding this may lead to appropriate intervention to improve adherence to the treatment regimen.

An overview of the areas in which the nurse can help the patient learn (including reinforcement of that taught by others), understand and apply knowledge about arthritis includes:

Knowledge about disease process—how the process applies to his individual case.

Medications—the identification, action (time as well as mode), dosage, how to take them, and the side effects to be alert for and what to do about them.

Quackery and unproven methods of treatment—recognition, susceptibility and how to deal with.

Rest and pacing—the reason for and how to do.

Posture and positioning—bed, sitting, standing and lying.

Heat and cold applications—the different modalities, their advantages and disadvantages, and the safety factors.

Home exercise program—its execution and incorporation in the daily schedule.

Joint protection—specific measures and how to problem-solve for other applications.

Work simplification—energy conservation.

The nurse can help the patient recognize how the disease process effects him. In learning about the inflammatory process, he can learn to recognize warmth, redness, swelling, and pain as signs of inflammation and take appropriate action such as resting the affected joint.

The practice of nursing in particular aligns itself with effective adult education principles. Not only is the nurse most apt to be the care provider present at the patient's "teachable moments" but she has the greatest opportunity to use patient-care times as a vehicle for her teaching. For example, while giving the patient his medications, she can check on his ability to recognize and identify his drugs.

The hospital provides an excellent environment for observation of the patient's ability to manage his medicines and to increase his ability to do so. Since most patients have been taking their own medications before they were hospitalized, and presumably will be able to do so after discharge, it seems reasonable for them to be on some sort of self-administered medication program while hospitalized.

To aid the patient in assuming responsibility and development of skills for continuity of the medication program, a graduated sequence in bedside medications can be used. First the patient learns about the medications through individualized instruction provided by the doctor on his rounds and the nurse while giving the drugs. The patient then takes responsibility for marking the time of the medication taken on a bedside record while demonstrating his knowledge about the drug by identification, dosage amount, mode of action, and reporting any side effects. From this step he progresses to having the medications at bedside and assuming responsibility for them himself under the supervision of the nurse. This allows for additional teaching as necessary, an evaluation of expected compliance, and prepares the patient for discharge.

Another area of patient teaching by nurses is that of quackery and unproven methods of treatment. Nurses frequently learn about the nonrecommended measures patients are using for their arthritis. The patient may be more likely to tell the nurse because she is less of an authoritative figure than the doctor, and she is more often present and available at the right time. Or, she may be told because the patient is looking for validation of his action and sees the nurse as an intermediary between himself and the doctor.

The nurse's attitude will determine the outcome of this interaction. If the nurse conveys shocked disbelief, uninterest, ridicule, or feelings that only persons of lesser intelligence would do such things, the results of her further intervention will be limited. If the nurse conveys a thoughtful nonjudgmental attitude and understanding, the chances of the patient resisting these unproven methods of treatment are greater. The most automatic, but often least effective , response is to inundate the patient with counter-information.

It is easier for the nurse and patient to recognize blatant quacks and questionable products because of their promise of "cure". Less easy to identify is the unproven method of treatment, or misleading (though not always incorrect) information. The increased role of the media makes information more widely available about unusual treatment and highly personalized accounts of supposed success.

Quackery should be seen as an effort on the part of the patient to seek additional health information, guidance, and assistance, and as such, should alert the perceptive care provider to ask "Why did that person try a special diet or special 'arthritis' medicine?" The reasons why intelligent, well-educated people are so gullible is complex. They may fear some aspect of conventional treatment without fully understanding the context of the information, such as that aspirin can make the stomach bleed. It may be fear of the consequences (such as crippling) of the arthritis itself. Ignorance may play a role. Patients may lack the ability to evaluate the purported claims. That the purveyors of do-it-yourself literature, drugs, vitamins, and health foods are better salesmen than the health professional, is evidenced by their multimillion dollar business. The patient may be on a continued search for relief of pain. The frustration of the chronicity of the disease or dealing with a fragmented care system may lead him to try a questionable practice. The expense of prolonged treatment can drive the patient to an even more expensive one if its promise is greater, quicker, or easier. The naive hope for a painless, quick, sure cure—a miracle, is often the reason for seeking an easy way out. For some, it may be lack of patience in sticking to the therapeutic program when observable results are slow to come. Grasping at straws may be the reason—"For my own peace of mind, I had to know I had tried everything possible." It is sometimes difficult to distinguish legitimate from illegitimate providers of information. Many of the "cure" books on arthritis have physician authors. The legitimate trial and error approach in individualizing treatment may shake the patient's confidence and make him feel like he is being used in an experiment. Human nature seems to drive the patient to look for a "natural" way, leading to fad foods and diets.

These reasons are played upon by the quacks who offer false security, thereby delaying the patient's seeking out or adhering to proper medical attention. The products or programs are usually worthless but may possibly be harmful, and certainly represent wasted resources and ill-gotten gain for the promoter. The common denominator for the patient's believing is delusion.

Patients need information so they can recognize unproven methods of treatment and quackery as well as being made aware of methods of validation. For instance, the patient needs to know to ask himself, "Is this harmful?" The answer is "Yes" even if it is the wearing of a copper bracelet, *if* it keeps the patient from seeking medical care, or causes him to discontinue regular treatment.

It should be realized that the care provider's behavior in itself may contribute to the patient's vulnerability. If the patient's needs are not met in his hope for cure or relief, he may seek a nontraditional method of treatment. Care providers need also to be flexible to allow for unorthodox and nonharmful or inexpensive approaches if they do not interfere with traditional treatment. A placebo effect may be gained.

The nurse may be the one most apt to recognize the patient's susceptibility to the unproven methods of treatment. She may be the care provider best able to guide the patient in his decision-making regarding this area.

The nurse's emphasis in teaching rest and pacing, posture and position, heat and cold applications, exercise program, joint protection, and energy conservation will depend on the availability and teaching role of other care providers. She may reinforce, supervise, and provide feedback, or she may be primarily responsible for content in these areas. There needs to be clear communication and common goals. If she is responsible for the teaching or supervision, she must know the exercises. If she is to reinforce joint protection techniques she should be using them herself.

If the nurse is to have a major role in teaching the patient, then opportunity must be provided for this. She must have the time, help in preparing herself for her teaching role, and available resources such as written and audio/visual materials.

It is difficult to assist a patient chronically ill with arthritis to understand his disease, to comply fully with instructions and to feel good about himself. It is not adequate for a diagnosis to be made, a plan of medicines, therapy and way of living given, and then to expect the patient to be able to follow the regimen successfully without a devastating struggle that may itself interfere with the treatment of the disease. Success comes almost as much from the supportive help during adaptation and change, as from the therapeutic regimen itself. This supportive help comes from all care providers but in particular from nursing.

COPING AND ADAPTATION

Chronic illnesses, such as arthritis, necessitate a great deal of emotional, psychological, as well as physical support in their management. A way of living must be found that will enable an acceptable but often compromised, lifestyle. An assessment by the nurse of how coping skills were used earlier may provide information that can be helpful at this time. It is difficult to maintain a healthy self image when faced with actual or potential crippling. This is compounded by frustration over "body failure" for long periods of time. The nurse uses her "active listening" skills as the patient ventilates his feelings.

A situational reactive depression is not unusual. The nurse can help the patient and family in understanding and dealing with this. She can play a part in its recognition, and can contribute information (number of times awake at night, anorexia, etc,) that may be helpful to the physician in determining the severity of the depression.

Anger at the disease may be displaced and expressed toward the nurse or other care providers. It may be displayed in the form of hostility or fault finding. Without the nurse being consciously aware of this possibility, she can easily find herself caught up in a responsive emotion triggered by a "difficult" patient. Anger on the part of the patient is difficult for a nurse to deal with as she tries to care for the patient. As the nurse recognizes the contribution of pain, frustration, fatigue, and chronicity to the anger, it becomes a less personally directed action.

The nurse can help the patient cope with living with his chronic disease. This includes living with the demands of the arthritis on an emotional level as well as living with it on a practical level. This counseling type of activity is an integral part of nursing care and of the educational process of the patient. It deals with problems of dependency, self image and sexuality. The patient's manner of coping can be evaluated by his ability to include elements of the treatment program such as rest and pacing and the substitution of other activities for those not compatible with his disease in his lifestyle. The ability of the patient to adapt to the desirable changes brought about by his disease is influenced by many factors and fluctuates with time.

The close contact between nurse and patient often makes sexuality a logical area of discussion. Sexuality is related to role change as well as physical changes caused by the arthritis. Patients with arthritis have the same basic needs as all human beings. Frequently the disease-related sexual problems that develop can be modified by improved communications between partners, patient and doctor, or other care provider. The partner may be afraid of hurting the patient or making the disease worse. The pain and fatigue that accompany arthritis can decrease libido. Particularly this is frightening in early disease and demonstrates the need for early discussion of the patient's sexual concerns.

Arthritis can necessitate that a person find alternative ways of positioning during sexual intercourse or different ways of sexual expression. Patients need information and sometimes permission to seek ways of meeting their sexual needs. The use of a warm tub bath or shower, loosening up exercises, and/or analgesics are activities that require planning prior to sexual intercourse. Consideration must be also given to the way lack of mobility can interfere with the patient's opportunities for socialization and affect their sexuality. Some of the rheumatic diseases (or their treatment) may require the nurse discuss family planning methods with the patient and spouse.

In different ways the nurse can help the patient gain control of the arthritis. One of these is in the recognition of his control. "When I rest I don't feel so bad." As the nurse helps the patient move from dependence to independence, to manage himself by learning to take charge of his disease, the patient will gain in his adaptation to the disease.

The hospital is conducive to these more comprehensive and coordinating roles of the nurse because of the prolonged and close relationship of the nurse and the patient in such a setting. To have an opportunity for such interaction requires adequate nurse/patient contact time, recognition of the value and expectation of it as a nursing function.

Another way the nursing care of the patient with arthritis may be approached is to look at the individual patient's problem and plan the nursing intervention from a selection of options of nursing intervention. This is more logical from a nursing standpoint and follows the nursing process of assessment, planning, implementation, and evaluation.

PAIN

Pain is a word of rather special connotation in arthritis. It is one of the most common terms associated with arthritis. Society's perception of pain is that it is something bad that should be completely eliminated. Yet in arthritis the nurse and patient must recognize that pain can be a helpful signal that something is wrong and indicate that action needs to be taken. Unfortunately, it is sometimes not possible to completely relieve all the pain and discomfort of arthritis. There is the dichotomy of realistic expectation that it may not be possible to eliminate all the pain of arthritis and yet it also may not be desirable to attempt to "tough it out." The nurse must help the patient recognize when there is a message in the pain and when it is something that is to be lived with as best one can after measures of relief have been taken.

The person whose knees are painful should not run up and down stairs, but should respect the pain and take an appropriate action such as resting the painful part by limiting weight bearing. Patients need to know guidelines, such as, pain that lasts approximately two hours or longer after an activity indicates the activity was excessive and should be limited in the future. They can then make individual determinations rather than blindly following lists of dos and don'ts. The patient can look at the activity and either cut down on the amount, eliminate doing it, or find another way which is less stressful.

The patient must be helped to distinguish between pain and stiffness. The patient with osteoarthritis can indeed "work out" the stiffness that may be present after maintaining a static position for a prolonged time such as sitting. The patient needs to understand that pain of bony origin is mechanical in nature and caused by movement in destroyed or damaged joints. Discomfort can then be avoided, at least temporarily, by not using the joint. This type of damage is irreversible and may require surgical intervention. This patient will most likely not have pain at night or while at rest, whereas the patient with soft tissue changes caused by inflammation will find the pain continuous and unrelenting. The latter patient needs to understand that more permanent relief will come with better control of the disease.

The nurse's careful assessment will not only identify the probable cause of the pain, but also the patient's perception of the pain. Intervention will include not only direct physical action on the part of the nurse but also teaching the patient practical methods for relief or modification of the pain, as well as an understanding of the pain itself.

Medications are often first thought of as a means of relief by patients and care providers alike. Because of the chronic nature of arthritis, the more habit-forming drugs are not used. The media's portrayal of the many over-the-counter drugs leads to unrealistic expectations on the part of many patients and families. Nurses and patients alike need to be aware of the role of both analgesics and antiinflammatory drugs in pain relief. There may be confusion between the physician and the patient in the amount of time needed in securing pain relief. The patient complains of pain, wishing for immediate relief, the physician sees relief more in terms of control of the underlying process which may take a longer period of time. This points to the need for patients to understand the quick but temporary results of an analgesic versus the longer lasting benefits of the antiinflammatory drugs and how they can use both optimally. Some antiinflammatory drugs have an analgesic effect themselves at the time of taking them and over a longer period of time in their control of the disease.

Nurses in their assessment of the patient and how he views and copes with chronic and acute pain should educate the patient about the appropriate and most effective use of analgesics. To be most effective, analgesics must be taken before the pain becomes unduly severe and the patient has tried to "tough it out." When he finally takes the analgesic, he finds it less effective than if it had been used earlier. Many patients are fearful of becoming dependent upon analgesic drugs, not realizing that the more habit-forming narcotics are rarely used, for that very reason.

Timing can also be important in the giving of an analgesic prior to a therapy session that has proven in the past to be painful. The therapist and patient are often able to accomplish better results with the use of a properly timed analgesic.

Other measures of relief from pain should be tried. Warm moist heat in its various forms (moist heating pads, hot packs, paraffin dips) can be effective and used at home as well as in the hospital. The weight of the heat application should be considered. If it is too heavy, additional discomfort may result. Cold can sometimes be equally effective. Often it is a matter of trial and error as to which works best.

Pain at night is of particular concern to the nurse, as it can add considerably to the patient's fatigue by interfering with restful sleep. There seems to be a difference between pain at night and day pain. In part, it may derive from the loneliness, darkness and lack of distraction at night. In some patients with arthritis, joints such as the shoulders and elbows become weight-bearing joints at night. Patients find it difficult to assume a comfortable position. Turning onto the painful elbow, hip, or shoulder causes further pain that awakens them.

Anxiety and/or depression may also cause wakefulness. Often a warm drink, warmed blanket, or a few minutes' conversation with the nurse will help the patient more than the hastily offered sedative repeat. Although medication in the form of a relaxing antidepressant can and should be used for long existing conditions, an opportunity to talk with the nurse may also be therapeutic.

The hospital is probably the best setting in which to teach the patient how to manage his pain. It allows a controlled environment with support and encouragement as well as supervision by the nurse. The nurse can provide the opportunity to the patient and engage him as an active participant in the process. The goal is a patient whose practices and behavior indicate knowledge of ways to avoid and manage discomfort with safety. The hospital is a good place to try different approaches to pain that can be duplicated in the home environment. Each case must be individually assessed. There is no routine for relief of pain. The options are many.

STIFFNESS

Stiffness is another patient problem in which nursing intervention can play an important role. Although it must be remembered by nurse and patient that the total therapeutic program as prescribed by the physician and followed by the patient will in the long run make the greatest difference with the control of the disease. By her careful assessment of the length of the morning stiffness in the patient with rheumatoid arthritis, the nurse can help the patient and care providers keep track of the progress in controlling the disease. This is not done by recording such vague terms as "more or less" but should be specific in terms of time. Care must be taken not only to how the question is asked, but when. The patient is asked, "How long is it from the time you awaken until you are moving the best you will for the day?" As this time decreases from 3½ to 3 hr, etc., all concerned are able to mark the progress. In the meantime, the use of warm moist heat in forms such as treatment tubs or pools, bathtub, shower, or hot packs, etc., early in the morning, can provide relief, as can the careful timing of the antiinflammatory or analgesic medication. The nurse can provide ample time for the slower movements that are necessary, and whenever possible schedule activities for the time when the stiffness has dissipated.

FATIGUE

The nurse can also help the patient deal with fatigue. The cause of the fatigue can be the chronicity of the disease, ever present pain, discomfort that prevents adequate restful sleep, or can result from psychological factors such as depression or anxiety. This knowledge about fatigue and people with arthritis, plus the recognized value of rest as a treatment modality, emphasizes the attention the nurse must pay to this aspect of patient care.

It is important that the nursing care in itself should not contribute additionally to the patient's fatigue. Careful attention to patient needs and the complete daily schedule with a planned pacing of activities can be very important.

First, the nurse must assess the cause of the fatigue. If it is known that the disease is in exacerbation (elevated sedimentation rate, increased joint involvement, etc.), then one can logically expect increased fatigue. When pain seems to be unrelenting (regardless of the intensity), fatigue can be expected merely from the effort of dealing with the continual discomfort. When the night nurse's documentation shows the patient is waking frequently and has difficulty in returning to sleep, one can be fairly certain that the quality of the sleep is diminished. Disturbed patterns of sleep such as insomnia and early morning awakening can be indicative of psychic disturbances. Fatigue can be caused by one or any combination of these factors. The more clearly the underlying cause can be identified, the more appropriate the nursing intervention can be.

Nursing action can be in the form of simple physical measures utilized to relieve or eliminate the underlying causes. Close attention to the therapeutic program should be given for greater control of the disease. The pain should be relieved or modified as has previously been discussed. The sleep environment should be comfortable and quiet. In addition to noise, light may need to be controlled. A more firm mattress may need to be provided. Temperature can also be a factor, as the patient should be warm without being weighted down by layers of blankets. If he is accustomed to wearing socks to bed at home to keep his feet warm, he should be encouraged to do the same in the hospital. A bedtime/sleep routine may be needed. This could consist of a "winding down" and deliberate preparation for sleep. It might include a warm bath, warm drink, or quiet music. These activities might be preferable over the usual "sleeping pill" so easily dispensed in the hospital. Patients are often fearful of becoming dependent on the sleeping pill and need very little encouragement to engage in substitute activities. However, there are patients who need the appropriate use of sleeping pills to aid them in breaking undesirable sleep habits. For the patient who wakes during the night (depending upon the cause) a warm bath, shower, or the application of hot packs may ease him enough to allow restful sleep for the remainder of the night. Sometimes a quiet chat with the nurse during which the patient unburdens himself or discusses his plans and/or thoughts may be adequate.

Obviously, the evening and night nurses' role can be extremely important in the care of patients with arthritis. The off-shifts of nursing need to understand the nature of the patient's problem, have appropriate orders from the physician, and hospital policies must allow them the flexibility and opportunity to tailor their intervention to the specific need of the patient.

Daytime rest must also be a concern of the nurse. In this respect, it is most important that she assume the recognized role of coordinator of the patient's time. The patient's daily schedule should provide for pacing of the activities. There should be planned times for rest. These rest periods should be regarded as part of the treatment program. If these are interrupted for the physician's visit or therapy, then it must be recognized that the rest period is not considered as a part of the treatment program. The focus must be on the patient's needs, not on the education program or care providers' schedules. Probably no other activity of the nurse requires greater skill in interpersonal relationships and sense of purpose than the role of coordinator of the patient's time while in the hospital.

CONTINUITY OF CARE

The nurse plays a major role in helping the patient make plans for his discharge. This is done through her teaching the patient skills needed in self-management. The nurse and the patient can review his situation for potential problems. She may provide the linkage of the patient with appropriate outside community agencies and resources. Because of her in-depth knowledge of the patient she is the one who is most apt to provide helpful information to care providers outside the hospital. Most certainly she will coordinate all the details making sure the patient and family are prepared for discharge and adequate arrangements have been made.

Conclusion

The hospital is the setting in which the nurse is the care provider with whom the patient has the most contact. Therefore it is essential that the nurse's contribution to the care of the patient with rheumatic disease be properly and adequately utilized.

Expectations of nurses caring for patient with rheumatic diseases will vary according to the density of patient population, the degree of expertise on the part of the nurse care provider and the specificity of care desired. They will be highly dependent upon the personal interest of the nurse, physician support and encouragement, supportive environment, the staffing ratio (including competition of the arthritis patient with the acutely ill patient for the nurse's time) and the accountability that is built in.

An overview has been provided of the nurse's role in physical care, data gathering, education about self-management of the chronic disease, coordination, support and caring for the patient with a rheumatic disease.

Three different nursing approaches to patients with rheumatic diseases have been described. These demonstrate the interrelated ways in which nursing can intervene. For instance, 1. medications as a *task* performed by the nurse; 2. patient education (in regard to the medication program) as a *function* of nursing; 3. pain (and its pharmacological intervention) as a patient *problem* addressed by nursing.

Nursing care during hospitalization can be the pivot upon which the treatment program can be based. It allows for intensive supervision, teaching coordination, and care. It can be a link in the continuity of care and extension into the community through adequate planning for discharge.

Understanding the role of the nurse in caring for the patient with arthritis with his unique physical and psychosocial needs will aid in providing quality nursing care of the population. Arthritis is not a new disease. However, the nursing care of these patients can present new challenges to developing new and creative ways to deal with old problems.

6

Rehabilitation Nursing and the Surgical Patient

MARY P. BRASSELL

Rehabilitation is a process to restore to a useful life—through education and therapy—a person who has been ill or handicapped. Because of the chronicity of many of the rheumatic diseases, it is inevitable that the patient's lifestyle will be affected. Therefore, it is imperative that the principles of rehabilitation be utilized in caring for the patient with arthritis, whether he is in the intensive care unit, general hospital, outpatient facility, or rehabilitation center. In the acute hospital setting, the life of the patient is saved, but because of a usual lack of rehabilitative procedures, the accompanying contractures, pressure sores, and loss of function bring the patient prolonged hospitalization and increased disability.

The rehabilitation nursing approach that will be presented in this chapter is based upon the team approach that has been part of the nursing philosophy at Moss Rehabilitation Hospital. The team includes a rheumatologist, surgeon, physiatrist, nurse consultant, floor nurse, occupational therapist, physical therapist, social worker, psychologist, and when necessary, a psychiatrist. Each team member works both individually and collectively to help the patient formulate realistic patient goals.

There are numerous excellent surgical textbooks (1, 2), periodicals (3), and journals (4) which illustrate, describe, and explain the various surgical procedures (5). There are equally numerous nursing tomes which explain the nursing care of the patient who must undergo extraarticular and intraarticular surgery. This chapter will dwell particularly on the practical aspects of the nursing care which are relevant to the patient with rheumatoid arthritis (RA). Since RA best exemplifies systemic rheumatic disease and joint problems, it will be used as the prototype

RA

RA is a disease which is characterized by synovitis which produces pain, swelling, heat, and redness over the involved joints. In addition, morning stiffness, fatigue, intermittent fevers, gelling, and night pains can be present.

Systemic complications include circulatory problems; viz., anemia, cardiac effusion, vasculitis, and pulmonary problems, including pleural effusion. Rheumatoid nodules may be found over the joints and in the lungs, brain, and heart in some patients. Inflammation begins in the synovium and, subsequently, destroys cartilage, bone, tendon, ligaments, and other surrounding structures. Deformity and disability follow.

Education of the patient, nurse, and all health professionals involved in caring for the patient with RA is the cornerstone upon which a realistic surgical outcome hinges. Both the patient and nurse must realize that arthritis surgery is done primarily to diminish pain, increase function, prevent deformity, and salvage whatever is possible. Arthritis surgery is never done for cosmetic purposes alone (6)! Arthritis surgery is, in most cases, an elective procedure.

Contraindications to arthritis surgery include the usual medical problems. local or systemic infection, and poor skin condition over the surgical site. Other major contraindications are *psychological* (e.g., the excessively depressed or abnormally overanxious patient who cannot be controlled with psychiatric intervention); *motivational* (i.e., lack of positive motivation, e.g., the patient who will not comply with an exercise program); and those based on *unrealistic expectations* (e.g., the patient who expects to play tennis daily after total knee replacement (7). Since the nursing staff sees more of the patient than any other team member, it is important that the nurse convey at once any evidence of the aforementioned contraindications to the surgeon and attending physician. Although there may be no medical contraindications to surgery, lack of positive motivation and unrealistic expectations are two major reasons for cancellation of a surgical procedure. The patient must be a willing and cooperative partner in his rehabilitation, so as to ensure maximum postoperative benefits.

Barring the usual postoperative problems that beset any patient who must undergo surgery, the following problems are indigenous to the patient with RA; viz., coping with painful morning stiffness or all day stiffness and/or gel syndrome, problems associated with immobility (particularly loss of function), prevention of contractures, cervical subluxation, and corticosteroid-influenced skin.

The hazards of immobility are well known and include pulmonary embolus, decubitus formation (8), and atrophy of structures. The patient with RA is certainly more prone to the hazards of immobility because motion is further inhibited by morning stiffness and gelling. A trite but relevant adage that we use frequently with patients is, "What you don't use, you lose." This explains simply to the patient and those who care for him that unless mobility is maintained in the nonoperated regions, complications will ensue. Using the example of the tennis professional or golfer who must train daily may help the patient understand the concept of preventing loss of motion or function. Using rehabilitation aids, such as pressure-alleviating mattresses (e.g., Eggcrate (Figs. 6.1 and 6.2)), Rochester bed, sheepskin, and of course, turning schedules, will aid in reducing problems of decubitus formation.

Cervical Myelopathy in RA

In a 1970 study of 100 patients with RA, atlantoaxial subluxation (AAS) was found in 36 patients. The study concluded that AAS was a common complication of RA and that its incidence correlated with the duration of the disease (9). AAS was not associated with progressive myelopathy and was not an indication for surgical intervention. However, in 1976, a follow-up study demonstrated that in 24 of the patients with cervical myelopathy, AAS occurred in 7 patients (38%). However, death was not attributed to cervical myelopathy. This study has several nursing implications for the patient with cervical subluxation. If upon nursing interview for assessment the patient complains of pyramidal tract signs (e.g., paresthesias in the upper or lower extremity, weakness, and instability), the nurse should immediately relay these findings to the physician in charge. It may be necessary to obtain new x-ray films immediately! If cervical myelopathy is present, the patient may be a candidate for cervical decompression and/or fusion to stabilize the cervical spine (10). Intubation of the patient with RA and cervical subluxation is difficult and dangerous, especially if the instability is below the C1 level or in the midcervical level. Preventing further

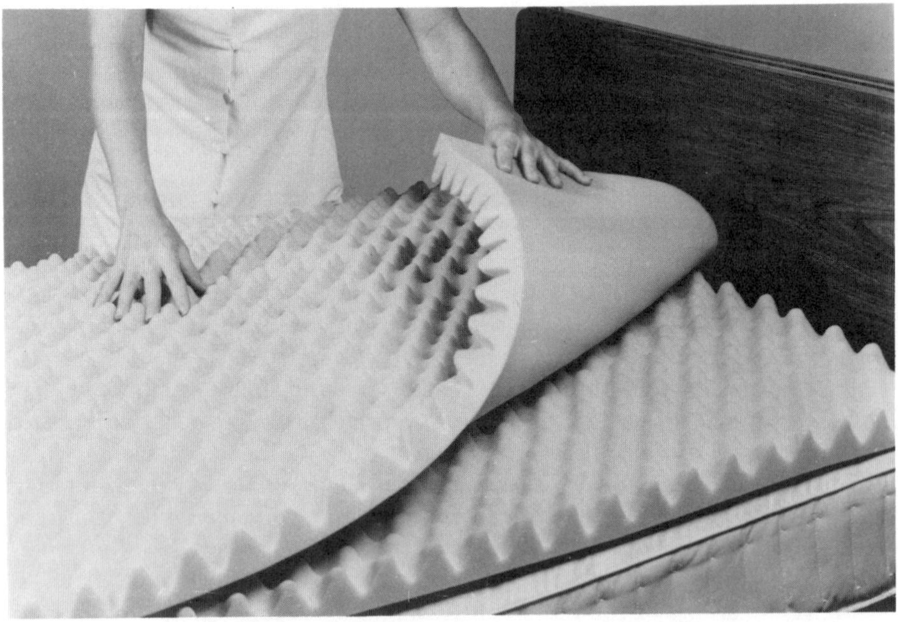

Fig. 6.1. An Eggcrate® bed pad—a pressure-alleviating mattress pad. (Figure provided courtesy of Bio Clinic Company, Media, Pennsylvania.)

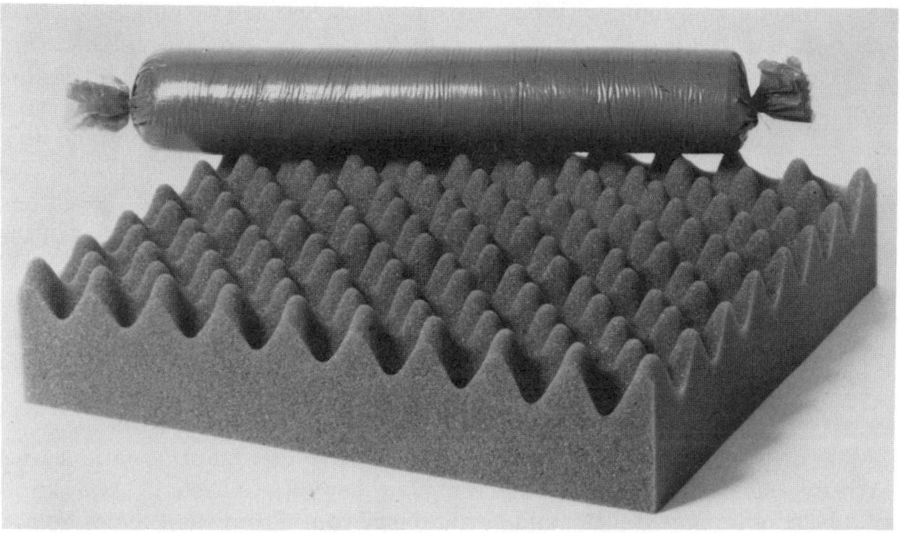

Fig. 6.2. A Puff Pak® wheelchair pad—a pressure-alleviating chair pad. (Figure provided courtesy of Bio Clinic Company, Media, Pennsylvania.)

subluxation becomes the primary goal once it is established that the patient has cervical myelopathy. The nurse or other allied health professional must secure from the neurosurgeon or neurologist immediate and specific orders regarding all phases of the patient's activities of daily living. The patient with symptomatic AAS must be treated like the acute-spinal-cord-injured patient! This patient is usually mobilized on a Stryker frame, Circoelectric bed, or Stokes-Mandeville bed, is placed in some form of skeletal traction, and probably will undergo cervical fusion. Joint surgery is now secondary to this life-threatening situation. However, the patient with asymptomatic AAS or AAS that is slight or moderate may be permitted to undergo the joint surgery.

Brattstorm and Granholm (11) advocate the use of some type of external support to aid in stabilizing the neck and attempt to prevent injury. A cervical collar is indicated if the patient has moderate long-tract signs. Usually, the patient is ordered to wear his prescribed collar to and during all therapeutic appointments, e.g., physical therapy, occupational therapy, perhaps even while in bed, and during sleep. This decision is best left for the neurosurgeon. The patient should be cautioned to wear the collar especially while in a moving vehicle, i.e., car, train, plane, bus, or boat. An abrupt stop can snap the head forward, with dire consequence.

The patient should wear his collar to the operating room, and the operating room team (anesthesiologist, surgeon, nurses, and transporters) should all be alerted to the patient with AAS. Induction of anesthesia may be difficult. It is strongly recommended that the patient be made cognizant of his role in complying with cervical collar restrictions! Placing a sign over the bed, which states "Cervical Precautions," is also advised, in the event that cardiopulmonary resuscitation (CPR) should be necessary. The cardiopulmonary team should be made aware of the cervical subluxation, so that the appropriate form of CPR be instituted to prevent further and life-threatening cord damage.

The patient with AAS who must undergo lower extremity surgery must be instructed that in moving from the foot of his bed toward the head of the bed, he *not use his head* as an anchor or pivot! Often, a patient will avoid bearing down on the operated extremity to avoid pain and will thus transfer the weight to his neck and head. This action, even with a cervical collar in place, can increase the chances of furthering AAS!

Corticosteroid-Induced Complications

The necessity of preoperative teaching is obvious when the patient with arthritis has been taking corticosteroids for some time. Usually, the skin is friable, fragile, ecchymotic, and tissue-paper thin. From the time of admission, wherever the patient goes, the skin must be protected against possible injury. For example, the x-ray technician must be warned either by a note in front of the chart or verbally that the patient has a contracture of the elbow or the knee, so as not to attempt forcible straightening. In transporting the patient, gentle unpressured movements must be used. A powerful grasp may be enough to cause ecchymosis and possible lacerations to the patient with corticosteroid-influenced skin. The operating room team can injure the patient! It has happened that while abducting a prosthesis, the grasp used by an attending resident resulted in a laceration at the distal femur. It is disconcerting to find two surgical wounds, instead of one, on the patient's return from the operating room. At New York's Hospital for Special Surgery, corticosteroid-treated patients are carefully wrapped in soft cotton batting, Webril, or other appropriate fabrics before a tourniquet is applied. This action prevents lacerations; however, ecchymosis is unavoidable. Once again, the importance of gentle transfer must be emphasized.

The healing process is much slower in most patients who have been taking corticosteroids; therefore, sutures and clips will be left in place longer.

When the patient is turned, extra precautions must be observed to prevent damage. If the patient is to be on continuous antibiotic therapy, avoid prolonged strapping of the patient to a rigid armboard. If it is necessary to immobilize the patient, do so, but release the board every 1 or 2 hr, as necessary, to prevent painful stiffness and circulatory problems at the intravenous site.

The nutritional status of patients who already have skin changes varies. Usually, the patient is undernourished even if the corticosteroids give a rounded appearance to the face. It is suggested that a dietary consultation be obtained so as to prevent negative nitrogen balance and to have the patient maintain a diet sufficient in minerals and vitamins that will enhance healing. Some physicians prescribe additional ascorbic acid supplements. If the patient is obese, it may be advisable to have the patient and dietitian confer about a low-calorie reduction diet. Sometimes, physicians will order reduction diet a week before surgery. The weight loss, if any, is negligible, whereas the added emotional and physical stress to the patient may be considerable.

General Guidelines for the Surgical Patient

Table 6.1 is a teaching guide for the arthritic patient. The guide can be used in any teaching situation involving arthritis and surgery. Table 6.2 lists the preoperative teaching checklist that is applicable to all arthritic patients who must undergo any surgical procedure. Both the nurse and the patient should review the guidelines, preferably together, to ensure patient understanding and cooperation and to aid in achieving a realistic postoperative outcome.

TABLE 6.1. *Teaching Guide for the Arthritis Patient*

General Guidelines

1. After the surgeon has discussed and explained the surgical procedure, allow the patient to ventilate his fears, expectations, and understanding of the surgery.
2. Give the patient some form of joint replacement literature to peruse so that he may formulate questions and gain further understanding of what will occur. Use the Joint Implant Surgery and Research Foundation pamphlet, Lilly illustrations, or other appropriate literature, to show simply the patient a reasonable and nonthreatening picture of the procedure (graphics are best) (see Table 6.1 insert).
3. A patient who has undergone a similar successful procedure may be of great help and a good resource.
4. When you have answered questions about the procedure, ask the patient to tell you his primary goals. If the patient has unrealistic expectations, relay them to the patient's surgeon and/or attending physician, so that he may clarify what is necessary (6).
5. If, at this point, the patient understands what is to occur, begin to give the patient specific instructions.
   a. Explain the necessity for urine culture and sensitivity and checking for the presence of minor infections, e.g., abscessed teeth, paronychia, urinary tract infection symptoms.
   b. Make certain the patient realizes the risk of joint infection postoperatively, if minor infections are present.
   c. Explain the need for deep breathing and coughing. Have the patient demonstrate deep breathing.
   d. Explain the need for vital signs and also add that analgesics may need to be withheld until signs are stable enough to prevent shock.
   e. Explain prophylactic antibiotics, the length of anticipated use, and the need to report redness, pain, and other signs of inflammation at the intravenous site to the nurse or doctor, immediately.

TABLE 6.1. —*Continued*

General Guidelines
f. Discuss the need for analgesics and the time span in which they are given. Assure the patient that effective pain relief will be provided. Be sure to instruct the patient to ask for the analgesic. (Many times patients appear to be sleeping, and the nurse may be unaware the patient is in pain.) Place the call bell next to patient.
g. Now begin explaining the specifics of the arthritis surgery and demand that the patient demonstrate what he will do postoperatively. If quadriceps setting exercises have been taught, have the patient give a return demonstration. Have patient explain the positioning; e.g., in a total knee procedure, the patient will have the leg elevated from above the heel to below the knee on two pillows or their equivalent (12). Explain that nothing will be under the knee unless the patient returns in a cast or posterior splint. (Emphasize that pillows or anything under the knee will build in contractures which will influence ambulation and take money and weeks to relieve.) Emphasize the importance of maintaining limb elevation (13) and the need to report at once a leaky ice bag!
h. Dressings: Ask the patient to place his hand on his dressings and to call the nurse immediately if they are damp or wet. Instruct the patient to call for the nurse if the dressings are soiled. Make the patient aware that soiled or wet dressings can become causes of infections!
i. Explain that the patient may be turned from side to side as long as a pillow supports the operated leg. (When turning, two people should assist. One will place the operated limb on the pillow and support it while the other assistant will help turn the patient.)
j. Tell the patient that he will not and should not receive any injections preoperatively in the site of the surgery.
k. Explain capillary refill, pedal pulses, or whatever else you will be checking. Explain to the patient to report numbness, tingling, and paresthesias.
l. If patient is to have a booster of corticosteroids prior to surgery, explain the rationale and need.
m. Explain the use of anticoagulants as simply as possible, also the importance of reporting burning or "pink" or bloody urine immediately. (If the patient is on any of the nonsteroidal antiinflammatory drugs, especially aspirin but also the various propionates, prothrombin time may be increased.)
n. Explain any aids that may be needed and their use and purpose, e.g., abduction, splint, Rochester bed, or Eggcrate mattress (Fig. 6.1).
o. Discuss physical therapy and/or occupational therapy instruction with the patient so that the nurse, therapist, and patient are all adhering to the same regimen.
p. Cervical precautions must be specifically explained to the patient. Use of the collar, turning, toileting, and feeding must be discussed preoperatively to ensure postoperative cooperation and prevent complications.

Surgical Candidates for Joint Replacement

The target population for joint arthoplasty is the arthritis patient population. Although synovectomy and osteotomy procedures are used, joint replacement is usually inevitable. Total joint replacements of the upper extremities include those for the shoulder, elbow, wrist, and thumb implant.

Information for Our Patients about Total Knee-Joint Replacement

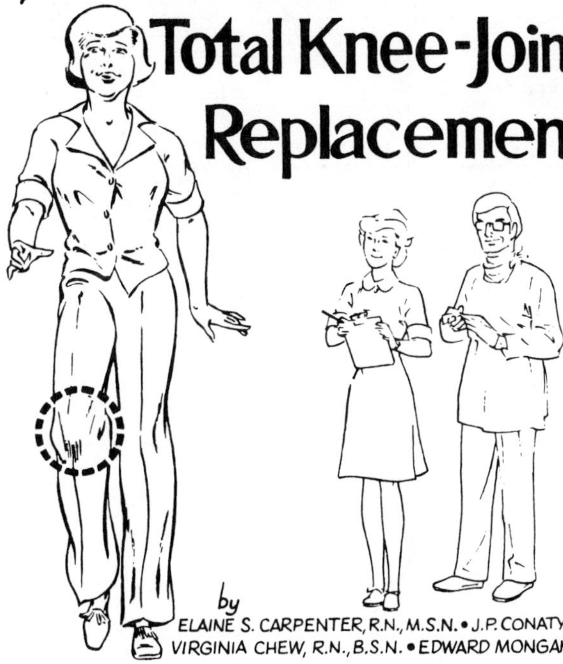

by
ELAINE S. CARPENTER, R.N., M.S.N. • J.P. CONATY, M.D.
VIRGINIA CHEW, R.N., B.S.N. • EDWARD MONGAN, M.D.

This book has been made available by sponsorship of

THE ARTHRITIS FOUNDATION
SOUTHERN CALIFORNIA CHAPTER
4311 Wilshire Boulevard
Los Angeles 90010
(213) 938-6111

Additional Copies • Apply to:
Ms. PAT GUSTAVINO, Rancho Los Amigos Hospital
Downey, CA 90242 or (213) 922-7111

THE ARTHRITIS FOUNDATION · **NATIONAL OFFICE**
1212 AVENUE OF THE AMERICAS • NEW YORK, N. Y. 10036

TABLE 6.1. *Insert*

TABLE 6.2. *Preoperative Teaching Checklist for Joint Surgery**

Subject	Patient Understanding	Comments
Urine culture		
Minor infections		
Surgical procedure		
Illustrations		
Patient questions		
Patient goals		
Skin preparation		
Vital signs		
Analgesics		
Respiratory therapy		
Anticoagulant therapy		
Positioning Pillow		
Bed (turning)		
Wheelchair		
Bedpan use		
Cervical precautions Collar		
Restrictions		
Dressings		
Steroid boost		
Capillary refill		
Reporting sensation		
Elevation of extremity		
Abduction device		
Bed		
Chair		
Sling		
Exercise regimen Knee		
Hip		
Hand, wrist, fingers		
Elbow		
Shoulder		
Sexual counseling Position		
Precautions		
Timing		
Other		

* Directions: Choose the term or terms which best describe the patient's understanding and acceptance of the surgical procedure. (unaccepted; poor; unrealistic; requires significant other adequate; excellent; appropriate; NA (not applicable)).

Lower extremity joint replacements include those for the hip, knee, ankle, and large-toe implant (14). Hemiarthroplasty is usually confined to the phalanges of the hands and feet (15).

The patients with RA, osteoarthritis, and traumatic arthritis comprise the largest number of patients for total arthroplasty. Indications for this type of surgery are pain, instability, and loss of function. However, surgery is only attempted after sufficient trials of medication, splinting, rest, and rehabilitation.

Total Shoulder Arthroplasty

Candidates for shoulder replacement usually complain of moderate to severe pain "like a toothache" (16). The pain is usually intensified at night. The secondary indication for shoulder replacement is to improve function so that the patient may perform activities of daily living (ADL). Contraindications to this surgery are infection, muscle paralysis, and neuropathy. Possible complications of this type of surgery are infection, loosening of bone cement, possible rotator cuff tears, and tears of the deltoid (see Chapter 11). Intraoperatively, in patients with traumatic arthritis, there is a possibility of nerve damage.

The patient is usually out of bed within 24 hr after surgery. Anticipated hospital stay is about 2 weeks, during which time the patient learns assisted motion exercises, isometric muscle strengthening for the noninvolved muscles on the 1st day, and on the 2nd day, hand and forearm exercises.

Total Wrist Replacement

Pain, limitation of movement, and instability are usually the prime indications for total wrist surgery (Fig. 6.3) (17). In 101 patients (18) who underwent wrist replacement, a triunion 3-part ball and socket joint was used and was held in place with methylmethacrylate cement. The wrist was immobilized for 1 week until edema decreased, then placed in static or dynamic splints for approximately 3 months to allow the soft-tissue swelling to heal. Guarded motion was begun within 1 week postoperatively (19). Patients with total wrist replacement are never permitted to lift more than 10 lb of weight and must avoid any type of impact sports, including golf.

Total Elbow Replacement

Pain relief and restoration of function are the primary indications for elbow replacement (8). The elbow serves as a link between the lower and the upper arm and aids in flexion and extension necessary to generate the force for lifting. All of the currently used prostheses provide satisfactory motion to carry out ADL. The largest majority of patients who undergo elbow replacement have RA, with traumatic arthritis secondarily (20).

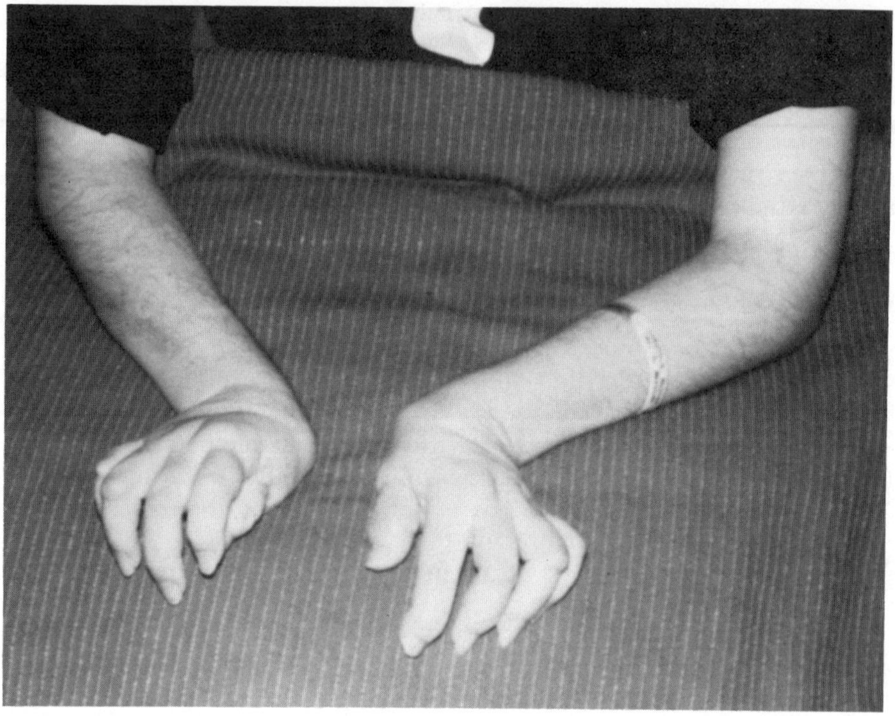

Fig. 6.3. Note bilateral bayonnet wrists and nodules on proximal interphalangeal joints. Patient is 25 years old with juvenile rheumatoid arthritis.

Total Hip Replacement (THR) and Resurfacing

In the late 1960s, when the Charnley low-friction total hip arthroplasty was introduced, it was hailed in the medical and lay world. Indications for total hip arthroplasty were pain, restriction of function, and increased disability (21). Contraindications to this type of surgery were infection, spasticity, or paresis of hip muscles. Some of the possible complications which can occur are thromboembolism (2), infection, dislocation, sciatic or femoral neuropathies, prosthetic loosening, and breakage (with newer designs this seems to be decreasing) (23).

In 1971, Paltrinieri and Trentani (23) of Bologna, Italy, reported that hip resurfacing could be an alternative to total hip arthroplasty if there was enough bone stock and an absence of significant deformity. The ideal candidate for this operation is the young patient with concentric hip disease. This operation is best utilized for patients with traumatic arthritis, osteoarthritis, aseptic necrosis of the femoral head with limited bone loss, and hip dysplasia. Ankylosing spondylitis (because it may lead to early postoperative fusion) and RA accompanied by significant osteoporosis are contraindications to resurfacing, as is the presence of an active infection. Although this surgery is intended for the younger population, with new design advances and follow-up, it may benefit others. One of the most frequent complications of this surgery is fracture of the femoral neck.

Total Knee Replacement

Pain, decreased functional ability, and the absence or presence of deformity constitute the indications for knee replacement. Not all patients with the aforementioned complaints may require total joint surgery. Pain relief and correction of deformity may be imparted by a high tibial osteotomy.

Patients who are grossly obese or extremely young are poor candidates for knee replacement. Currently, there are three types of knee prostheses. Gunston's polycentric knee is a minimally constrained design which is limited only to the tibiofemoral joint since the stability of this knee is provided by the ligamentous and capsular structures. The ICLH, geometric, UCI, and total condylar (24) knees are examples of partially constrained prostheses, and they constitute the largest number of total knee implants. The Walldius, Guepar, and Shiers are examples of the fully constrained arthroplasties. The postoperative complications include infection, mechanical failure, loosening of the cement fixation, neuropraxia of the peroneal nerve in the presence of severe contracture deformities, and delayed tendon ruptures (7).

Upper Extremity Surgery (Hand, Wrist, Elbow)

Prior to surgery of the hands, wrist, elbow, or shoulder, check the preoperative teaching guide (Tables 6.1 and 6.2) and begin to instruct the patient and explain the need for cooperation with postoperative management. The patient must demonstrate understanding, and questions about the procedures are encouraged.

When the patient returns from the operating room, all phalanges should be visable. If necessary, cut or trim Webril or other materials that may interfere with observation and result in compromise of the circulation.

Elevation of the operated limb is one of the most critical care issues in upper extremity surgery (25). If the patient has undergone hand, wrist, or elbow surgery, it is vital that the standard orthopedic rule be followed: Elevate the hand higher than the wrist; the wrist, higher than the elbow; and the elbow higher than the shoulder. Although some inexperienced orthopedists or house officers order that the limb be elevated on two pillows, it is more expedient to use an alternate method of assuring that the limb of a sedated patient will not slip off the pillows inadvertently. The resulting edema could produce circulatory and/or neutral complications which would affect function adversely. A suspended stockingette, commercial sling, or a pillow case can be used to cradle and suspend the extremity. Commercially available small icebags may be applied. It is important not to use heavy icepacks since their weight could add pressure to the incision and perhaps inhibit circulation. Latex or vinyl gloves partially filled with ice may be substituted.

Preventing damage to the ulnar nerve from pressure while the extremity is supported on the elbow can be achieved by applying either a commercial foam elbow protector or by filling a rubber glove one-half to two-thirds full of air, fastening the glove with a rubber band several times, and placing it directly under the elbow.

If the patient must use a posterior splint or cast postoperatively, it must frequently be checked for signs of pressure, edema, and infection. Teach the patient to sniff the cast to detect odors which may signal infection. Should the fingers seem severely blanched or even moderately cyanotic, notify the orthopedic surgeon or his surrogate immediately. A cast cutter should be available and if the cast must be split, maintain alignment of the limb, loosen the cast, and apply an ace bandage over it to prevent dislocation. It is much easier to reapply a cast than to correct damage to the limb caused by compression.

Should the patient return with Kirschner wires through his fingers, the nurse should protect both the patient and staff from possible injury from protruding wires or pins. Sometimes, the surgeon will cover the ends of the pins with cork. If cork is not available, applying a rubber stopper from a test tube will give adequate protection if it is fastened securely with tape. Often the orthopedic technician will apply a plaster circular arch from thumb base to the base of the little finger, if the patient has a cast. This plaster arch also will prevent snagging of the pins. Checking for infections or drainage around the pin should be done on every tour of duty (26). Postoperative dressings are maintained until edema is decreased to the surgeon's expectations.

The patient with hand surgery will require preoperative and postoperative instructions or suggestions concerning ADL. Usually, during the first 24 hr, the patient may require more assistance since it is a period of adjustment to a state of one-handedness.

Sometimes, various types of splints (6) may be ordered for the patient, to aid in restoring and improving function. Some of these splints are discussed in Chapter 11. If one is blessed with an occupational therapist who understands the surgeon's expectation of what the splint is to accomplish, the therapist should instruct the staff and the patient on its application and use. The occupational therapist is an excellent resource person for information about hand function. If there is no trained occupational therapist available, it is incumbent upon the nurse to consult with the surgeon about both the use and the application of the splint. Since the nurse is the most constant professional with the patient, the nurse will have to teach the patient its use.

The patient will need to learn how to adapt to one-handedness. Food preparation, dressing, and toileting may present problems and must be anticipated by the nurse so that assistance may be provided when necessary

(4). During the initial 48 hr after surgery, the patient will constantly require reminders to remember to keep the extremity elevated. Encouraging the use of attractive scarves as slings may help some of the more fastidious patients adhere to their elevation regime!

Unless contraindicated by the surgeon, the patient may be allowed out of bed on the day of surgery upon return to the room. The elevation can be maintained by simply moving the intravenous pole with the patient. When the patient is permitted out of bed, the arm should be suspended in a triangular cloth sling, a commercial sling, or a stockingette arrangement (4). If the arm is suspended in a triangular sling, *do not fasten the sling at the neck*! Many patients with RA have asymptomatic involvement of the upper cervical spine, even subluxation of the 1st or the 2nd vertebra. Pressure from weight may cause damage, and fastening the sling at the base of the neck can contribute to worsening of subluxation of the cervical spine. The

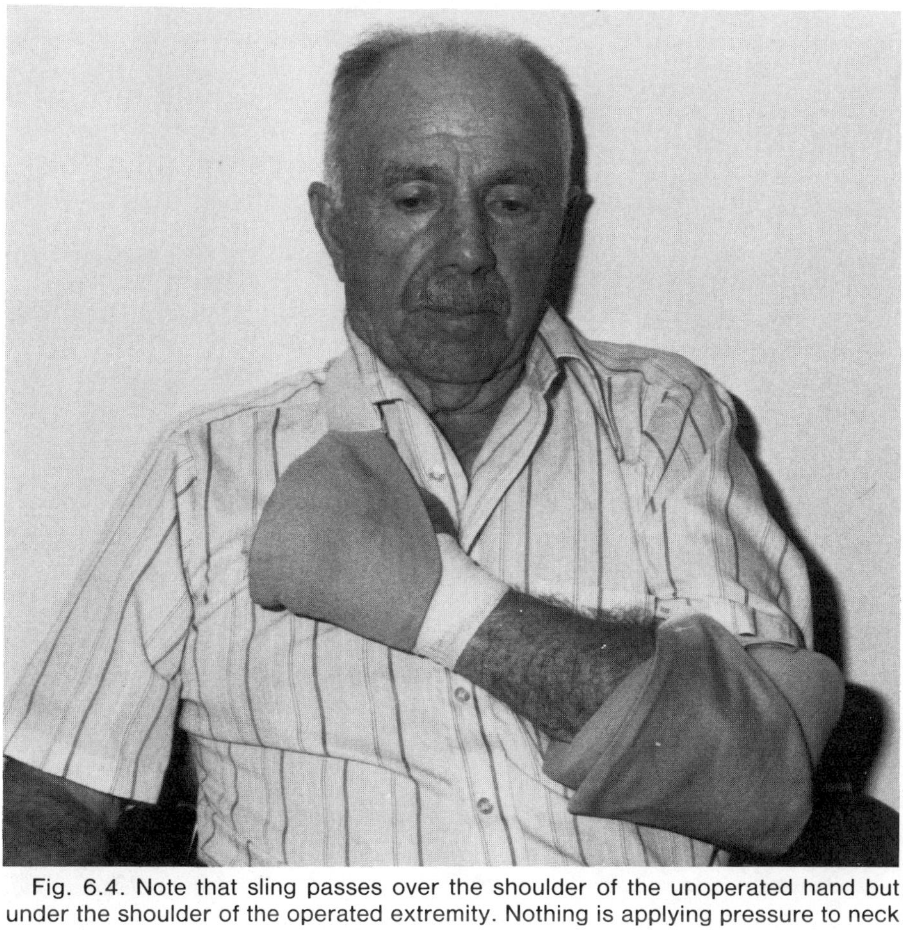

Fig. 6.4. Note that sling passes over the shoulder of the unoperated hand but under the shoulder of the operated extremity. Nothing is applying pressure to neck area.

sling should be passed under one shoulder and over the other and fastened over the scapula. The patient must be reminded to maintain high elevation of the upper extremity; dangling of the operated limb should be avoided. The method of elevation are seen in Figures 6.4–6.7.

Edema of the hand can persist from 3 to 10 days. The patient must be reminded frequently to keep his hand elevated. If for some reason a sling is not worn, the patient should place the hand between the 2nd and 3rd button level of the shirt or robe, to prevent edema (Fig. 6.6).

It is suggested that the patient who has any type of hand, wrist, elbow, or shoulder implant have vital signs checked every 4 hr for 48 hr and then that the temperature be taken every 8 hr and other vital signs be ordered during the length of the patient's hospital stay. Monitoring the condition of the dressing should continue, and if the patient is to be discharged with dressings, the patient or a companion should continue to check for infection, capillary refill, and edema, until the orders are discontinued by the surgeon.

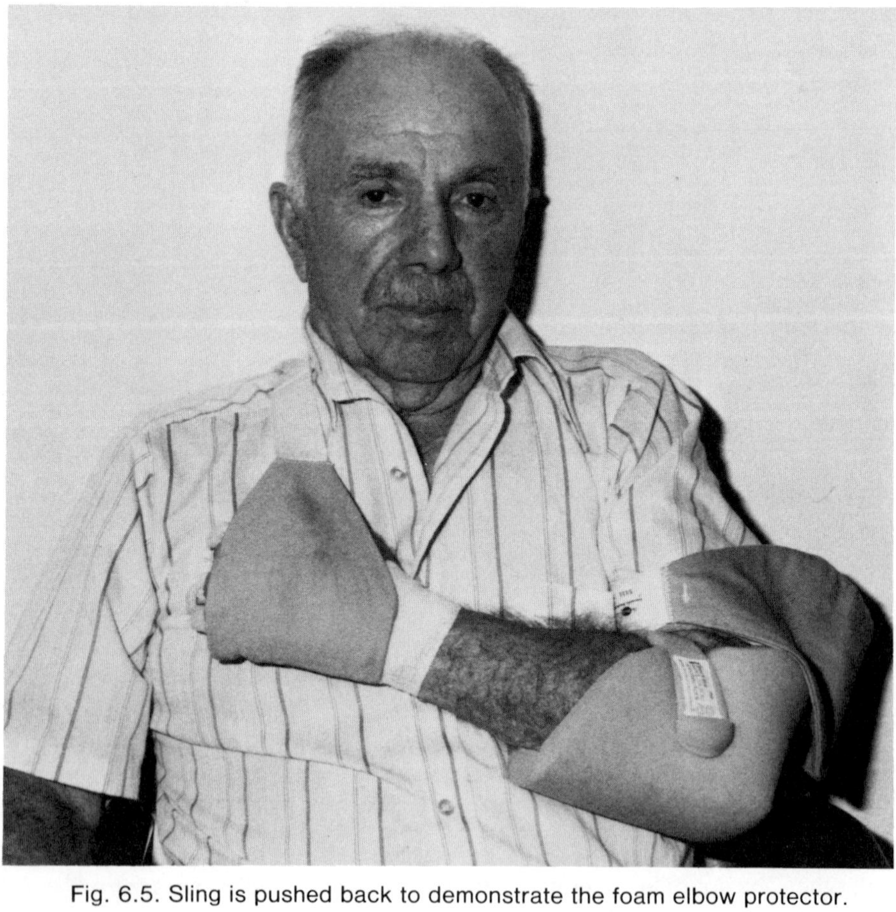

Fig. 6.5. Sling is pushed back to demonstrate the foam elbow protector.

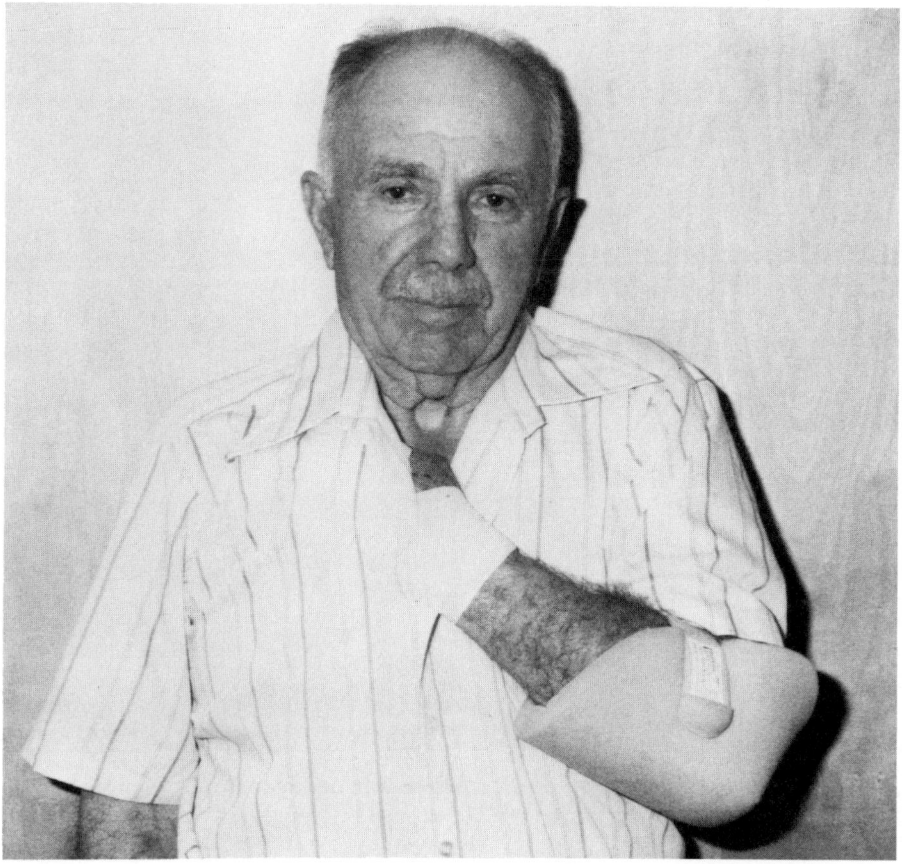

Fig. 6.6. Maintaining elevation without sling.

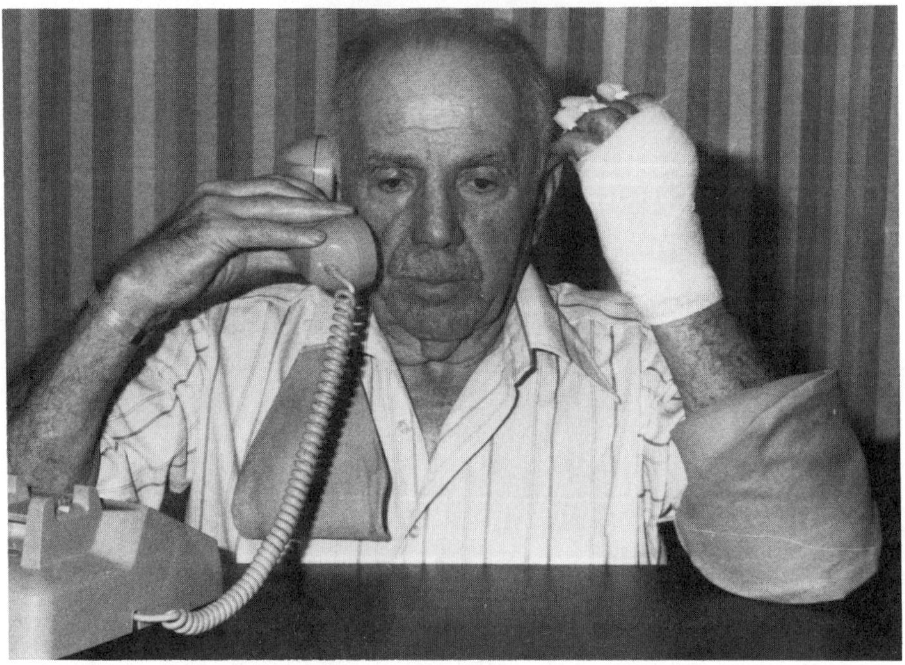

Fig. 6.7. Avoiding pressure on ulnar nerve with use of foam elbow protector.

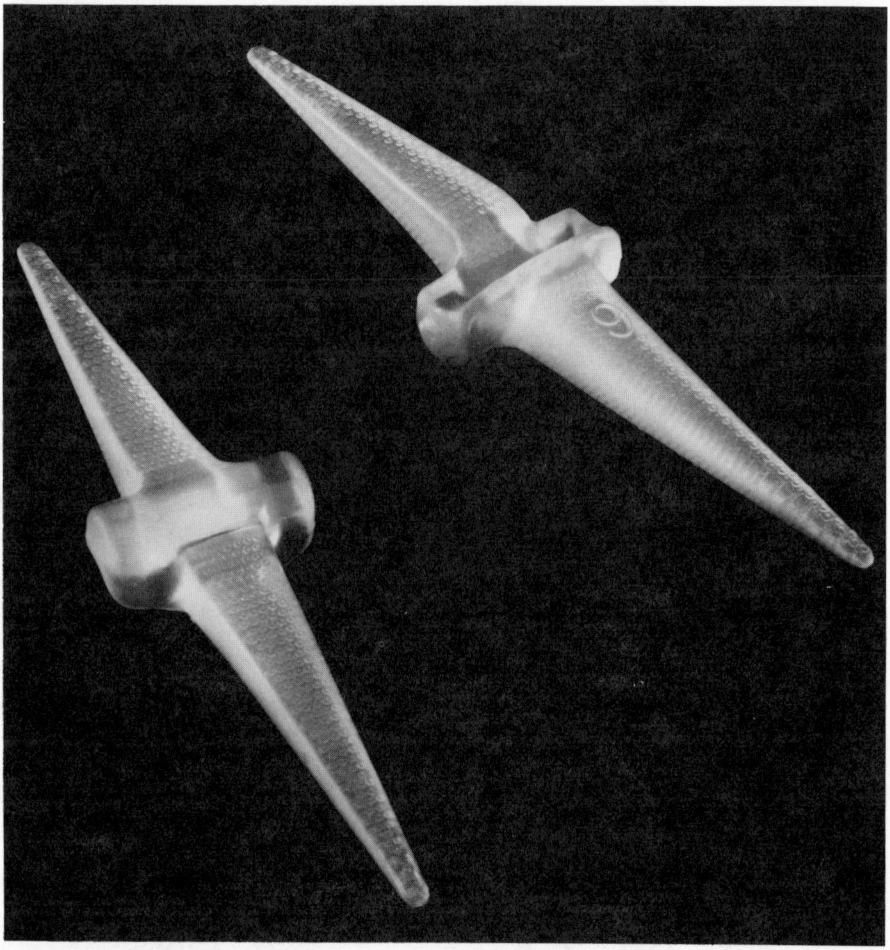

Fig. 6.8. Silastic finger joint implant HP(Swanson design). (Figure provided courtesy of Alfred B. Swanson, M.D., F.A.C.S.)

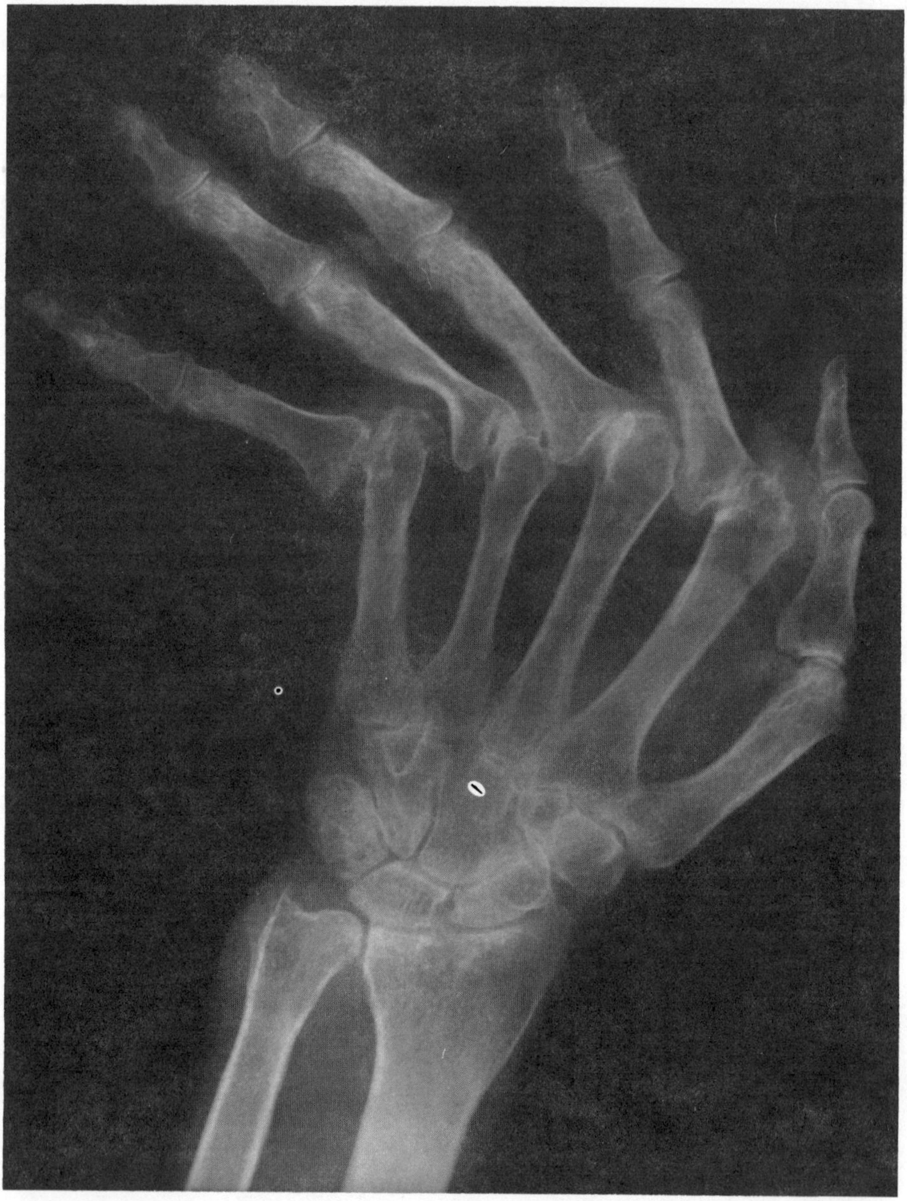

Fig. 6.9. Preoperative RA hand. (Figure provided courtesy of Alfred B. Swanson, M.D., F.A.C.S.)

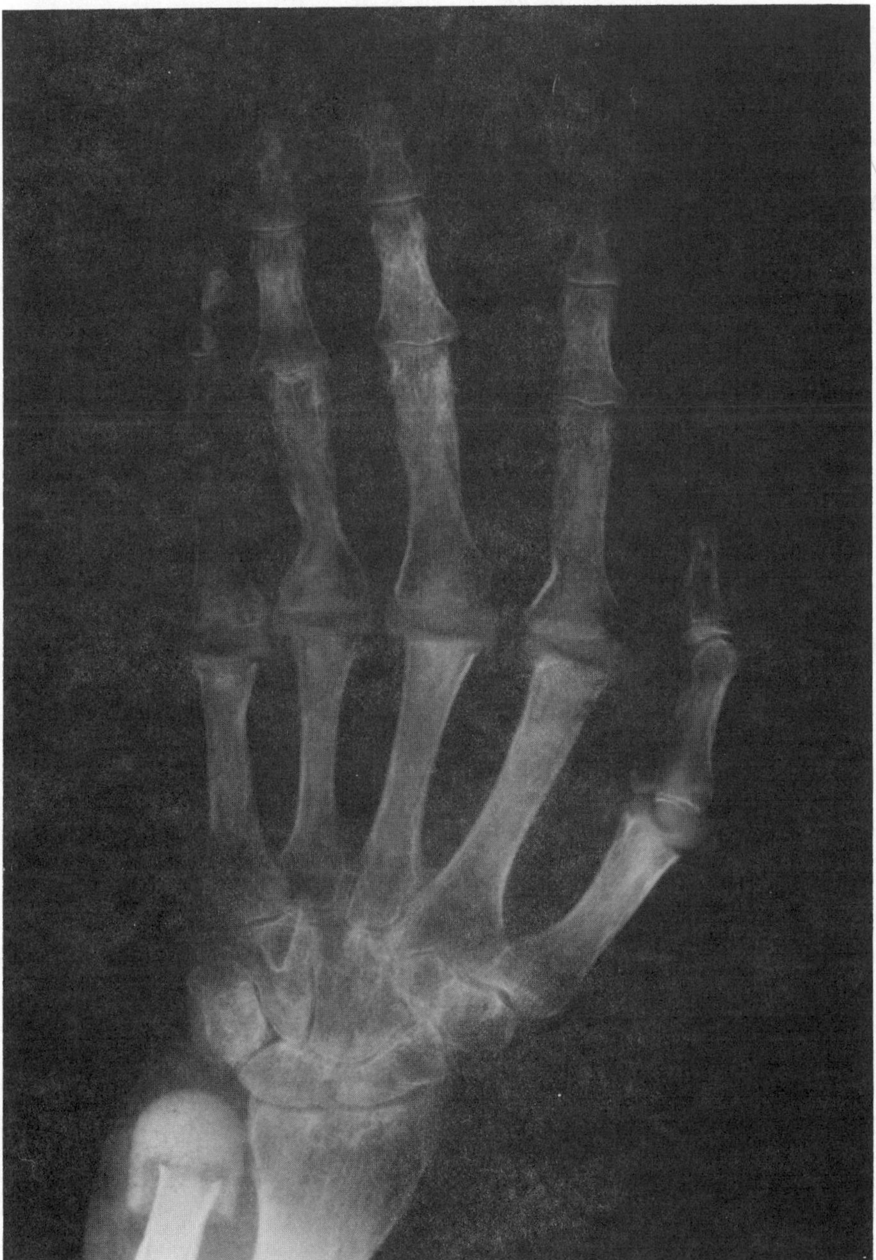

Fig. 6.10. Postoperative 3-year follow-up of RA hand in Fig. 6.10. (Figure provided courtesy of Alfred B. Swanson, M.D., F.A.C.S.)

Shoulder Arthroplasty (Total Joint Replacement)

The patient who undergoes shoulder replacement usually returns from the operating room with the elbow at right angle at slightly above waist level, with the shoulder incision swather in postoperative bulky dressings and a Velpeau type of dressing application, which may or may not be suspended in a sling (5). Care should be taken that all the phalanges are exposed so that capillary refill can be checked. The usual postoperative nursing care should be observed. Numbness or any type of paresthesia should be reported immediately to the surgeon since it may indicate circulatory embarrassment. The dressings remain in place from 48 hr or until the surgeon orders them to be removed, so that gentle and prescribed range of motion can be started by the surgeon, physical therapist, and nurses. The patient is permitted out of bed as desired, usually by doctor's orders within 24 hr postoperatively, unless there are contraindications. Dressings should be checked for signs of drainage. Teach the patient, postoperatively, to use the unaffected hand to check the dressings for wetness and to call the nurse immediately if drainage is present (see Table 6.1).

Table 6.3 illustrates one type of nursing plan that can be utilized in caring for the patient with lower extremity replacement. It can serve as a care plan for the patient with upper extremity surgery also, with minor revisions. These care plans were designed for use by nursing assistants, practical nurses, and registered nurses. Samples of the physical therapy approaches to upper and lower extremity arthritis surgery are illustrated in Table 6.4.

Total or Partial Knee Replacement

The patient should have total or partial knee replacement instructions before the operation, and the postoperative regime should be explained. However, a very crucial aspect of nursing care for the patient with RA, which begins immediately upon the patient's return from the operating room, concerns positioning. Usually, the patient may return with a muff-type dressing that includes surgical dressings (Hemovac, Webril, or other appropriate padding) and ace bandages from groin to toes. Make certain all toes are exposed and accessible for capillary refill. Checking pedal pulses is not possible since they are relatively inaccessible because of the several layers of dressings. The operated limb must be placed in extension or the equivalent (35). *No pillows are permitted under the knee* unless the patient has returned with either a posterior splint or cast, which automatically prevents flexion! *Pillows should extend from above the heel to approximately 4 inch below the knee*! Patients with RA can develop flexion contractures within 24 hr. Releasing those contractures may require 2 weeks of additional hospitalization and financial expense. The heels of these patients should be checked every shift and moistened with lotion, to prevent pressure sores. Foam or Posey-type booties which have been sprinkled

TABLE 6.3. *Moss Rehabilitation Hospital Department of Nursing Service*

POSTOPERATIVE NURSING CARE PLAN FOR John Smith RA, C1 C2 Subluxation DATE 8/24/79

SURGERY Total Knee Replacement (R) ANESTHESIA Spinal

1. Vital signs every 15 min × 4; then every 30 min × 3; then every 1 hr × 2; when vital signs are stable, take every 4 hours until ______
2. Check dressings for tightness, bleeding, drainage, edema, etc. If hemovac is present, check hemovac output every 2 hr. *IF MORE THAN 300 ml IN THE FIRST 6 to 8 HR* notify charge nurse, supervisor, and orthopedic resident. STAT. Include Hemovac output every 8 hr on intake and output sheet.
3. Check capillary refill of each toe. (Squeeze toe until it becomes white, then let go. If normal, toe should turn red immediately.)
4. Check toes for sensation of numbness, tingling, *warmth*, etc. (Compare coolness of operated foot to unoperated foot.)
5. If patient returns with a cast or posterior splint, *DO NOT COVER CAST*! Allow to dry exposed!
6. If patient has had INNOVAR, give only one-third to one-fourth of prescribed narcotic for 6 hr postoperatively (i.e., on return from the operating room) or as directed by surgeon or anesthesiologist.
7. Position of operated limb: If total or partial knee arthroplasty, elevate limb on two pillows or the equivalent of two pillows, *but nothing under the knee.*
   Casted or posterior splinted limb may be placed on two pillows with knee supported. (This is permitted because patient cannot flex knee in cast.)
8. Ice bags to cast or superiorly on dressings IF COLD CAN PENETRATE DRESSINGS. Make certain ice bag does not leak!
9. Patient may be turned from side to side as long as operated limb is supported during turning by personnel or on pillow and back is supported by pillow.
10. Check patient's voiding. INTAKE AND OUTPUT for 48 hr or until discontinued by physician.
11. Encourage patient to cough and deep breath every 2 hr while awake. (IPPB/SPIROCARE as ordered.)
12. Remember—Ask patient if he is having any discomfort or pain. Offer analgesics.

OTHER: Ice chips only.
CERVICAL COLLAR ON AT ALL TIMES! Folded Washcloth under occiput.

TABLE 6.4. *Physical Therapy Approaches to Upper and Lower Extremity Arthritis Surgery*

Types of Surgical Procedures	Definition	Indications
1. Arthrodesis	Bone fusion, where severe deformities affect weight-bearing joints (pips, wrist, elbow, knee, ankle, rarely the hip) (see Figs. 6.10 and 6.11)	Failed arthroplasty, septic joint, gross destruction and instability
2. Arthroplasty	Building an artificial joint, either partly (hemiarthroplasty) or the entire joint (TJR) using either metal or metal and plastic components (fingers, elbows, shoulders, wrist, hips, knees, ankles, toes) (14, 27–33) (see Fig. 6.8)	Pain, deformity, stiffness, RA
3. Carpal tunnel release	Surgical release of the carpal ligament and median nerve	Entrapment of median nerve
4. Darrach procedure	Resection of the distal ulna; may be accompanied by dorsal tenosynovectomy	RA, synovitis
5. Osteotomy	Correction of a deformity by surgically inducing a fracture; realignment of bone to heal with the aid of internal fixation devices (e.g., screws, plates)	RA, osteoarthritis, deformity, impaired function, pain
6. Tendon transfer	A redirection or transfer of an intact tendon from one functional position to another (34)	Prevention of tendon rupture, improvement of function, synovitis
7. Tenorrhaphy	Repair of a tendon	Prevention of tendon rupture, improvement of function, synovitis
8. Tenotomy	Incision of a tendon (analagous to osteotomy)	Relieve contractures
9. Tenosynovectomy	Removal of synovium from tendon sheaths and bursae	Improve function, prevention of nerve entrapment, synovitis, effusion, beginning deformity in a joint
10. Synovectomy	Surgical removal of part or all of the synovium	Persistent unresponsiveness to 6 months of medical treatment, local corticosteroids

lightly with talcum powder can cut down friction rub. If the patient's operated limb tends to go toward external or internal rotation, it would be wise to secure an order for a Bunny Boot, sandbags, or trochanter rolls to maintain the foot and leg in a neutral position, i.e., the toe pointing toward the ceiling.

Helping to alleviate stiffness of upper extremities can be accomplished by gentle range of motion when giving the patient back care or assisting with position changes. Patients may be turned as long as the operated limb is supported from toes to groin by either pillows or personnel.

During the first 24-hr postoperative period, the patient will be confined to bed (36). The next day, unless contraindicated by the surgeon, the patient should be out of bed and in a wheelchair. Early mobility will aid in preventing contractures, alleviate painful stiffness caused by inactivity, and lessen the chance of pulmonary complications.

Usually, the patient with an arthroplasty (37) is ready to begin physical therapy in the gymnasium within 3 to 5 days postoperatively, as ordered by the surgeon (38, 39). Before going to the gym, the patient should have received bedside therapy. Since the patient is usually transported in a wheelchair, the operated limb should be elevated in extension and secured with soft restraints or towels which have been fastened under the leg rest. This measure prevents sudden jarring or dropping of the operated limb and will protect the patient from unnecessary pain. Fear of pain may prevent patient compliance with therapeutic exercises and program. The patient, nurse, and physical therapist can best judge when the patient should receive his analgesic. Giving the analgesic 30 min before going to therapy may give the patient a sufficient edge of comfort so that he may cooperate more fully. Some patients may prefer to take the analgesic upon their return from therapy. The patient, nurse, and therapist can choose the most effective time slot for individual patient medication routine.

One method of eliciting patient cooperation and enhancing positive motivation of the patient's compliance with his program is to give the patient a "number" goal. A patient who can flex 40° one day and can achieve 60° of flexion 48 hr later will be encouraged to greater adherence to the regimen and achievement. If this patient is not achieving the desired degree of flexion and/or extension, his number goal will serve as an indicator for manipulation under anesthesia. Should the need for manipulation occur, the patient will have a better comprehension for its need.

Patient, therapist, and nurse should continue to check daily for signs that the patient's wound may be draining. If there is any type of serosanguinous drainage, pus, or synovial fluid, a culture should be taken immediately and reported to the surgeon. (At Moss, any nurse may take a culture and then report the action to the physician, without a written request, as part of our infection control system; regulations vary in different institutions.) Reporting to the surgeon and/or attending physician is necessary, to prevent infection and possible subsequent loss of the prosthesis. Often, a patient will have no dressings over his wound if the area and incision are clean and dry. Some surgeons will allow the patient to attend pool therapy with sutures in place, whereas others prefer to allow the patient to ambulate in the pool when the sutures have been removed and the incision is healed.

It is during this time span that the nurse and other team members should be alert for signs of poor positioning. A patient who places a pillow or folded towel under the knee while in bed or wheelchair must be cautioned that the flexion contractures which will ensue can adversely affect the surgical outcome. Often, patients who have had severe flexion contractures preoperatively will inadvertently revert to the habit of sitting in bed or in a chair with the knee flexed. This must be brought to the attention of the surgeon since it may necessitate application of a posterior splint whenever the patient is not actively performing exercises. Sometimes, a flat 1-lb sandbag weight is sufficient to serve as a reminder to avoid flexion.

In addition to attending physical therapy in the gymnasium, a patient after arthroplasty or synovectomy (40) may be ordered to perform knee-sling exercises. The knee sling is usually a soft-felt canvas piece or sheepskin material that is placed under the patient's thigh, above the knee, *not over the knee wound itself.* It is fastened on either side of the sling to a spreader bar, with a central portion connected by a rope that extends over two pulleys spaced sufficiently apart. The handle which the patient must grasp is over the first pulley, which is over the knee. The patient is instructed to pull the handle slowly, which in turn causes the knee to flex. The patient is instructed to perform this task 10 to 15 times every hour. If the patient has poor hand function or is unable to make a closed fist, the handle should be padded and built up to accommodate the patient's grasp. If the patient has weakness or inability to perform the exercise, the nurse or significant family member must help the patient perform the exercise since it is necessary for the return of optimum range of motion. Patients who require assistance include those with poor hand grip or weakened or destroyed wrist joints; they may also need platform crutches and/or a walker-with-wheels to aid in ambulation. Very often, lower extremity surgery can be delayed in the patient with hand or wrist involvement until the hand and/or wrist are able to aid in walking. A patient with evidence of impending tendon rupture may require tendon transfer and healing before lower extremity surgery is performed. It is imperative that the patient fully understand the need for one surgery to precede the other. Often, a patient will reject the hand surgery stating, "I came here to walk. There is nothing wrong with my hand." This is the patient who must be convinced of the need for functional upper extremities to achieve the goals of lower extremity surgery.

If the patient is not capable of adhering to this program of proper positioning and exercises, make certain that a companion be brought to teach how the program is to be continued after discharge. Both the patient and the companion must fully comprehend what is expected for successful rehabilitation.

Sometimes, patients will require the use of a knee stabilizer if, at the time of surgery, the knee was unstable. There are many types of knee braces which can be used temporarily, as well as permanent braces tailored to individual patient's needs. Instruction in the application and use of the brace may be necessary.

Total Hip Replacement (THR)

The development of a polyethylene acetabulum, a metal ball and stem prosthesis (usually Vitallium steel), and the use of methylmethacrylate cement have afforded almost complete pain relief to many patients with arthritis (42). Although the primary effect of THR has been dramatic pain relief, the secondary effect has been improved walking or other lower extremity use in a great majority of patients (43). Since one of the greatest risks to joint implant surgery is infection, it is imperative that during nursing and physician assessment, the patient is carefully screened for any signs of minor or major infections (44). An abscessed tooth or paronychia of toenail or fingernail can cause an infection at the prosthesis (inert materials promote infection). Patients taking long-term corticosteroid therapy are particularly at high risk since corticosteroids mask infections (Table 6.2). Postoperatively, the guard against infection must continue, especially when dressings are changed. Aseptic technique and prompt disposal of dressings must be enforced. Dressings should not be discarded in the patient's room.

The careful monitoring of vital signs of patients who have corticosteroid-attenuated skin can cause ecchymosis from sphygmomanometer cuff pressure. Health team members, as well as the nurse, must be aware of the flexion or extension deformities of RA patients so as not to injure the patient. If the patient is receiving anticoagulation therapy and has been taking corticosteroids for some time, the patient must be treated gently and carefully to prevent further injury.

The patient with THR will return from the operating room with some type of abduction device. It may be a leather wedge pillow, foam-lined abduction splint, or foam pillow (45). Although there are numerous types of abduction devices, their purpose is singular—to maintain abduction. The abduction device adds to the patient's discomfort, increases painful stiffness, and enforces immobility. Patients with THR usually do not complain of pain in the hip joint, except when being turned or undergoing position changes (42). Most THR patients receive mild analgesics, e.g., acetaminophen with codeine or a propoxyphene-acetaminophen combination, after the first 24 hr postoperatively. But patients will complain of the effects of the decreased mobility of the upper extremities, knees, ankles, feet, and even the back. Guiding the shoulders through gentle ranges of motion and releasing arms from intravenous boards greatly relieves stiffness.

Patients usually wear some type of antithromboembolic thigh-high stockings (46). These stockings should be removed every 8 hr so that the heels may be checked for signs of pressure areas. Applying lotion to the heels and using some type of foam or sheepskin booties will prevent pressure problems, especially in patients with steroid skin. The patient should have been taught, preoperatively, to report any sensation of burning or heel pressure immediately to the nurse. Keeping the operated limb in neutral position is vital. Both internal rotation and external rotation should be prevented. Using the rolled towels at the trochanter and along the leg will help. A Bunny Boot will also maintain the leg in neutral position effectively.

Unless contraindicated by the surgeon, most patients with THR are permitted out of bed within 24 hr. RA patients with upper extremity involvement are fearful of moving; therefore, it is advocated that sufficient staff be present to reassure the patient. If the abduction device is to remain in place, the task is easier. Two staff members should aid the patient in his first transfer, to ensure safety (47). If the abduction device has been removed, abduction must still be maintained when moving the patient from the bed to the edge of the bed and also while in the chair. A raised chair or wheelchair should be available before attempting to get the patient out of bed. A wheelchair should have the appropriate equivalent of pillows of Puff Pak to prevent increasing the flexion of the hip beyond 90°. The patient should be brought to the edge of the bed, the operated limb carefully placed on the floor, and the patient's weight placed on the unoperated leg. If an osteotomy of the greater trochanter has been performed, no weight bearing is permitted on the operated limb. The patient may touch the toes but without bearing weight on the operated limb and must be assisted to take short steps to the chair. When seated in the chair, a rolled towel, small pillow, or partly inflated beach ball may be used to maintain abduction. When weight bearing is permitted, the patient may take short steps to the chair and/or bed. Patients should not sit at a 90° angle during the immediate postoperative period since it can encourage increased flexion of the hip and possible subluxation. The wheelchair should be angled at about 100°. During meals, if the patient is in bed, he should eat while in a slightly more than semi-Fowler's position.

It is suggested that preoperatively a patient be given an inkling of the postoperative cooperation regarding positioning, transfers, and eating that will be required. Postoperatively, the patient should receive some written instructions that can be consulted, to remind him of his restrictions.

The patient with THR should have a trapeze overhead so that both patient and nurse can assist in transfers. If the patient has limited hand function or is unable to use the trapeze, the nurse or other team member will have to help the patient with position changes. Patients with AAS must be cautioned against using the head and neck as a fulcrum when attempting to change positions, e.g., when going from the foot of the bed toward the head of the bed. These patients must be cautioned not to use the neck as a pivot point of transfer. Some patients perform this action because they fear that pressure on the buttocks may cause hip pain. These patients will attempt to shift the weight to the neck. The nurse must emphasize to any patient with AAS, that the nurses will assist in turning or changing the patient's position. Using a sheepskin or turning sheet is the safest method of going from the foot of the bed towards the head of the bed.

Within 3 to 5 days postoperatively or whenever the surgeon orders, the patient is taught how to use the knee sling. While the leg is in abduction at all times, a knee sling is set up over the operated leg. The patient is taught how to do the knee-sling exercises as ordered. Patients with poor hand function will have to have the handle adapted to their particular needs. If the patient is unable to perform this function, the nurse, physical therapist, and/or patient's family will have to help. Currently, the use of sheepskin slings under the thigh decreases the usual discomfort that can occur when a canvas sling is used. Patients with fragile skin must be protected. If a sheepskin sling is not available, wrapping the patient's thigh with several layers of Webril will help cut down on friction or pressure rub.

Often, within 2 or 3 days, the postoperative dressings may be removed by the surgeon if the incision is dry and free from any drainage. The patient's skin should be checked frequently for signs of infection around sutures. If the dressings are kept in place, soiled or wet dressings should be changed immediately. Part of the preoperative patient preparation should have stressed the importance of reporting the condition of the dressings to the nurse.

When the patient is permitted to walk and to use the bathroom, a raised toilet seat should be provided. Most hospital facilities have low seats which can encourage increased flexion of the hip, which can cause dislocation. The patient should be taught how to transfer with assistance by utilizing grab bars and an assistant, until the nurse has deemed it safe to allow the patient to transfer independently and safely.

No patient who has undergone THR should be allowed to place himself on the bedpan. There have been documented cases of patients who dislocated the hip by flexing the operated hip inadvertently. No patient should be allowed to turn unattended until the nurse and physical therapist are certain that the patient is capable of placing a pillow between his legs and safely turning independently. Many patients with RA are too weak and incapable of turning. Patients should be instructed to call the nurse when they wish to turn. Lower extremity dressing precautions must be enforced during the first 3 months postoperatively, until the surgeon deems otherwise. Patients must be instructed that they cannot put on slacks, shoes, socks, stockings, etc., for 3 months postoperatively. The patient is permitted to do lower extremity dressing only if the occupational therapist has instructed the patient in the use of the dressing stick and stocking donner and has ascertained that the patient is capable of safely carrying over the appropriate techniques. Patients must be instructed that they may not pick up items off the floor or stoop to check shoelaces, etc., since all of these actions are most conducive to dislocating the new hip. Crossing the legs, whether in bed or while seated in a chair, is prohibited. Patients need constant reminders. It is suggested that the families or companion also be instructed in postoperative total hip precautions.

No patient with RA who has undergone THR is discharged from the hospital unless he uses some type of rehabilitation aid, e.g., cane, crutches, or walker. He must be instructed to avoid walking on uneven ground and to always be alert to avoid wet floors and other slippery areas.

The instructions which have been presented are applicable to patients who have undergone hip resurfacing.

Transportation and Lower Extremity Surgery

Patients with total knee replacement are permitted to drive when the surgeon feels the patient has comprehension and sufficient strength to be independent in driving. However, a severely involved patient with RA with accompanying upper extremity disabilities may not be able to drive for 6 months or until whatever time period is deemed safe enough for the patient and "others" on the road.

Sexual Counseling

Since sexuality is part of ADL and the patient's lifestyle, patients with lower extremity surgery should be counseled so as to prevent possible prosthetic dislocation or injury (48). The patient who has undergone synovectomy or total knee replacement should be advised to support the operated limb on a pillow during intercourse. The pillow supports the knee joint and reduces stress to the operated area. However, it must be emphasized to the patient that the pillow must be removed immediately after sexual activity. Pillows left under the operated knee can cause flexion contractures.

The patient with THR or total hip resurfacing must be advised to avoid intercourse for 6 to 8 weeks postoperatively, since it takes approximately that length of time for the internal capsule to heal. Abduction precautions must be maintained so as to protect the operated hip during intercourse. Side-lying positions and posterior approach positions are contraindicated, as are any positions which increase hip flexion. The recommended position is with the patient supine and the legs in abduction. If the patient has been on long-term steroids or has undergone osteotomy prior to the THR, the patient should also be told to caution his partner to avoid falling on the operated extremity. There have been reported cases of patients who suffered linear fracture of the femur at the osteotomy site. Reverting to positions other than those described must be cleared by the orthopedic surgeon after the 3-month postoperative checkup.

Patients who have accompanying Sjögren's syndrome should be advised to use a water-soluble lubricant, such as K-Y jelly, and to avoid vaseline since it predisposes to infections.

It is important that the health professional offer sexual counseling to patients who have undergone lower extremity surgery (49). Patients are often too embarrassed to ask for assistance, but patients feel the physician and/or nurse or other health professional should offer the counseling (50) (Tables 6.5 and 6.6).

Discharge Planning

The greatest risk to any type of joint implant is infection (51). While the patient is in the hospital, the nurse should use every opportunity to teach the patient of the need for ensuring continued success of the prosthesis, by teaching the patient to be ever on the alert for any signs of minor infection. All infections, no matter how minor, should be reported to the surgeon or family physician so that appropriate antibiotic therapy may be instituted.

Conclusion

Since patients with RA have systemic disease as well as joint problems, the nurse and the health professional caring for the patient should remember to integrate methods of relieving stiffness of the nonsurgical areas. Special

TABLE 6.5. *Moss Rehabilitation Hospital Physical Therapy Department Rheumatology Service*

Guidelines for the Physical Therapy Treatment of Postsurgery Arthritis Patients: Upper Extremity

Reminder:

Check the order on the chart before initiating therapy on any postsurgery patient. Consult directly with the orthopedic surgeon regarding precautions or contraindications concerning the treatment of the operative joint. Include the type and date of surgery in the physical therapy progress note.

Respect pain! Do not exceed the patient's tolerance. Observe the patient performing his own passive range of motion (PROM) and notice what is happening with the nonsurgical wrist and hand, i.e., whether it is going into ulnar deviation.

Hands and wrist

A. Avoid ulnar deviating forces acting on hands:
   1. Prolonged static grasp; this generally tends to produce muscle fatigue and instability of an arthritic hand.
   2. Weight bearing on metacarpophalangeal joints (fists) in transfers.

TABLE 6.5. —*Continued*

Guidelines for the Physical Therapy Treatment of Postsurgery Arthritis Patients: Upper Extremity

B. Be aware of precautions regarding patient's thumbs. For example, if wrist extension is absent or severely limited, the supine patient doing push-ups with a weighted cane may be supporting total weight with thumbs rather than palm of hands. These forces are destructive to a vulnerable thumb; it is then recommended that a substitute exercise be used.

C. The arthritic wrist may require splinting for stabilization and protection against pain and stress. Foam or crutch grips enlarge and soften surfaces, on canes, pulleys, trapeze, etc. They decrease stress on hands, increase patient comfort and ability to perform, and teach joint protection techniques.

D. Due to the excessive stress placed on the structures of the wrist and hand, it is contraindicated postoperatively to place wrists and hands on overhead reciprocal pulleys or weighted pulleys.

Hand exercises

1. To reduce swelling and decrease stiffness, active range of motion (AROM) of finger joints should be encouraged.

2. When the patient reaches the limits of his active finger range of motion, therapist should complete the motion passively. PROM should be done gently but firmly with support provided proximally and distally to each joint.

3. Instruct patient that keeping wrists and hands in dependent position will increase edema.

Wrist exercises

1. AROM and PROM: flexion, extension, pronation, and supination (gently but firmly).

Elbow prosthesis (or osteotomy)

Patient may have a postoperative resting splint provided by the occupational therapist or the surgical team. Positioning is usually 90°, with forearm in neutral and supported to the wrist. Again, instruct patient to avoid dependent position. Check with surgeon or physician regarding weight-bearing status of elbow and observe patient's method of transferring.

Exercises: AAROM: flexion, extension, supination, pronation

Shoulder prosthesis

As soon as sling is removed, encourage patient to position arm on wheelchair arm rest or in arm trough in as much abduction as is tolerable.

The total shoulder prosthesis is fairly recent; its primary purpose is *pain relief* with some improvement in mobility and stability. Preoperative muscle power, condition of joints, and other upper extremity involvement will dictate therapy and progress.

Exercises: assisted active range of motion for all motions—gently. Initially Codman's pendulum exercises may be the least painful and provide the greatest amount of motion.

TABLE 6.6. *Moss Rehabilitation Hospital Physical Therapy Department*

*Home Instructions for THR Patients**

Precautions
1. Do not raise your knee higher than your hip level because this will cause your hip to bend too much.
   a) Acquire a raised toilet seat
   b) Do not put your foot on a stool when sitting
   c) Put cushions on low chairs
   d) Avoid bucket seats in cars
2. Use crutches or a cane as long as you have a limp.
3. Avoid sitting for more than 1 hr at a time at home or when traveling in an automobile. (This decreases the chance for dislocation.)
4. Lie on your stomach 2 to 3 times per day to prevent hip flexor tightness.
5. Do not cross your legs (operated leg over nonoperated leg).
6. No squatting for 6 months.
7. Do not bend forward to put on shoes and socks because this will cause your hip to bend too much.
8. Do not roll leg inward.
9. No bicycle riding.

Exercises†
1. On your back: bend your hip and knee.

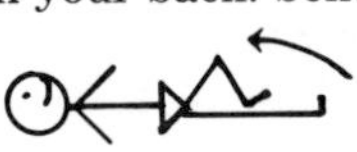

2. On your back; place rolled towel or blanket under your knee, then press down.

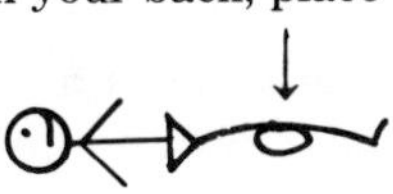

3. On your back: squeeze buttocks together.
4. Sitting: move ankles up and down.

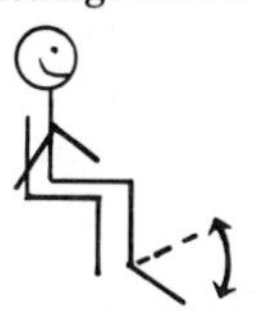

* When doing home exercises, remember that over exertion is the most frequent cause of pain and that muscle soreness and stiffness that is not relieved by rest or aspirin is a sign of overactivity.

† These exercises are designed to help you continue to regain your strength after surgery and prevent joint tightness. Your therapist may give you additional exercises to meet your particular needs.

precautions must be considered in preventing pressure problems in all patients but particularly in those with steroid skin. The patient with AAS must be protected from encountering cord problems that can occur if specific instructions regarding collar use, limitations of activity, etc., are not adhered to by the patient and the nurse and other health professionals. Preventing further injury is important in all patients with RA who have either steroid skin, osteoporosis, AAS, etc.

Both the preoperative and postoperative preparation and teaching of the patient will be the major stepping stones to effective discharge planning and patient compliance.

Any patient who undergoes any type of major joint replacement must be taught to be forever on guard against any minor infection. Paronychias of the toes or fingers, infected teeth, urinary tract infections, boils, carbuncles, etc., are all foci for seeding the new joint with an infectious process. Pharyngitis, if untreated, may cause the loss of a prosthesis and/or septicemia. Recently, it was documented that a patient visited his orthopedic surgeon for her postoperative 3-month follow-up visit. She neglected to mention to the surgeon that she had an infected 2nd digit. Within a week, the patient developed hyperpyrexia (103°), inflammation, redness, and tenderness of her total knee replacement. The patient had to be admitted to the isolation unit where she underwent antibiotic perfusion and intravenous antibiotic therapy. The prosthesis had to be removed and knee fusion followed. Not enough emphasis can be placed on the importance of making the patient aware of the need for constant surveillance of signs of fevers, infections, etc. It is of great help if the patient can be given written instructions to take home with him. Any patient who has undergone implant surgery must be made aware of the necessity of reporting any minor infection so that appropriate antibiotic therapy can be instituted. Physician follow-up must be emphasized as well. Checking upon the home adaptations prior to discharge must be attempted in sufficient time to allow for various rehabilitation aids; e.g., raised toilet seats, grab bars, tub seats, shower heads, etc., can be available for the patient's use, before he goes home, so that inadvertent injury can be avoided. All of the patient's questions should have been answered before the patient leaves the hospital. At Moss, it is the policy to telephone the patient within a week after discharge to help the patient adjust to his home environment, allay separation anxiety, and answer questions regarding unforeseen problems which may occur. If necessary, a home visit is made if the patient's problems warrant it or a community agency is asked to visit and intervene. The patient is also encouraged to call his primary nurse or nurse specialist if the patient has any questions regarding his surgery, medications, etc.

In patients who undergo arthritic surgery, it must be made clear to them that the most important member of the team is the patient himself. The patient's cooperation, understanding, and compliance are essential to achieving realistic postoperative goals.

REFERENCES

1. Larson, C. B. and Gould, M. *Orthopedic Nursing.* C. V. Mosby Co., St. Louis, 1974.
2. Brunner, L. S., Emerson, C. P., Ferguson, L. K., and Suddarth, D. S. *Textbook of Medical-Surgical Nursing Education.* J. B. Lippincott, Philadelphia, 1975.

3. Olson, E., and Johnson, B. J. Hazards of immobility. *Am. J. Nurs., 67:* 781, 1967.
4. Bowden, S. S. New surgery for arthritis hands. *Nursing, 76 6:* 468, 1976.
5. Cresswell, P. M. Total shoulder replacement. *Nurs. Times, 70:* 593, 1974.
6. Katz, W. A. *Rheumatic Diseases, Diagnosis and Manageme.* Lippincott, Philadelphia, 1977.
7. Peterson, L. F., Fitzgerald, R. H., and Elner, J. A. Total joint arthroplasty— the knee. *Mayo Clin. Proc., 54:* 564, 1979.
8. Moury, B. F., and Bryan, R. S. Total joint arthroplasty—the elbow. *Mayo Clin. Proc., 54:* 507, 1979.
9. Shaw, D. A., and Cartilidge, N. E. Cervical myelopathy in RA. *Acta Neurol. Scand., 76:* 279, 1976.
10. Detenbeck, L. C. RA of the spinal column. *Orthop. Clin. North Am., 2:* 679, 1971.
11. Brattstrom, H., and Granholm, L. Atlanto-axial fusion in RA. *Acta Orthop. Scand., 49:* 611, 1976.
12. Shiers, L. G. Total replacement of knee joint. *Nurs. Times, 69:* 1477, 1973.
13. Thomas, B. J. Total knee—new surgical miracle. *RN, 36:* 36, 1973.
14. Swanson, A. B. Flexible implants in orthopedics. *Orthop. Digest, 4:* 15, 1976.
15. Comey, W. P. Total joint arthroplasty—introduction to the upper extremity. *Mayo Clin. Proc., 54:* 495, 1979.
16. Cofield, R. H. Total jo'nt arthroplasty—the shoulder. *Mayo Clin. Proc., 54:* 500, 1979.
17. Linsheid, R. L., and Peckenbaugh, R. D. Total arthroplasty of the wrist to relieve pain and increase motion. *Geriatrics, 3:* 48, 1976.
18. Beckenbaugh, R. D. Total joint arthroplasty—the wrist. *Mayo Clin. Proc., 54:* 513, 1979.
19. Ranawat, C. S. Anatomical considerations and design features of total wrist joint. *Orthop. Nurs. Assoc. J., 2:* 56, 1979.
20. Dobryns, J. H., Bryan, R. S., Lundscheid, R. L., and Petersen L. F. A. The special problems of total elbow arthroplasty. *Geriatrics, 31:* 91, 1976.
21. Coventry, M. B. Total joint arthroplasty symposium. Introduction to the lower extremity. *Mayo Clin. Proc., 54:* 557, 1979.
22. Harris, W. H., Salzman, E. W., Athanasoulis, C. A., Waltman, A. C., and DeSantis, R. W. ASA prophylaxis of venous thromboembolism after THR. *N. Engl. J. Med., 297:* 1246, 1977.
23. Cabanela, M. E., Campbell, D. C., and Henderson, E. D. Total joint arthroplasty—the hip. *Mayo Clin. Proc., 54:* 559, 1979.
24. Insall, J., Scott, W. N., and Ranawat, C. S. The total condylar knee prosthesis. *J. Bone Joint Surg., 61:* 173, 1979.
25. Helal, B. Replacement of fingers. *Nurs. Times, 70:* 1348, 1974.
26. Orthopedic Nurses Association. *Manual of Orthopedic Nursing Care Plans.* ONA Inc., Atlanta, 1973.
27. Swanson, A. B. Implant arthroplasty for disabilities of the distal radioulnar joint. *Orthop. Clin. North Am., 4:* 51, 1973.
28. Swanson, A. B. Flexible implant arthroplasty and other items of interest in hand surgery. *Orthop. Rev., 59:* 67, 1976.
29. Swanson, A. B. Silicone rubber implants for the replacement of the carpal scaphoid and lunate bones. *Orthop. Clin. North Am., 1:* 299, 1970.
30. Swanson, A. B. Flexible (silicone) implant arthroplasty of the metacarpophalangeal joint of the thumb. *J. Bone Joint Surg., 59A:* 362, 1977.
31. Swanson, A. B. Flexible implant arthroplasty for arthritic disabilities of the radiocarpal joint. *Orthop. Clin. North Am., 4:* 384, 1973.
32. Swanson, A. B. Flexible implant arthroplasty for arthritic finger joints. *J. Bone Joint Surg., 54A:* 435, 1972.
33. Swanson, A. B. Porous implant systems for prosthesis stabilization. *Clin. Orthop., 89:* 220, 1972.
34. Flatt, A. E. *The Care of the Rheumatoid Hand.* C. V. Mosby Co., St. Louis, 1974.

35. Townley, C., and Hill, L. Total knee replacement. *Am. J. Nurs., 74:* 1612, 1974.
36. Shoemaker, R. R. Total knee replacement—procedure and results. *Nurs. Clin. North Am., 8:* 117, 1973.
37. Laskin, R. Total knee replacement. *Orthop. Clin. North Am., 10:* 223, 1979.
38. Manske, P. R., and Gleeson, P. Rehabilitation program following polycentric total knee arthroplasty. *Phys. Ther., 57:* 915, 1977.
39. Dow Corning Corporation. *New Life for Old Hands.* Dow Corning Corp., Midland, Mich., 1977.
40. Marmor, L. Synovectomy of the knee joint. *Orthop. Clin. North Am., 10:* 211, 1979.
41. Nills, S. A. Knee flexion Mobiliser. *Physiotherapy, 64:* 264, 1979.
42. Jennings, K. R. The cheerful operation: total hip replacement. *Nursing, 76 6:* 32, 1976.
43. Mallory, T. H. Total hip replacement—a comparison study. *Ohio State Med. J., 43:* 123, 1978.
44. Sculco, C. D., and Sculco, T. P. Management of the patient with an infected total hip arthroplasty. *Am. J. Nurs., 76:* 584, 1976.
45. Meyers, J. M., McNelly, D. B., and Nelson, K. Total hip replacement— A team effort. *Am. J. Nurs., 78:* 1485, 1978.
46. Johnson, C. F., and Convery F. R. Preventing emboli after total hip replacement. *Am. J. Nurs., 75:* 804, 1975.
47. Feinstein, P. A., and Haberman, E. Selecting and preparing patients for total hip replacement. *Geriatrics, 32:* 91, 1977.
48. Ehrlich, G. E. *Total Management of the Arthritic Patient.* J. B. Lippincott, Philadelphia, 1973.
49. Brassell, M. P. *Who Should Mention Sex?* Arthritis Center, Moss Rehabilitation Hospital, Philadelphia, 1972.
50. Brassell, M. P. Arthritis nursing. In *Rheumatic Diseases, Diagnosis and Management,* edited by W. A. Katz. J. B. Lippincott, Philadelphia, 1977, pp. 1000–1010.
51. Fitzgerald, R. H. Prevention of wound sepsis in joint replacement surgery. *Geriatrics, 31:* 81, 1976.
52. Rodman, G. P. *Primer on the Rheumatic Diseases,* Ed. 7. AMA, Chicago, 1973.
53. Coventry, M. B. Probable place of total hip arthroplasty in RA involving the hip. *Orthop. Clin. North Am., 10:* 191, 1979.
54. Kaye, J. J., Kimmelfarb, E. Knee arthroplasty. *Orthop. Clin. North Am., 10:* 51, 1979.

7

Complications from Arthritis Surgery

MARK KAUFFMAN

The only situation worse than a stiff, malaligned, unstable, painful arthritic joint is a *postoperative* stiff, malaligned, unstable, painful arthritic joint. Few situations in rheumatology are so hopeless or threatening to the patient as a grossly failed arthroplasty.

The ego strength of a chronically arthritic patient leaves little reserve with which to cope with surgical failure. When a patient who has been suffering with chronic progressive pain, unrelieved by medical and physical modalities, agrees to undergo surgery, that patient believes that this is the last resort. By agreeing to surgery, he has admitted failure of conservative treatment and now embarks upon the surgical phase of his treatment, with renewed hope for relief. There is patient admiration for modern medicine, the surgeon, and euphoric expectations of appropriate and sometimes inappropriate pain relief and increase of functional capacity. Although complications and risks of surgery are thoroughly explained to him, he hears not. Patients hear and retain only what they desire to hear. Understandingly, and not without merit, full faith and expectation are placed in the surgeon, his ability, and the procedures recommended.

When this stored-up faith and expectation is shattered by surgical failure, the chronically ill patient may not be able to cope. Despair ensues, and a doomed feeling that even the "last resort" treatment has failed (which may well be true). A patient, normal in all other respects (as, for example, after an acute fresh fracture) who needs revision from surgical failure, is better able to cope than the patient who is chronically ill and has already faced multiple failures from previous therapy.

In considering the complications that can arise from surgical reconstruction, one must not lose sight of the fact that far in the majority of instances progress is smooth and uncomplicated, resulting in a pleasant, satisfactory, beneficial result. Often it is only a surgical procedure which can give significant, if not complete relief of symptoms, and return a patient to a normal lifestyle and increased life space.

While it is true that there is little as unfortunate as a disastrous surgical result, it is also true that to be aggressively conservative and withhold the chance of symptomatic and functional relief to an arthritic patient is a medical practice to be strongly condemned.

Specific indications (not in the province of this chapter) should be met, and if so, surgery offered (Table 7.1). *The lack of a contraindication does not in itself make the indication*, and each patient as a whole and the involved joint or joints specifically should be considered. Appropriate preoperative evaluation is an absolute necessity to reduce complications (Table 7.2).

The complications in arthritis surgery fall into two areas, general and specific.

A. General complications
   1. General complications inherent in any operative procedure.
      a. Intraoperative
      b. Postoperative
B. Specific complications inherent to joint surgery
   1. Intraoperative
   2. Early postoperative
   3. Latent postoperative

General Complications of Surgery

The discussion of general complications of any surgical procedure in any patient is not germane to the present chapter. Any general anesthesia or local anesthesia and operative procedures have inherent risks. Cardiac arrests, myocardial irregularities, intubation complications, bleeding complications and their sequelae, transfusion reactions, postoperative phlebitis, atelectasis, myocardial infarctions, drug reactions, etc., are well known to every physician. Detailed discussion herein is not indicated. What should be pointed out are the areas of greater risk to the arthritis patient as compared to the general population.

TABLE 7.1. *Contraindications for Surgical Reconstructions*

Absolute	1. Sepsis in joint. 2. Systemic septic condition. a. Urinary tract b. Paronychia c. Bronchitis 3. Insurmountable medical problems.
Relative	1. Anemia 2. Cardiovascular deficits 3. Respiratory deficits 4. Debility 5. Lack of motivation. 6. Systemic factors.

TABLE 7.2. *Considerations for the Preoperative Evaluation*

History	Physical Examination	Ancillary Studies	Preoperative Orders
Allergic history	General examination	Complete blood count (anemia!)	Correct severe anemia
Medications	Vital signs	Electrocardiogram	Type and cross-match for blood
Local anesthetic	Cardiorespiratory	Urinalysis (culture if indicated)	Surgical skin preparation
Medication history	Decubiti	Chest roentgenogram	Operative consent
Corticosteroids, past year	Peripheral vascular	Joint roentgenogram	Anesthetic consent
Antihypertensive medications	Focus of infection—teeth, decubitus gastrointestinal, liver	Blood urea nitrogen, creatinine	Corticosteroid supplementation
Gout medications	Anesthetic examination	Bleeding and clotting times	Preoperative antibiotics if indicated
Tranquilizers	Subluxation of cervical spine	Prothrombin time	
Narcotic usage	Stiff cervical or lumbar spine from spondylitis/osis	Erythrocyte sedimentation rate	
Anesthetic history	Dental considerations	Lateral cervical spine in flexion	
Past difficulty	Loose teeth	Serology	
Intubation problems	Carious teeth		
Post spinal anesthetic sequelae	Temporomandibular joint stiffness		
Surgical history			
Bleeding difficulty			
Slow healing			
Decubiti			
Transfusion history			
Reactions			
Hepatitis			
Cardiorespiratory history			
Diabetes mellitus			
Hypertension			
Anemia			

General Complications to Surgery Likely to Occur in the Arthritis Patient

The arthritic patient, usually (but not necessarily) being older, is more likely therefore to develop complications of surgery in general. There is frequent anemia in rheumatoid arthritis, thus often requiring a greater amount of blood replacement in major reconstruction and, it follows, a greater risk for transfusion reaction and serum hepatitis.

Chronic corticosteroid administration produces skin and subcutaneous atrophy making a postoperative decubitus problem more likely. The corticosteroids also produce capillary fragility with resultant soft tissue ecchymosis. Skin atrophy from chronic steroids can lead to a "tissue paper thin" skin with an increase in the skin fragility. This may cause large macerations of the skin and lacerations during operative manipulation of the leg, or even due to relatively minor postoperative trauma.

Wound healing is also a greater problem in the rheumatoid patient than in the normal population. This is attributed to poorer skin healing which is known to occur in the rheumatoid patient as well as greater wound stress required by early mobilization of operated joints (to prevent postoperative stiffness). Corticosteroid therapy may also contribute to this problem.

Carious teeth and atrophy of dental pulp can lead to anesthetic difficulty and intubation problems. Anesthetic loss of teeth is not unusual from a difficult intubation, and occasional nasal intubation may be required. The cervical spine may be so rigid as to make general anesthesia impossible.

Spinal anesthesia may also be more difficult in a patient suffering from multiple joint arthritis, and proper positioning may be impossible due to greater pain on the part of the patient. Axillary anesthesia may be impossible if arthritis of the shoulder joint prevents appropriate abduction.

Intraoperative hypotension following the use of methylmethacrylate bone cement has been known to produce problems in the older patient. Osteoporotic bone from disuse and chronic corticosteroid administration can lead to fractures during transfer of the patient to and from the operating table and during the procedure itself. The presence of wide tissue dissection, excessive bleeding, and the large amount of foreign body inserted by using bone cement and prostheses increase the risk of infection.

Mental aberrations can and do occur after surgery/anesthesia in the rheumatoid arthritic patient. This is more frequent than in the osteoarthritic patient who only has one or two joints involved. Postoperative depression from self-pity is frequent. Early inappropriate disappointment can also lead to or may magnify this depression. The realization that multiple subsequent procedures will be required may also lead to depression. Conversion hysteria appears to be more prevalent in the rheumatoid patient than in the general population.

Specific Complications

These complications fall into three categories. Intraoperative, early postoperative, and latent postoperative. The early postoperative complications are taken to mean the immediate postoperative period, usually the first 3 to 6 weeks. There are, however, latent postoperative complications that can, and indeed do, occur. These latent complications are directly related to the patient having undergone surgery. They may ensue any time from discharge from the hospital throughout the patient's entire life.

Intraoperative Complications for Joint Surgery

These complications exclude those which can arise from any operation. They are specific complications for arthritis surgery. Excessive bleeding, cardiac arrest, and intraoperative drug reactions, are examples of complications occurring during surgery that can occur during any operative procedure, not specifically a procedure involving joint reconstruction.

Fractures are a common complication during surgery (Table 7.3). Arthritic patients are osteoporotic from the disuse of the extremity or the body as a

TABLE 7.3. *Examples of Intraoperative Complications for Hip Arthroplasty*

1. Fracture
   A. Shaft or femur
   B. Greater trochanter
   C. Acetabulum
2. Malposition (leads to instability)
   A. Cup anteversion
   B. Cup retroversion
   C. Cup valgus
   D. Cup varus
   E. Femur anteversion
   F. Femur retroversion
3. Length—pelvic trochanteric muscles too tight (lead to flexion contractures and decreased range of motion and increased wear)
   A. Neck length too long
   B. Flexion contracture of iliopsoas or abductor muscles—pelvic trochanteric muscles too loose (leads to instability and possible dislocation)
   C. Neck length too short
   D. Acetabulum reamed too deeply
4. Soft tissue complications (injury to vital structures). Femoral nerve laceration, sciatic nerve laceration or contusion, femoral artery or vein laceration, bladder contusion, excessive blood loss.
5. Acetabular floor secondary to excessive reaming, acetabular floor may wander into the pelvis
6. Methylmethacrylate
   A. Hypotension
   B. Loose fragments
   C. Excessive intrapelvic extravasation with bladder impingement

whole, enforced by chronic arthritis. This is magnified, frequently by long-term corticosteroid therapy. During insertion of prostheses, especially total hip and total knee replacements, strong and sometimes vigorous manipulation or traction on the extremity is required. It is during this time that a fracture can, and not uncommonly, does occur.

The most common example of this is a fracture of the greater trochanter during reaming of the femur for acceptance of the femoral component.

A fracture during an arthroplasty may vary from an incidental occurrence to a disastrous complication. A greenstick fracture of the greater trochanter only requires the postoperative patient to use a cane in the opposite hand for 4 to 6 weeks, to allow the trochanter to heal. A fracture of the shaft of the femur during total hip replacement, however, requires bold and drastic internal fixation leading to complications that can stagger the imagination.

While reaming the acetabulum during the total hip replacement, the osteoporotic bone can be overzealously reamed, causing penetration of the acetabulum into the pelvis. This may cause bladder damage and vascular injury to the intrapelvic structures.

Fractures of the patella and distal femur during total knee replacement have been known to occur.

Soft tissue complications can occur by injury to vital structures. During total hip replacement, femoral nerve, femoral artery, and the sciatic nerve are vulnerable to injury by retractors and surgical instruments. During total knee replacement the popliteal vessels and peroneal vessels have been damaged leading to poor or disastrous results. Ankle arthroplasty is associated with posterior tibial artery and nerve damage while shoulder arthroplasty may lead to an axillary nerve injury. The ulnar nerve is most vulnerable when arthroplasties of the elbow are performed.

In many of these surgical procedures, the at-risk vital structure is dissected out and inspected under direct vision to avoid their trauma.

Malposition of a prosthesis is a definite complication. During total hip replacement, the cup can be anteverted, retroverted, placed in excessive valgus or varus as well as the femur being anteverted, retroverted, or placed in excessive valgus or varus. The combinations of malposition from these eight variable factors can individually and collectively lead to further complications of decreased range of motion, excessive wear, and subsequent dislocation.

The malposition is not confined to total hip replacements, but is inherent to each and every joint reconstructed. A ten degree error in insertion of a total knee prosthesis, can lead to an unsightly genovalgus, or flexion contracture. This will also cause excessive wear from the abnormal stresses caused by the malposition.

The length of the extremity can be affected by improper prosthesis insertion. The leg can be lengthened or shortened as clinically required by using variable sizes in prostheses. As much as one inch can be lengthened or shortened by prosthetic choices and by varying the depth of reaming. Flexion contractures, particularly about the knee, can be corrected if arthroplasty is properly carried out. If unskillfully, however, the postoperative extremity can remain just as deformed.

There are some complications inherent to the use of methylmethacrylate. One is the hypotension produced by methylmethacrylate, particularly when placed about the hip. This is not a problem in the knee, ankle, elbow, or wrist as these procedures are performed under tourniquet, and the toxic substance is, therefore, fixed to the tissues. Later, when the tourniquet is released, hypotension does not ensue.

Early Postoperative Complications

Loose fragments of bone cement can be inadvertently left in the joint, acting as a "joint mouse" and leading to excessive wear of the prosthesis. The bone cement can extravasate through the acetabulum to protrude on the bladder; a vital artery in the pelvis could be burned during the exothermic curing process. Therefore, care must be taken to avoid excessive intrapelvic extravasation of methylmethacrylate.

Dislocations of prostheses can occur, particularly in hip arthroplasty. Ankle, elbow, and knee prostheses are more constrained and less likely to dislocate, although the problem with knee dislocations is not unheard of. A hip prosthesis will dislocate usually secondary to abnormal insertion. An acetabular cup, which is placed in retroversion, with a retroverted femoral component, is more likely to dislocate and require subsequent revision.

Complications from reaming the bones for insertion of prosthesis may be another cause for fractures. There can also be penetration of the stem through the confines of the cortical bone. This stem may migrate subcutaneously and give the patient a painful bursa. This usually occurs with posterior penetration of the stem during total hip replacement or anterior penetration of the stem during a Waldius knee prosthesis. Stem penetration may lead to weakening of the bone and subsequent femoral shaft fractures.

This can only be prevented by obtaining x-rays in two planes during the operative procedure to check that the stem has not penetrated the cortical bone. A single anteriorposterior x-ray is not sufficient, and lateral x-rays are mandatory to discover this complication.

Complications of wound healing may occur, particularly if large prostheses are inserted just below the skin, with poor subcutaneous covering. One of the most common areas of prosthesis penetration is total elbow replacement. If the patient has had multiple operative procedures prior to joint arthroplasty, the surgery must be carefully planned so as to retain a vascular cutaneous supply. Incisions which cross at 90° to a previous scar are prone to poor tissue healing.

Intraoperative revision is not a procedure to be denied. Improper positioning of a prosthesis and anticipated poor results from an arthroplasty cannot be accepted. It should be revised during the same anesthetic, should the complication be recognized.

Postoperative phlebitis can be discouraged by anticoagulants administered prophylactically and by early mobilization, elevation, and external pressure dressings. With all of the prophylactic measures mentioned above, postoperative phlebitis and pulmonary embolism still remain significant postoperative complications.

Postoperative infection is the greatest cause of concern to the orthopedic surgeon. Prophylactic antibiotics should definitely be used in any reconstructed joint, especially when foreign bodies are implanted, such as a prosthesis and bone cement.

Ideally, prophylactic antibiotics should be used several hours prior to the operation, and a sufficient clinical dose of the surgeon's choice of antibiotics should be used for 3 to 5 days postoperatively.

Despite prophylactic antibiotics, infections do occur and the results may be disastrous. They should be treated aggressively, once discovered, with large doses of antibiotics as deemed indicated by deep tissue cultures, surgical drainage, and rest of the part. If the infection cannot be controlled, the prosthesis must be surgically removed together with the implanted cement and involved debris.

Latent Postoperative Complications in Reconstructed Joints

Once the patient has gained the maximal use of his reconstructed joint there are complications which may arise from that day on throughout the rest of his life.

The most common latent complication is a latent infection (Table 7.4). Any bacteremia, such as that produced by an abscessed tooth, a urinary tract infection, or bronchitis can seed bacteria adjacent to the inert prosthesis and cement and initiate a deep-seated joint infection. Every potential bacteremia-producing condition should be vigorously treated with antibiotics. Should a latent infection occur, it should be surgically drained and vigorously treated with antibiotics for a sufficient length of time. Usually, unfortunately, this is a lost cause as once the joint is infected, surgical removal of the prosthesis is almost universally required.

TABLE 7.4. *Latent Postoperative Complications in Reconstructed Joints*

Latent infection
Fracture of bone
Loosening of implant
Wearing of bone stock
Wearing of implant stock
Fracture of implant stem
Disarticulation of implant
Dislocation of implant
Migration of component
Ischemia distal to arthroplasty

The fracturing of a bone is another complication. The bone is likely to fracture at the tip of an intramedullary stem (the stem of a total hip femoral prosthesis or the stem of a Waldius knee prosthesis). This is because the bone tensile strength is more elastic than the rigid metal and all lines of force are magnified at the tip of the prosthesis. This is not at all an uncommon complication. These fractures may have to be surgically repaired by bone plates or intramedullary fixation.

Implant loosening is another common complication which is occurring increasingly. The bond between the metal and the cement, or the cement and the bone, can loosen from the trauma of daily use. As the patient

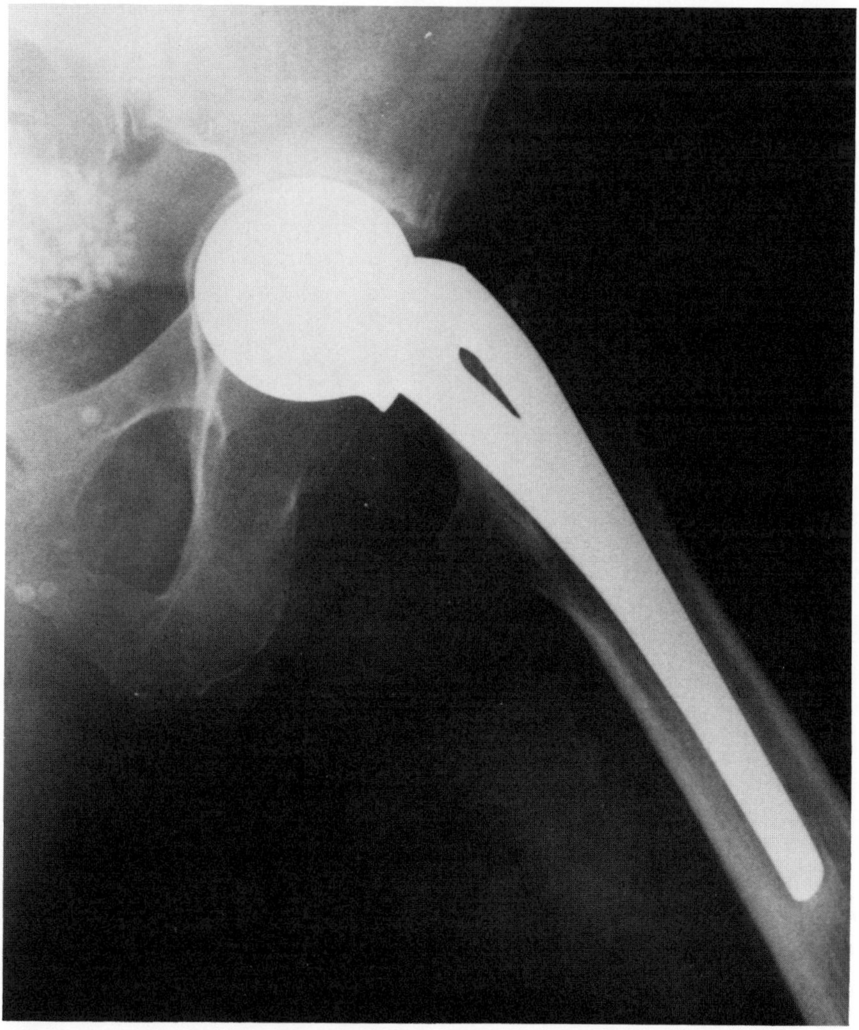

Fig. 7.1. Wearing away of acetabulum; note the very thin layer of bone over the prosthesis, which is migrating into the pelvis.

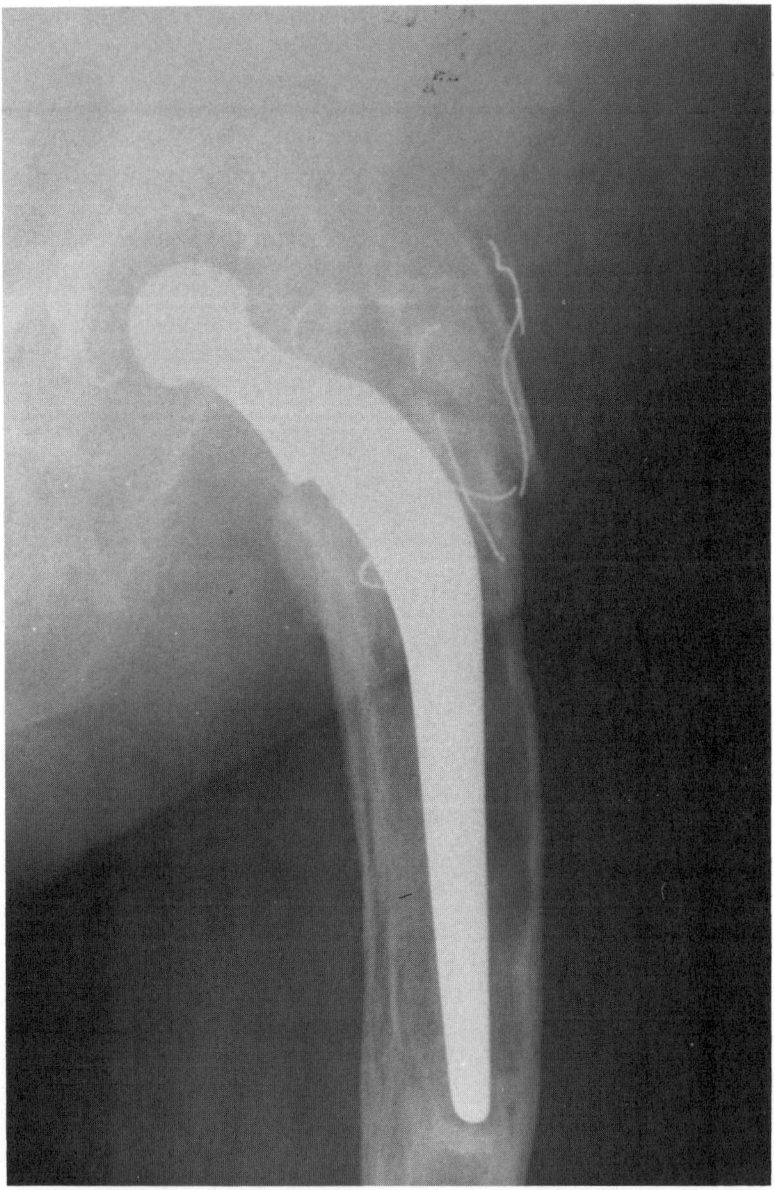

Fig. 7.2. Infection of the hip after surgery. Note lysis about the stem.

continues to use his rebuilt extremity, further loosening ensues and, ultimately, revision of this prosthesis is required.

Wearing of implant stock and bone stock can also occur. The implant will certainly wear with time. This can be anticipated to a much higher incidence in the weight-bearing knee and hip, but also occurs in finger and elbow prostheses.

With further fatigue and overuse, the implant, though it is metal, may fracture. There are innumerable cases of fractures of the stem of femoral prostheses after total hip replacement (especially in heavy active men) as well as silastic implants in metacarpophalangeal arthroplasties.

Dislocation, particularly of the hip, is another potential complication. The longer the postoperative interval, the less likely is a dislocation, as a new capsule is formed which assists in stabilizing the hip.

Components in the arthroplasty may migrate. Proximal migration of the greater trochanter (sometimes associated with fracture-dislocation) may occur. Early postoperative ischemia (or even late ischemia) of the extremity operated upon may occasionally occur. Vascular surgery or sympathectomy may be required to remedy the situation.

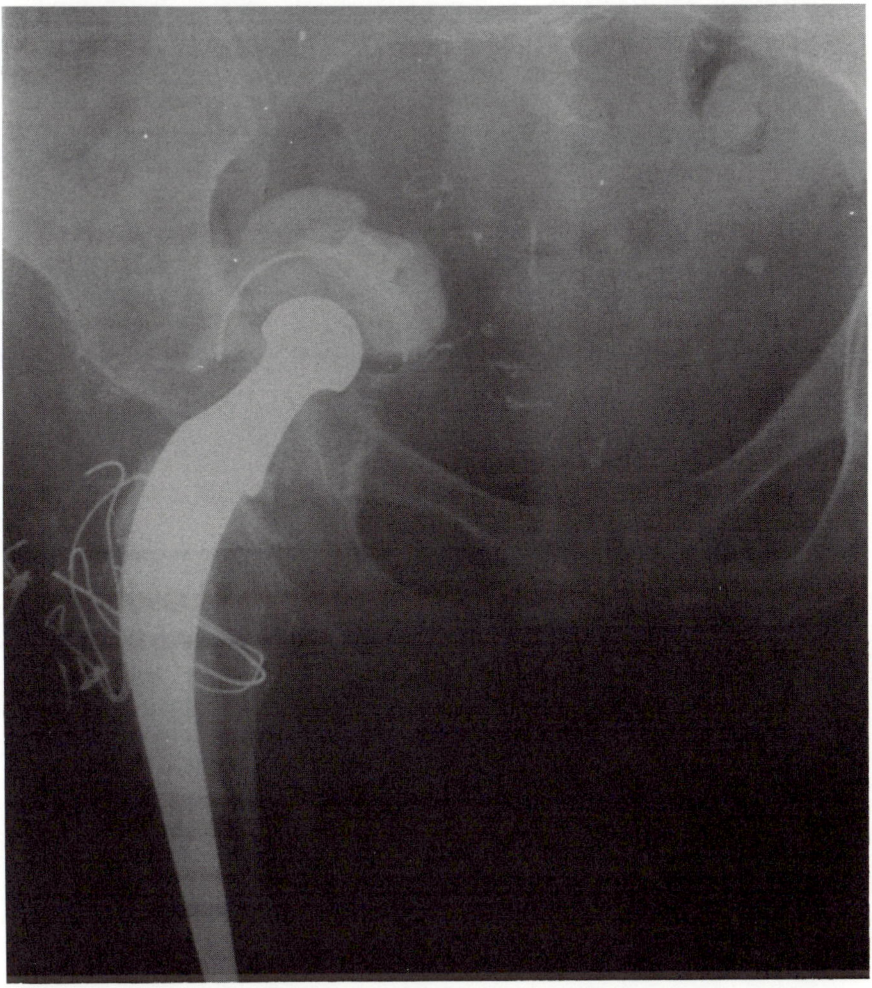

Fig. 7.3. Fracture of acetabulum, with Charnley cup extruded into pelvis.

Paralysis of nerves coursing past surgical sites have been recorded. This may be a complication of hematoma accelerated by anticoagulation. Operative decompression can lead to recovery; irreversible nerve damage could occur otherwise.

Illustrations of operative complications are seen in Figures 7.1–7.23.

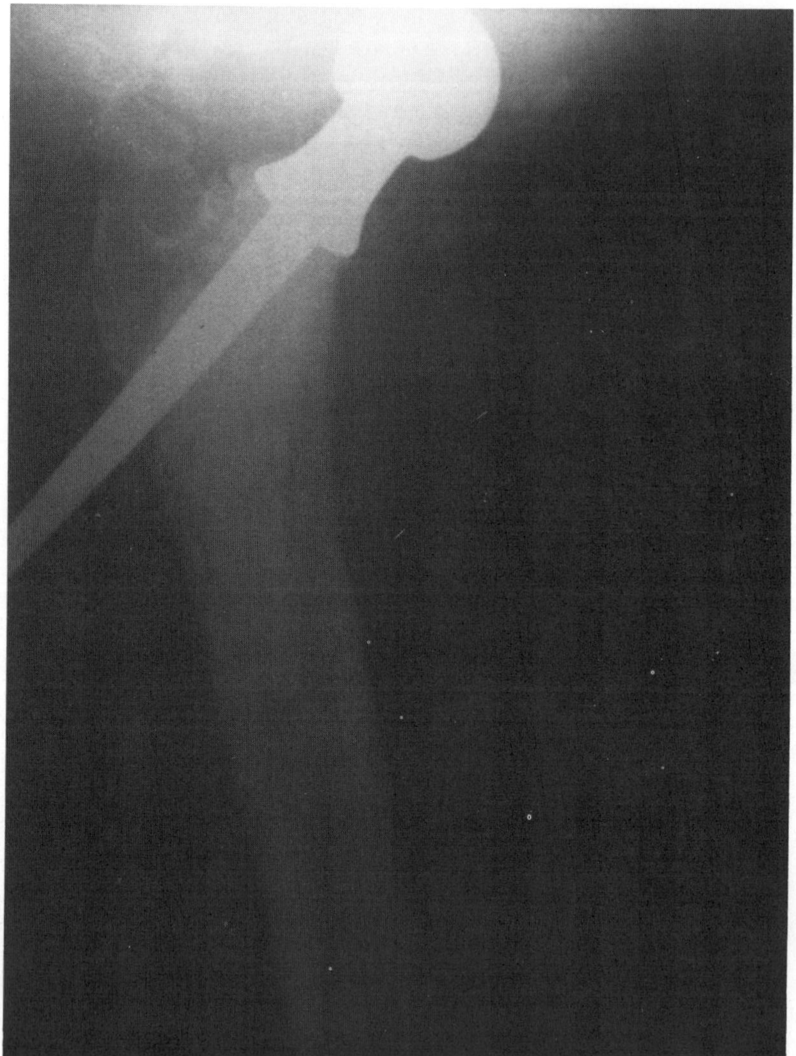

Fig. 7.4. Prosthetic stem is not in the femoral canal. Dislocated total hip is the inevitable result.

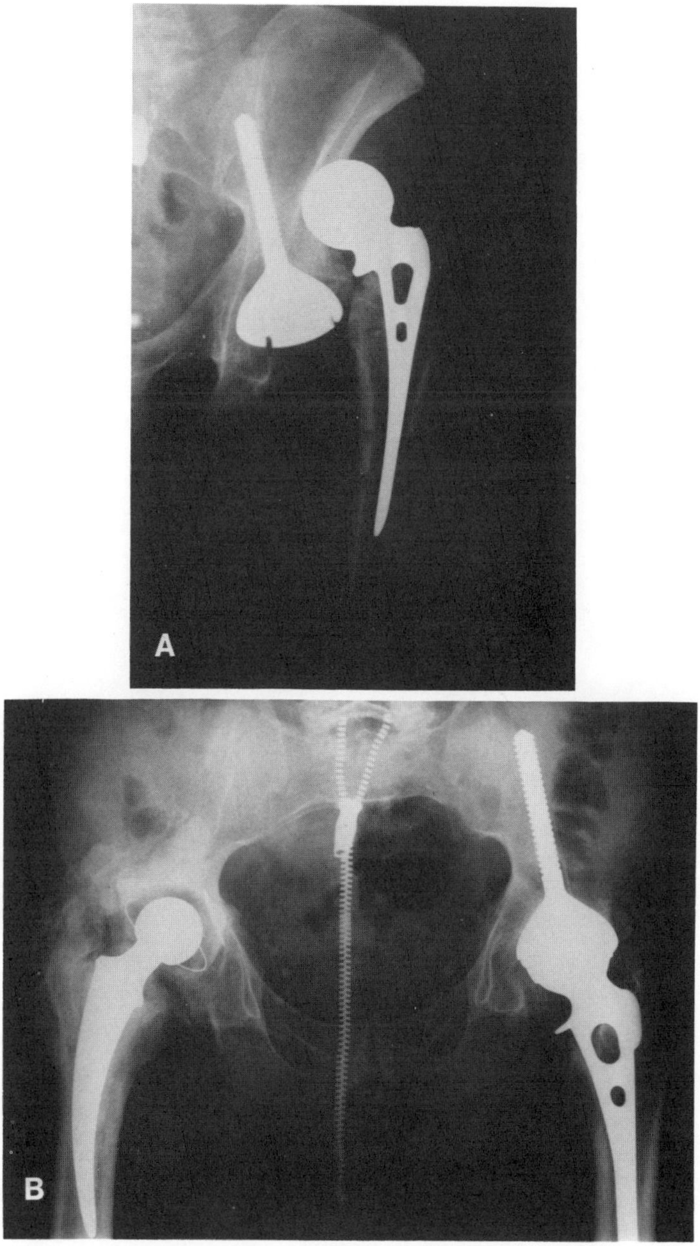

Fig. 7.5. (*A*) Dislocation of Ring prosthesis; (*B*) relocation.

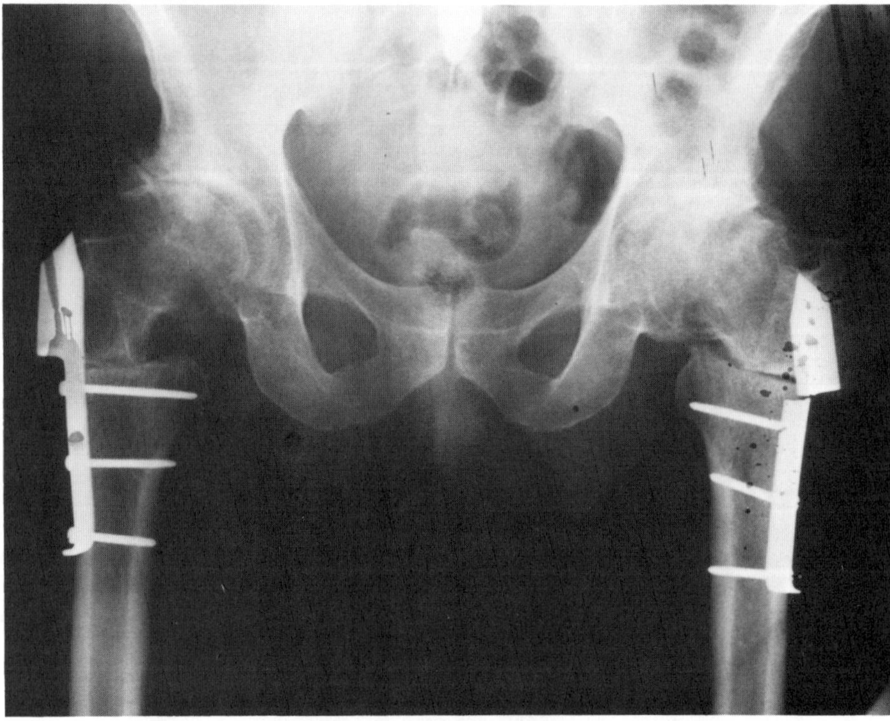

Fig. 7.6. Breakage of nail after osteotomy, with nonunion.

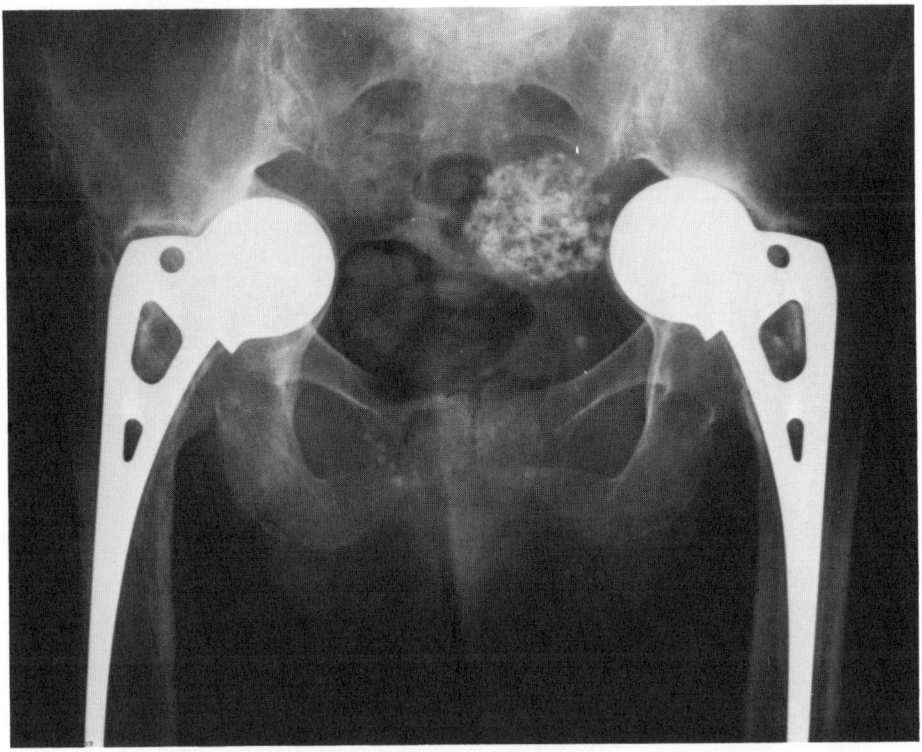

Fig. 7.7. Prosthesis sinking into pelvis.

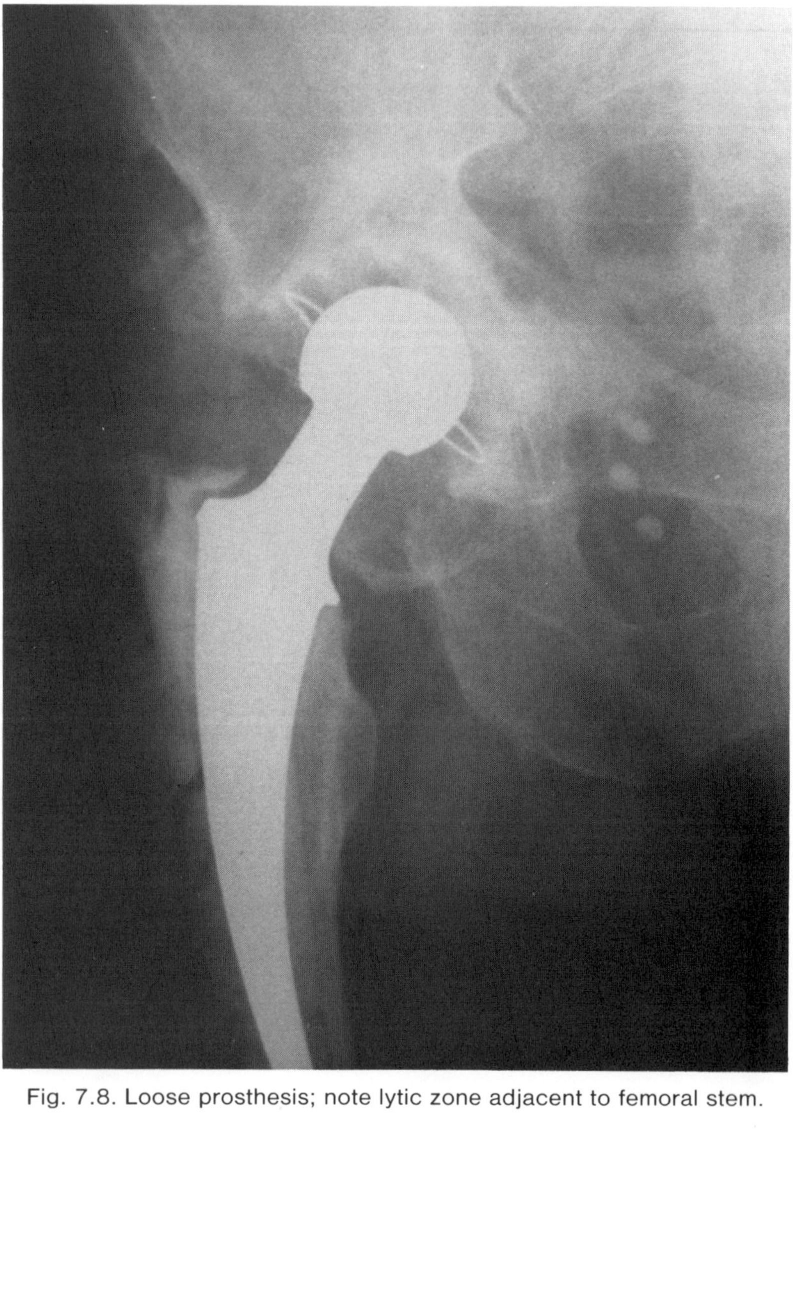

Fig. 7.8. Loose prosthesis; note lytic zone adjacent to femoral stem.

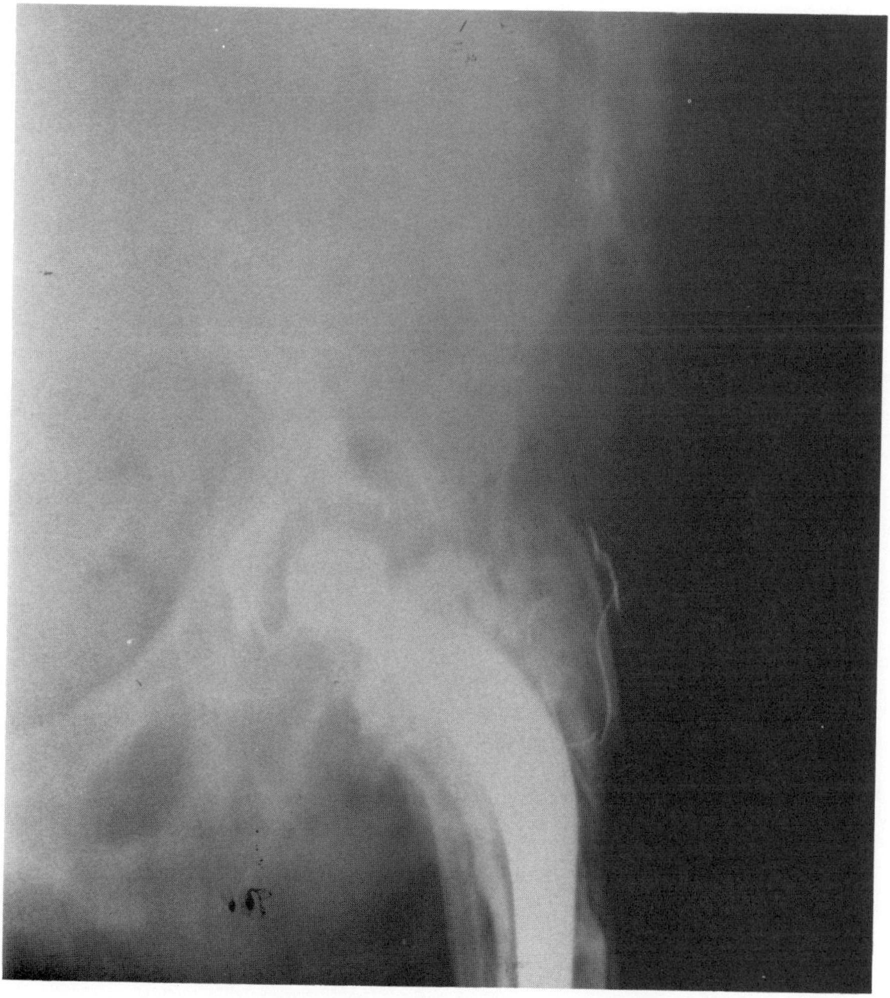

Fig. 7.9. Charnley prosthesis sinking into femur.

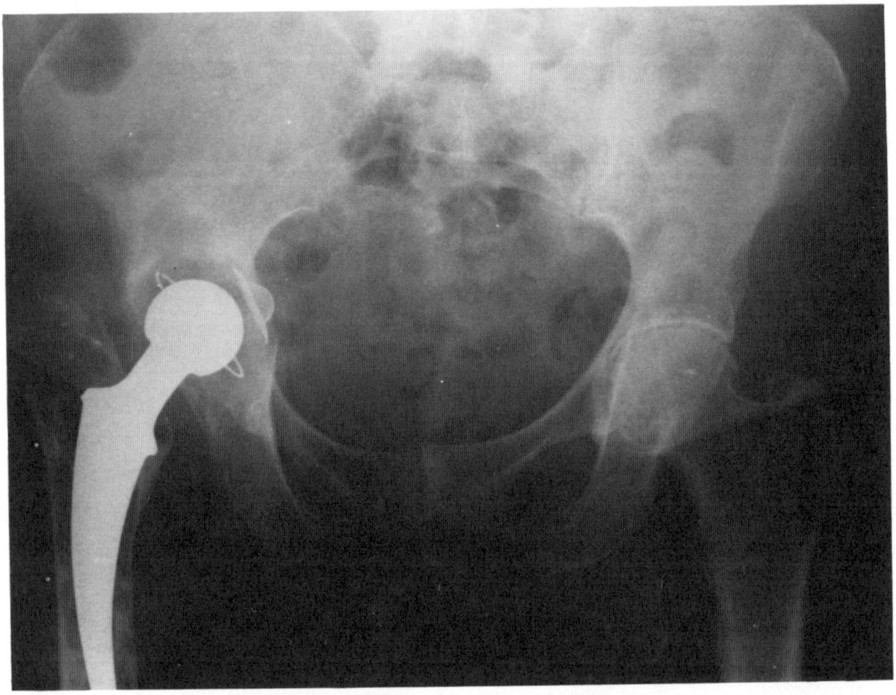

Fig. 7.10. Loose total hip prosthesis; note lysis adjacent to femoral stem.

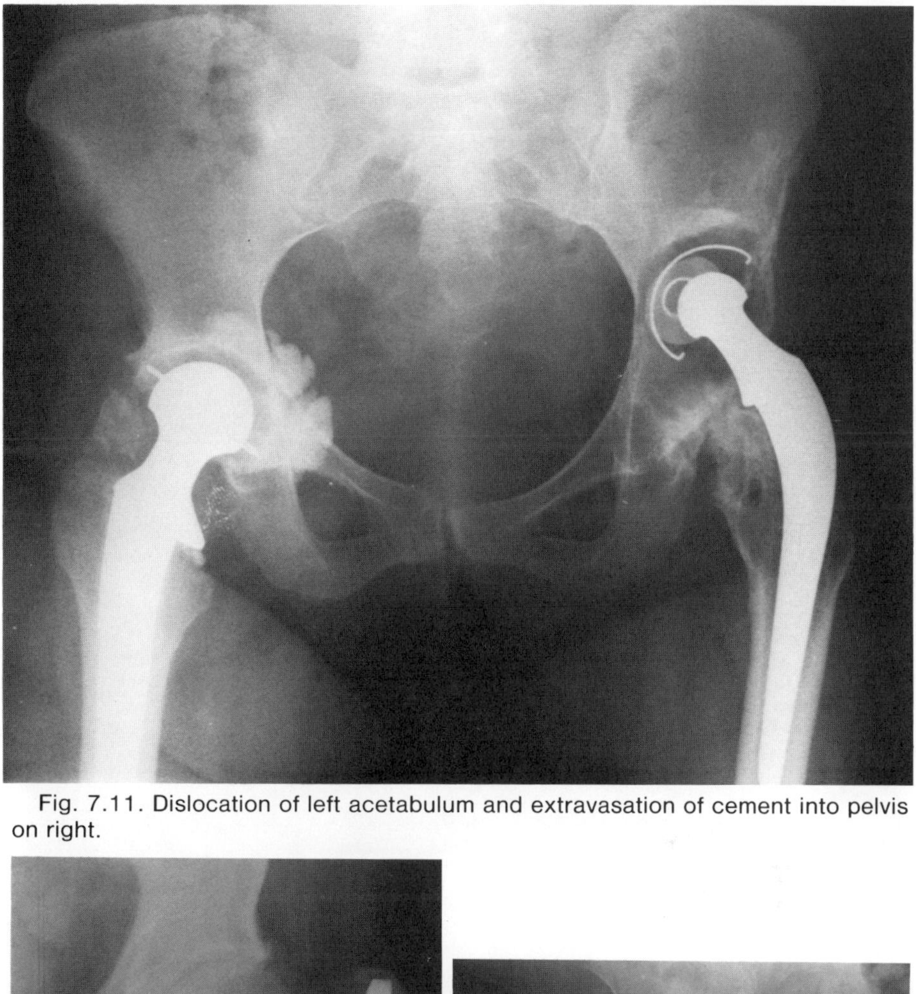

Fig. 7.11. Dislocation of left acetabulum and extravasation of cement into pelvis on right.

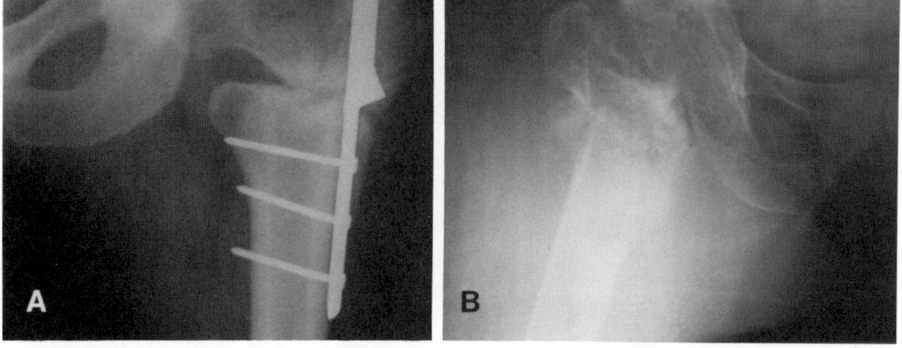

Fig. 7.12. (*A*) Nonunion of osteotomy of hip; (*B*) after removal of hardware.

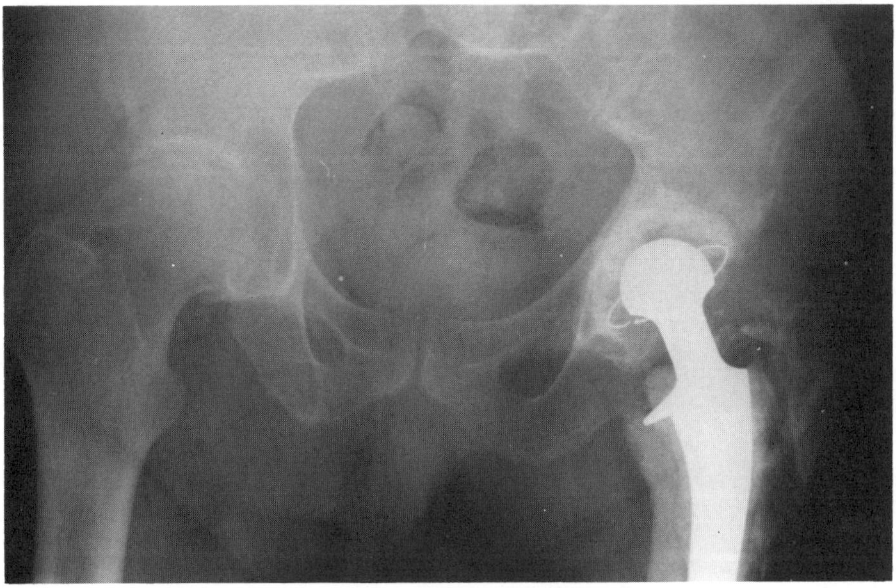

Fig. 7.13. Fracture of acetabular component.

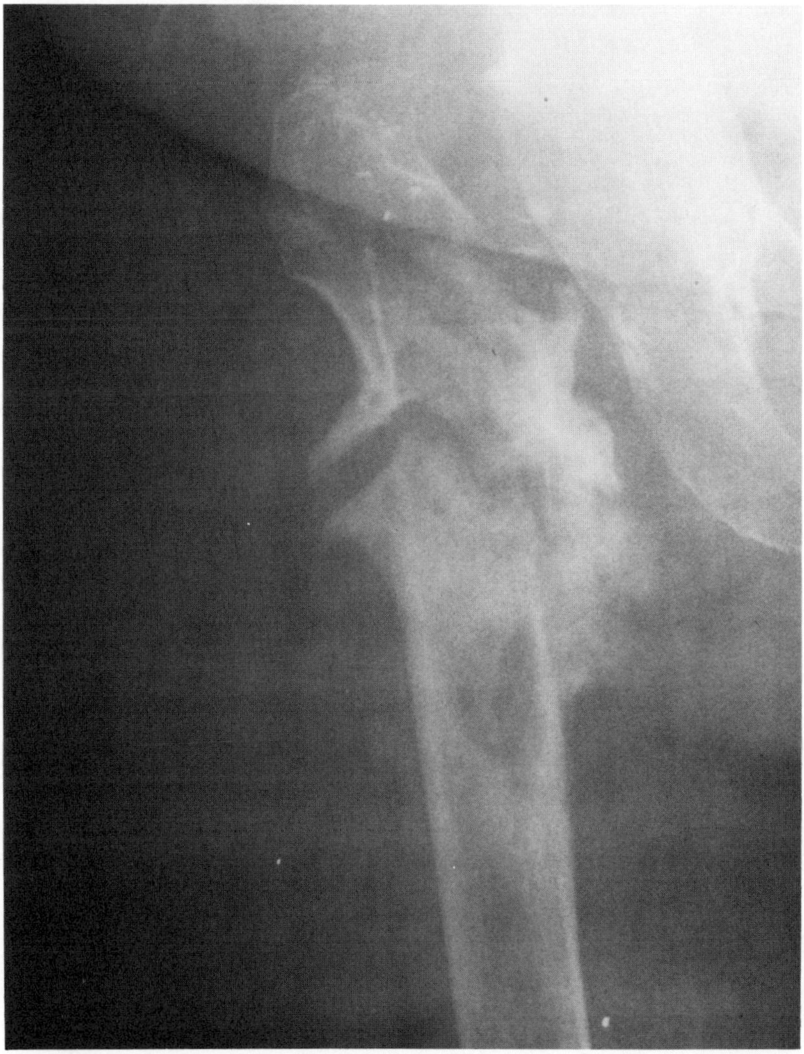

Fig. 7.14. Removal of infected total hip component and subsequent fracture.

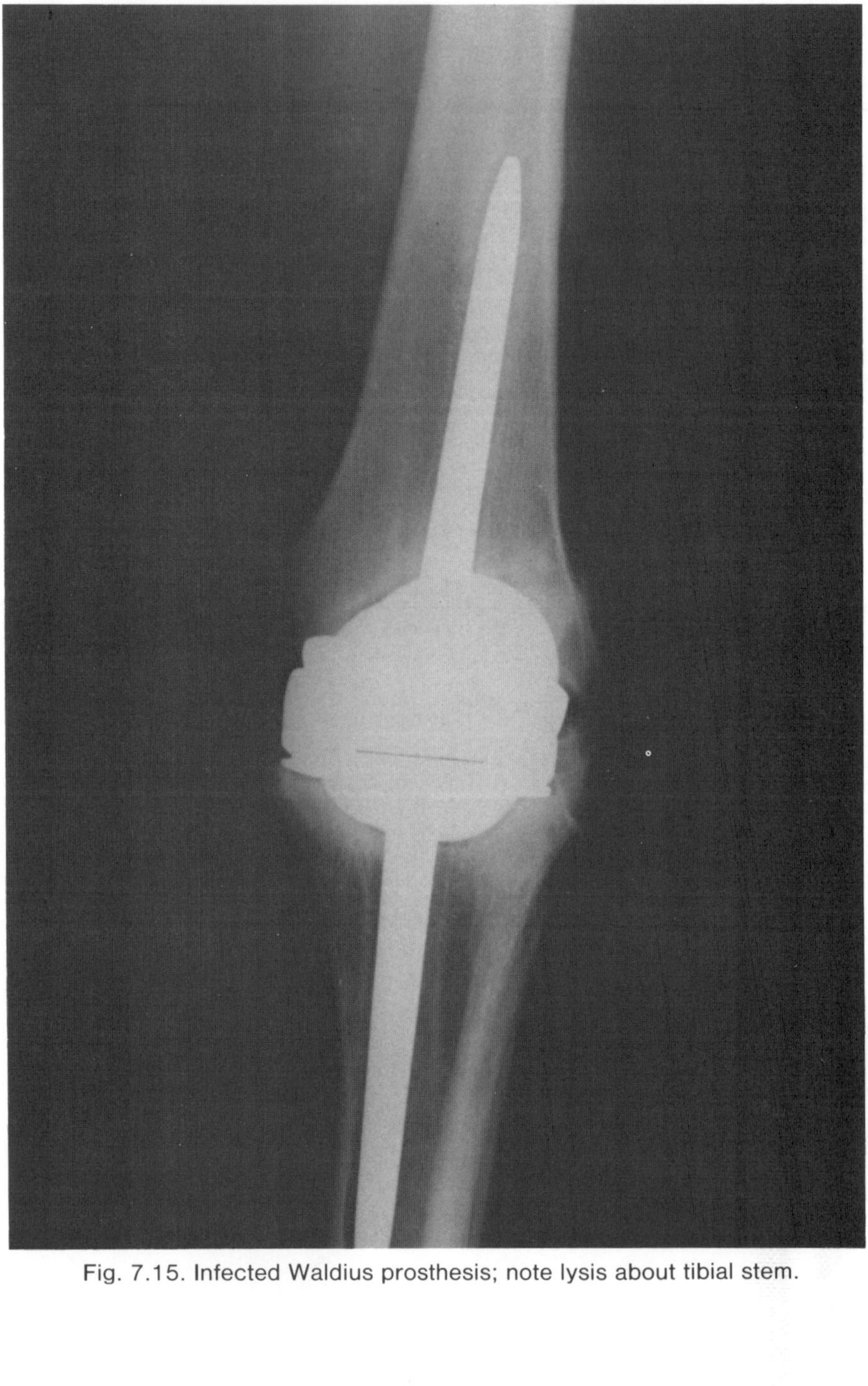

Fig. 7.15. Infected Waldius prosthesis; note lysis about tibial stem.

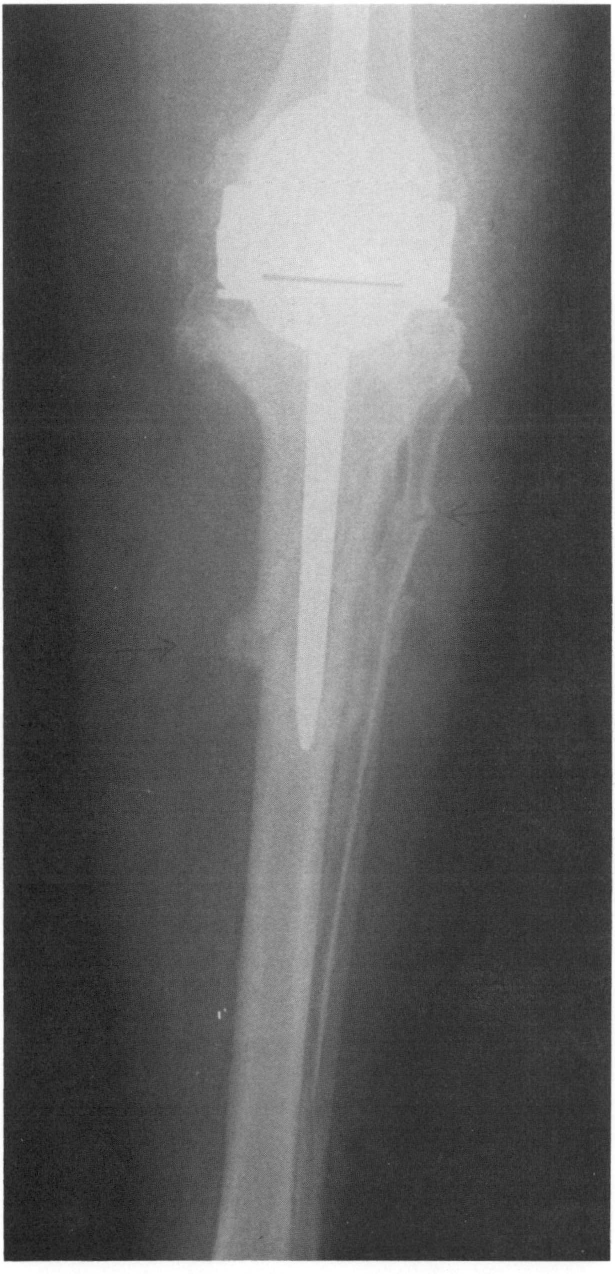

Fig. 7.16. Fracture of tibia and fibula under a Waldius prosthesis (healing).

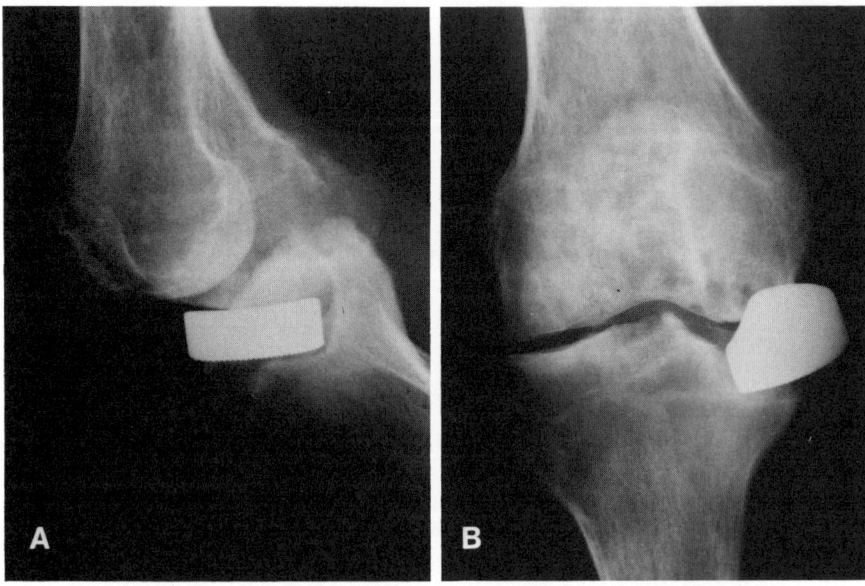

Fig. 7.17. (*A* and *B*) Examples of loosened tibial prostheses.

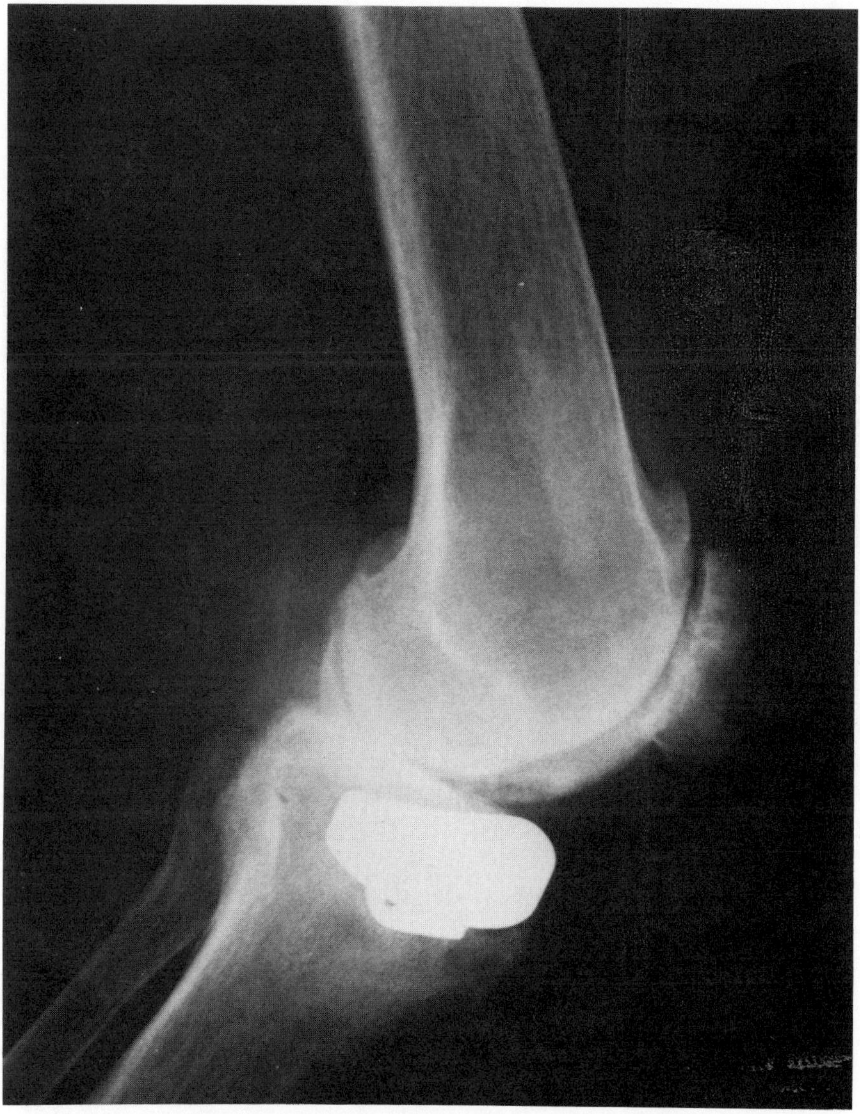

Fig. 7.18. Sinking of tibial prosthesis into tibia.

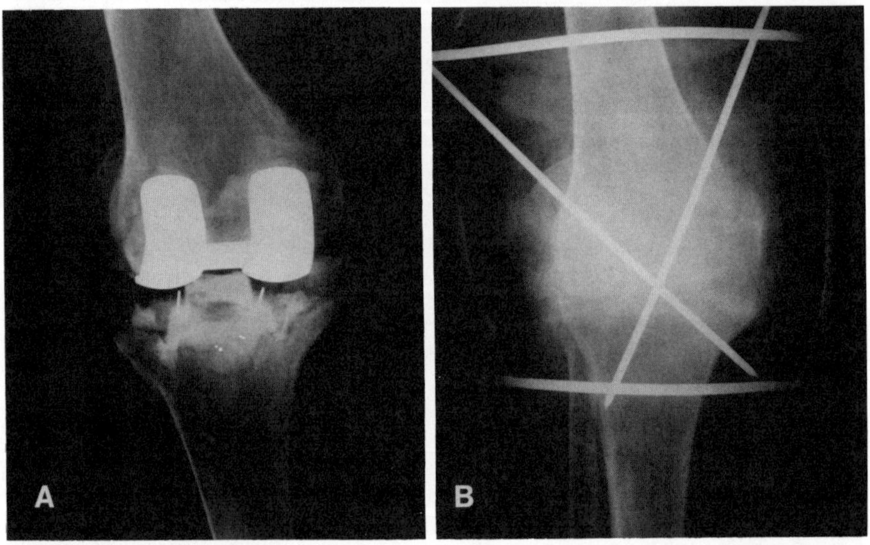

Fig. 7.19. (*A*) Loose total knee prosthesis (geometric)—note lysis under cement; (*B*) removal of prosthesis, and fusion.

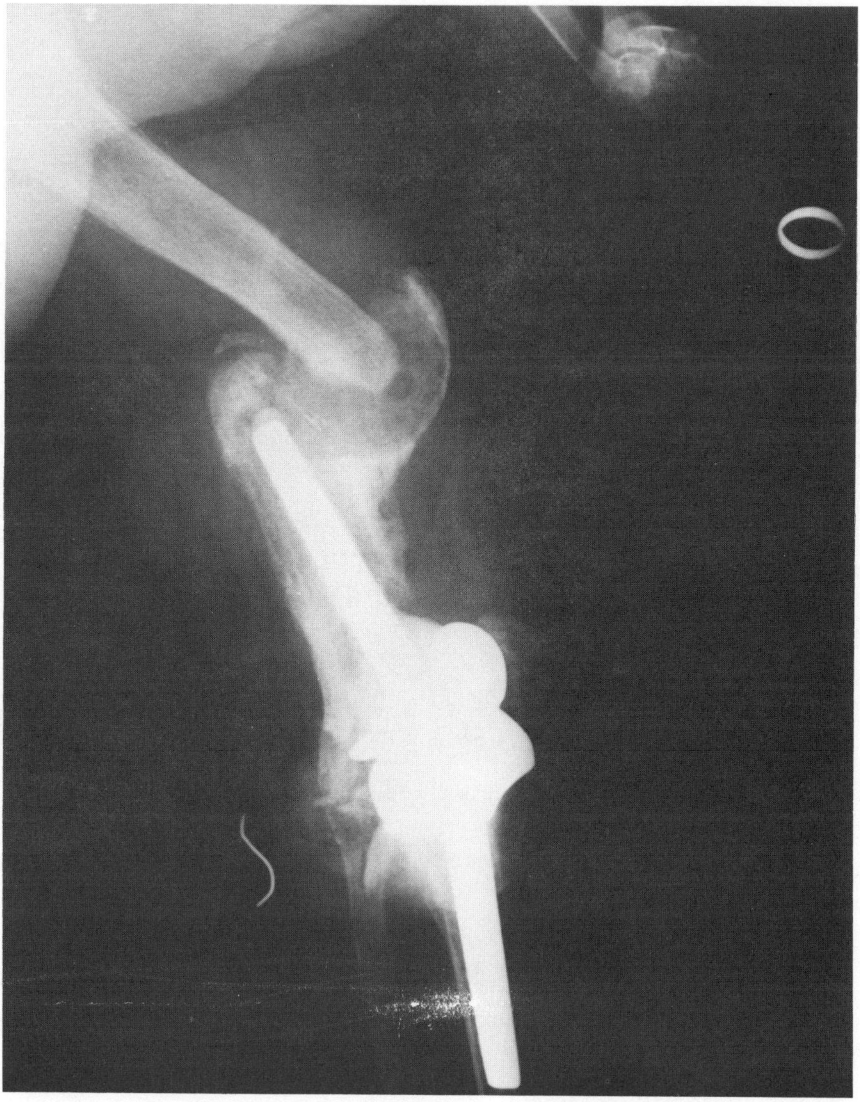

Fig. 7.20. Fracture of femur over Waldius prosthesis.

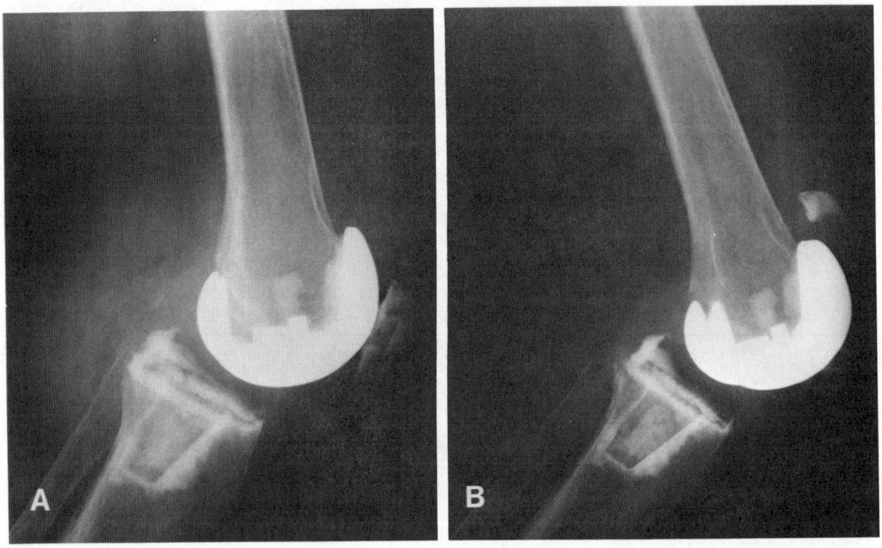

Fig. 7.21. Fracture of patella after total knee replacement: (*A*) before, (*B*) after.

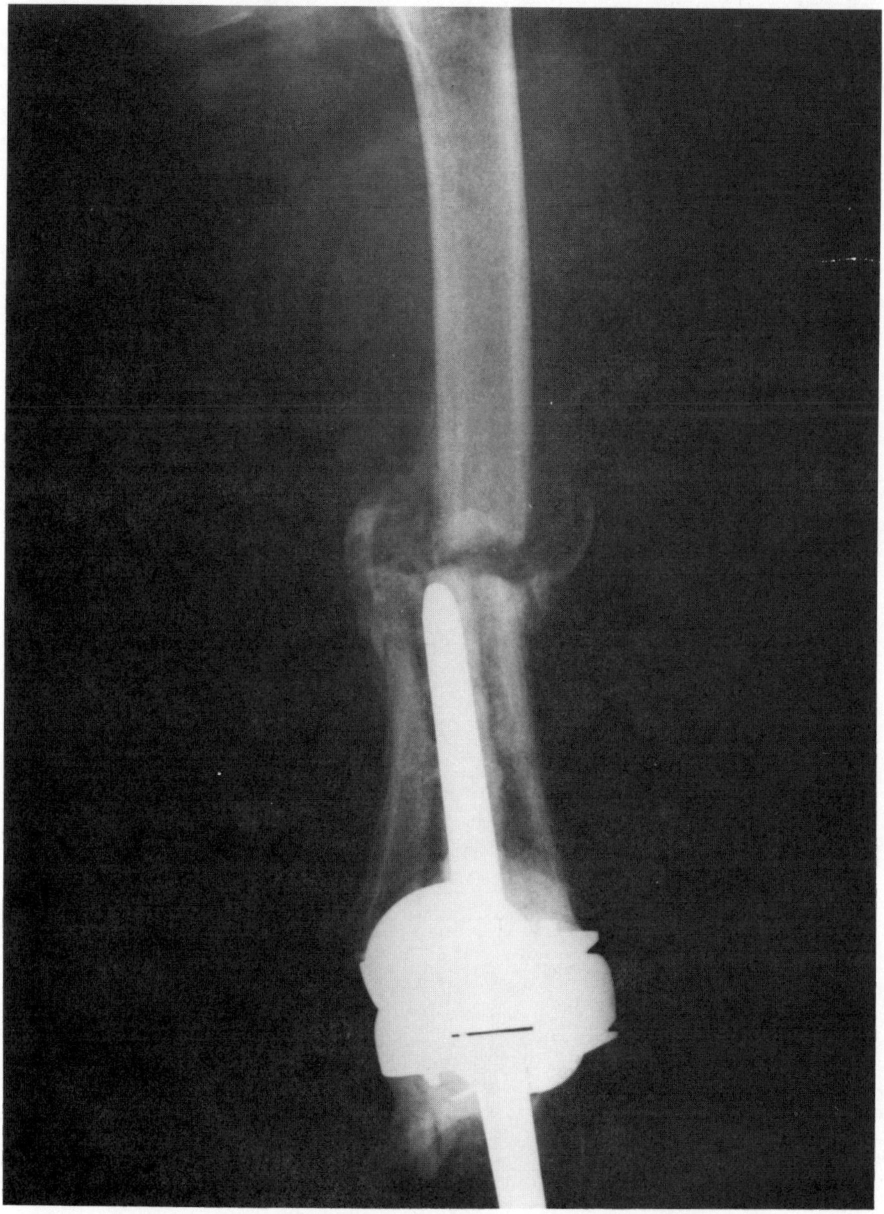

Fig. 7.22. Fracture of femur over Waldius prosthesis.

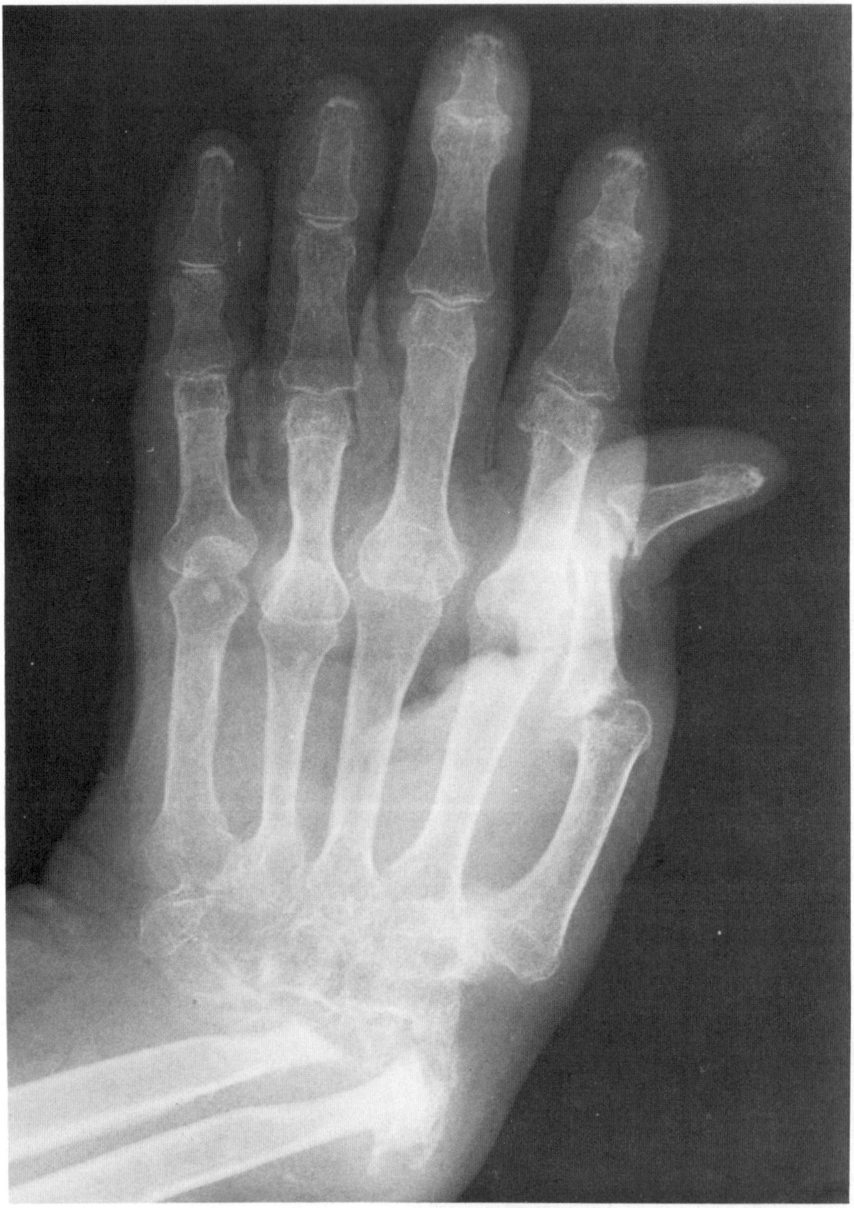

Fig. 7.23. Failed wrist fusion.

Summary

With the protean number of complications that can ensue from joint reconstruction, one may be discouraged and adopt the attitude of "why bother". This attitude is not justified by the facts. It is not amazing that so many and varied complications can and do occur, but it is more amazing that most arthoplasties are successful and without any of the aforementioned complications. By and large, most arthroplasties, successfully chosen and planned, skillfully carried out, and intensively followed during the postoperative course, lead to a successful result.

There is no surgery which gives to the surgeon a higher rate of satisfaction or a greater depth of despair as joint replacement. In no surgery can a result be as dramatic as an eminently successful joint replacement. Having a patient rise from the depth of pain and immobility to a state of normality is as satisfying as anything in medicine. However, treating the treatment, or treating the complications of surgery, can lead the surgeon to frustrating disappointments.

Therefore, both the surgeon and the patient must enter the reconstructive, elective procedure with eyes open. The patient has the right to be informed and the surgeon should make his recommendations without undue pressure on the patient to accept this procedure. The combination of a radical rheumatologist, a conservative surgeon, a cooperative physiatrist and physical therapist, and an informed motivated patient should lead to the best combination of results obtainable in the present state of the art, and reduce the incidence of complications.

8

The Role of the Social Worker in the Rehabilitation of Rheumatic Disease Patients

JUDY L. ERFLING

There is a series of roles for social workers in the rehabilitation of patients with rheumatic diseases. The seriousness and universality of the impact of chronic illness, the infancy of comprehensive care, and the lack of understanding by the general public require the social workers to define their roles not only for the patient and the immediate family but also within the institution providing the care and in the community itself.

The tasks in which the social worker engages, whether with the patient, family, institution, or community, can be grouped into five basic areas. This chapter will focus on the roles of evaluation, education, counseling, communication, discharge planning, and community referral as being descriptive of the function and process of the social worker's participation in the rehabilitation of patients with rheumatic disease.

Why a Social Worker?

Before beginning a discussion of the roles of a social worker involved in the rehabilitation of rheumatic disease patients, it seems appropriate to address the question of why patients or other staff members need a social worker on the treatment team. The answer lies in the fact that almost all rheumatic diseases are chronic illnesses. The implications of the word "chronic" are enormous, perhaps as enormous as for the word "terminal". For the patient it not only means "no known cure yet," but more importantly, it means that the patient will adapt, adjust, or in some way change lifestyle, attitudes, and relationships with other people. The changes brought on by living with chronic illness not only affect the patient but also family, friends, employers, and congregately, the community.

Social workers by profession are trained to not only deal with the "total person" (someone who has an identity other than his illness), but also to understand and work with the total person in his environment. Social workers have skills in psychosocial assessment, counseling, communication, individual, marital and family therapy, discharge planning, and community referral and organization.

If the change produced by living with chronic illness is to be more than a negative reaction to increasing disability, then the treatment team should include someone whose focus with the patient and the family is on adjustment to illness. Social workers have the skills needed to increase patient and families' abilities to cope with chronic illness and the orientation to try to further institutional and community understanding and responsiveness to the needs of those with rheumatic disease.

Evaluation

As a member of the treatment team the social worker's first role with the patient is to do a psychosocial evaluation. A complete evaluation which becomes a part of the patient's record can serve as an aid to the social worker, patient, and other members of the treatment team. For the social worker, doing the evaluation serves several purposes. It helps begin a relationship with the patient. It helps to delineate potential problem areas for the patient. It defines a plan for participating in the patient's care or rehabilitation. And it may be an opportunity to begin a contract with the patient for further areas of discussion and problem solving. For the patient, the broad content of the interview reassures him that he is going to be treated as a total person. The interview allows the patient time to express (in an unhurried atmosphere) his anxieties, concerns, and priorities. And it begins or reinforces an awareness that living with a chronic illness produces change and requires adaptation in many areas of one's life. For other members of the treatment team, an evaluation, especially if it is written out and put in the patient's chart, efficiently transmits the picture of the patient as a whole person, delineates the patient's priorities and concerns, and summarizes the social workers' impressions and planned points of intervention.

There are probably as many styles of doing psychosocial evaluations as there are social workers. However, in the area of rehabilitation, the framework of role functioning as a basis for evaluation of the patient is useful. If rehabilitation focuses on the restoration or maintenance of functioning, then an analysis of the patient's prehospitalized level of role functioning not only helps provide baseline data, but also helps set functional goals which are important to the patient. A role-functioning evaluation not only tells the team what the patient has been unable to do recently, but it also identifies what elements it is crucial to regain for the maintenance of self-identity and emotional well-being.

The major roles which patients fulfill are those of homemaker, breadwinner, independent adult, parent and/or grandparent, spouse, and enjoyer of life.

In doing a role-functioning evaluation, a good place to start is with the role of homemaker or with home responsibilities. Beginning with a discussion of the type, size, and arrangement of living quarters and then the patient's responsibilities in his/her home is useful for several reasons. First, it is usually a nonthreatening topic for the patient. Most patients can easily discuss whether or not they are doing the cooking, laundry, cleaning, or shopping. They have little trouble sharing their difficulties with yard work, handyman chores, or housework. From this topic you can usually find out: 1. if the living arrangements are physically suitable (manageable size of house and yard, general degree of physical barriers, amount of maintenance required, proximity to stores and services), 2. if the patient is having difficulty with any specific homemaking or handyman tasks, 3. if the patient sees the performance of any of these tasks as crucial to his self-esteem, and, 4. if any family members, friends, or community agencies are helping the patient in these areas.

A second closely related role is that of independent adult. Here the social worker and the patient are discussing changes in self-care skills and independent functioning. Is the patient able to dress, feed, and bathe himself? Does he take his own medications? Can he drive a car or use public transportation? Is he financially independent? If not, who helps the patient in these areas and how does he feel about this help?

In addition to many potential entries on a problem list, covering these two areas of role-functioning helps to begin formulating the short- and long-term treatment plans. Short-term goals might include arranging home health and homemaking services, educating family members in areas where the patient does and does not need help, information or referral for income supplementation, and/or seeking an occupational therapy referral from the physician for further evaluation of the patient's self-care potentials. Long-term goals might include the discussion of possible changes in housing, means of transportation, or home responsibilities. Or a goal might focus on more intangible things such as discussing the patient's attitude toward expectations for himself and his ability to seek and accept help from others.

Although "arthritis" is usually thought to be a problem of an elderly population and identified chiefly as degenerative joint disease, the reality is that many rheumatic disease patients are within the usual ages of the working population. Certainly the most obvious cost of rheumatic disease to society is the millions of dollars lost through sick and disability pay. However, the role of breadwinner has not only national significance but also much personal significance for the rheumatic disease patient. For most men and many women, much of their self-esteem is based on the successful performance of their role as breadwinner. The other immediate concern for patients is the effect which their illness may have on their family's economic well-being.

In the evaluation, then, one needs to discuss many aspects of the patient's employment. One would want to ask questions concerning the number of jobs a patient is holding? What are the hours? What problems are being encountered at the job? How stressful is the job? What do employers and fellow workers understand about his illness? What is their attitude toward the illness? How important is the job to the patient? And what does the family think about the work? Some of these areas may be covered more thoroughly by the occupational therapist during a job evaluation. However, the social worker may want especially to tune in to the patient's degree of emotional involvement in work activities, the amount of stress connected with the job, and whether the patient believes it would be feasible to change jobs or responsibilities if necessary. At the patient's request, it may also be useful for the social worker or occupational therapist to talk with the employer and explore his perception of the problem and the degree of flexibility available to the patient.

Short-term goals might include those of: 1. reduction of excessive work patterns, 2. techniques for avoiding or dealing with stressful work conditions, or 3. teaching the patient ways of communicating with employers and/or fellow workers regarding the nature of the illness and needs for assistance. Long-term goals usually revolve around referrals to vocational rehabilitation for retraining and job change, or to social security for disability income.

In evaluating the role performance of the rheumatic disease patient, one looks at the situation in two ways. The primary focus concerns the manner in which the disease process has altered the patient's ability to perform his role. But the second perspective concerns the manner in which the role performance of the individual is affecting the disease process. Certainly the fastidious housewife and the driving businessman or woman can physically push themselves to the point of exacerbating their symptoms. In the next few role categories, we will also be looking for the potentially negative effects of role performance which can come from the more intangible problems of worry, tension, and stress.

Patients who have rheumatic diseases must also be able to fill their roles as parents or grandparents. Many rheumatoid arthritis patients are women in the child-rearing ages whereas in the degenerative joint disease population many patients are involved with grandchildren or great-grandchildren. In evaluating rheumatic disease patients in this area, first it is good to find out the ages of the children around the home and the amount of physical care that they require. Is there a friend, relative, or spouse available to assist or relieve the mother? If there are older children in the home, are they being asked to assume responsibility for some of the household chores, and if so what is their attitude about increased responsibility? Has the parent lost some of the companionship activities with the child? Does the parent feel guilty, inadequate, or isolated in the family because of the changes in style and capabilities as a parent?

Grandparents may also be assuming responsibility for small children, and one needs to evaluate whether this is appropriate. Another focus in evaluating the older patient is the question of whether family problems are adding stress to the already difficult task of living with a chronic illness. Worry over divorce, illness, death, financial and child-rearing problems of grown children or other family members can interfere with the rheumatic disease patient's functioning and ability to participate in rehabilitation and recovery.

Short-term goals might range from arranging some alternative child care for a young mother to helping with nursing home placement of the rheumatic disease patient's own parents. Education of family members as to the needs of the rheumatic disease patient is a task often shared with the other staff members.

Long-term goals might focus on development of new companionship activities for parents and children or on helping the rheumatic disease patient recognize his strengths as a parent despite his physical limitations. Another area of intervention in the family might concern working out a realistic plan for sharing the responsibilities that the parent who has a rheumatic disease is no longer able to handle alone.

The interview now moves into the patient's functioning as a spouse. Although this can be a sensitive area of discussion, by now the patient is probably more at ease and is starting to grasp the concept of discussing role performance. Questions usually cover three basic areas: 1. changes in companionship activities, 2. changes in sexual functioning, and 3. the partner's attitude toward the patient's illness and the amount of support the partner is able to provide. Marital roles can be catagorized as maintenance, companionship, and sexual behaviors. Maintenance behaviors are those tasks which must be accomplished to run a household, etc. Usually the discussion of homemaking or household responsibilities fairly well delineates the distribution of maintenance behaviors. Companionship behaviors are usually activities the couple enjoy doing together such as bowling, dancing, fishing, traveling, visiting family, etc. The discussion should focus not only on whether their illness has interfered with their activities but also on whether the couple has developed any alternative companionship activities.

The symptoms of rheumatic disease may or may not affect the patient's sexual functioning. However, since sexual functioning is not only an important factor in a marital relationship but is also important in maintaining one's identity, the patient should be given the opportunity to voice concerns over this aspect of functioning. There certainly is no hard-and-fast rule as to which member of the treatment team is most qualified to evaluate sexual functioning. It may be the physician, nurse, occupational therapist, or basically anyone who is sufficiently knowledgeable and comfortable to answer patient's questions and make appropriate referals for treatment. However, the area of sexual functioning does fit very easily into a discussion of the patient's functioning as a spouse. Although the patient has a right to be given the opportunity to express concerns in this area, he also has the right not to discuss this area of functioning and/or to not regard this aspect of his or her functioning as being of major concern.

If the patient indicates that sexual functioning is a problem there are several basic questions to explore. Do the difficulties seem to be directly related to rheumatic disease symptoms, e.g., problems with fatigue, positioning, weight bearing, and joint immobility? Briefly what was the nature of the relationship prior to the onset of chronic illness? In other words is this a long-standing problem indicating the partners had never achieved a satisfying sexual relationship? Are there any potentially physiological difficulties, e.g., impotence or vaginismus which suggest the need for further medical evaluation? It may be more appropriate to save this discussion for a second interview when one can assure sufficient privacy and time to explore the problem.

It is also appropriate to give nonmarried patients an opportunity to discuss their concerns regarding sexual functioning. Many single people do have regular sexual partners and so may be experiencing sexual problems. Also it is not unusual to find older men and women who are considering remarriage but are apprehensive about their abilities to be good sexual partners.

By the time one has discussed maintenance, companionship, and sexual behavior, one should have a good idea about the degree of support the spouse is giving the patient. There may or may not be the need to ask the patient directly about the spouse's attitude toward the illness. The other perspective in looking at the patient's marital relationship is that of trying to determine if the relationship is a source of continual stress rather than support for the patient.

The potential short- and long-term goals stemming from this area of discussion could be many. Short-term goals might include trying to involve the spouse in the education program, helping the couple develop new companionship activities, or doing some short-term counseling. Long-term goals would probably focus on further evaluation of problem areas and then referral for outpatient counseling.

Rheumatic disease often first interferes with an individual's "ability to enjoy life" in the sense that it hampers the enjoyment of many forms of recreation. If one asks a rheumatic patient the question "What do you do for fun'" a majority of them will quickly answer "nothing!" Fatigue and problems with ambulation and joint functioning can limit or even eliminate the rheumatic disease patient's ability to dance, bowl, hunt, fish, travel, play golf or tennis, etc. Not only are active forms of recreation affected, but many patients loose their ability to participate in groups and organizations. Often architectural barriers or inability to sit in one position for any length of time can exclude rheumatic disease patients from attending churches or participating in organizations. In addition, the rheumatic disease patient may not only eliminate recreational activities but may lose friendships associated with these activities and companionship with family members and friends.

Short-term goals might well center around mustering the talents of various team members to maintain important recreational activities. Occupational therapists, for example, might adapt the handles of golf clubs or fishing rods to enable the rheumatic disease patient to continue those activities despite weakened or damaged hands. Long-term goals probably focus on helping the rheumatic disease patient develop new recreational activities and become reinvolved in community activities.

By the time one has finished an evaluation of the patient's role functioning, a picture of the external sources of stress and support for the patient has emerged. The next major area to evaluate is the patient's internal sources of stress and support. In other words, what are the primary emotions the patient is experiencing and what are the thoughts, fears, and expectations concerning rheumatic disease? Frustration, anger, and depression are feelings which are common to the experience of living with a chronic disease. The question then becomes, how does the patient cope with these feelings? Are any of these emotions overwhelming? There may be a proportion of rheumatic disease patients for whom it is necessary to arrange psychiatric consultation because of depression or anxiety.

In addition to all the data about the patient's adaptation to his illness, it is also useful to find out what the patient's thoughts are regarding the illness. Has he known someone else with the same illness? Does he spend a lot of time trying to answer the question "why me" and if so what is his answer? Is he optimistic about the future? Is he afraid of being crippled? What are his treatment goals?

Finally one may need to ask some practical questions about financial resources and insurance coverage, etc. By the end of the interview one should know if there are any obvious problem areas which might require assistance. An effort can be made to form a contract with the patient, focusing energy on solving specific problem or working toward specific goals. Again, there will always be a proportion of patients who are managing well, have little external or internal stress, and have good support systems. One may not identify any initial goals with these patients, but the social worker has been identified as one concerned with their total functioning and at some future date some of these patients may need and seek assistance.

A written evaluation (similar to a consultation) that is typed and is attached to the patient's chart is the most efficient way of communicating to other team members. The written evaluation can be a summary of the patient's problems and strengths in role functioning, along with social work goals and any impressions or suggestions that might be useful to others. If the evaluation is brief or has a summary section, other team members will read it, thereby enhancing their concept of the patient as a total person.

An article by Doremus (1) and a self-instruction manual developed by Kaufman and Samuels (2) offer two other ways of handling psychosocial evaluations.

The preceding evaluation outline is aimed at adults, but of course there are children and young adults with rheumatic diseases such as juvenile rheumatoid arthritis or ankylosing spondylitis. For children and young adults the role of student is one of their primary identities. One would want to know if they are having attendance problems, difficulty with access to classrooms, whether school personnel are supportive and understanding, and what are the attitudes of their peers toward their disease and possible limitations.

Interviewing parents would also be important in evaluating young rheumatic disease patients. It is important for the staff to know the parents' feeling about the child's illness and their approach to his limitations. As with other childhood illnesses, it is often difficult for parents to encourage appropriate independence, effectively discipline the child, or prevent the illness from becoming a manipulative tool. Helping parents set realistic limits on their child's behavior and on their own "helping" behavior would almost always be appropriate goals for working with parents.

Another area for evaluation with the pubescent or teenage patient concerns the question of when should the adolescent begin taking responsibility for his or her care and treatment goals? At some point the physician and other staff should identify the adolescent as the primary client to be consulted for decisions and cooperation rather than going through the parent as is necessary with young children.

The child or teenager's variety of roles may be more limited but this only adds to the importance of the roles he has as a child, student, family member, recreator, and friend. He is having not only to meet the challenge of adaptation to chronic illness but also to face the routine problems of growing up. Adolescence is often an age when individual differences are not well tolerated and so there is an increased importance in maintaining the young rheumatic disease patient in his normal roles. The social worker who is working with young rheumatic disease patients has more of a duality of identified clients. There is not only the challenge of identifying needs and setting goals for the patient, but also there is also a need to provide support and guidance for the parents.

Before leaving the topic of evaluation, one should broaden the social worker's role. Just as it is necessary to treat the "total person" when treating a disease, so too it is necessary to put that total person in the context of the institution where he is receiving treatment and in the community in which he lives. As an evaluator then, it is also important to ask whether the institution and community are meeting the needs of the rheumatic disease patient. Social workers are not alone in this task but find that other medical personnel and community members are asking the same questions. Nevertheless, one's particular experience with rheumatic disease patients might allow one to identify needs in patient care and community resources not readily perceived by others.

Education

Reducing the role of the social worker to the simplest terms, it becomes the task of identifying the needs of the patient and then helping him meet them. Since we have covered evaluating the needs of the rheumatic disease patient, the remaining material will be devoted to helping rheumatic disease patients meet their needs. There are a variety of approaches to helping patients meet needs including education, counseling, communication, and community referral and discharge planning.

Not enough can be said about the importance of educating the rheumatic patient *and his family* about his disease, prognosis, medications, and total treatment program. Families need to be especially cognizant of symptoms, suggested limitations, and the emotional stress of living with rheumatic disease. Again, none of these would be quite as important if the illness were not chronic. But chronic illness requires adaptation by the patient and understanding and appropriate help from the family.

But what is the role of the social worker as an educator? Normally information about the disease, prognosis, medications, and treatment program come from the physician, nurses, and therapy staff. However, patients will ask social workers questions about all these areas. Rather than ignoring these questions a reply of "What did your doctor say about that?" can be useful and safe. In listening to the patient's answer, one discovers whether the patient is taking his questions to the appropriate people and whether he is understanding and retaining the information they are giving him. So here we are evaluating again, but in this case the evaluator can also be the educator. Having a patient repeat and explain information is a way of reinforcing knowledge the staff is trying to impart.

One role, then, is to reinforce information given by the medical staff. In addition, however, there is some basic information regarding rheumatic disease and its care that a social worker and any other team member should know if they are going to be facing the public formally or informally. One should know the incidence variety of rheumatic disease. One should be familiar with the basic symptoms of rheumatoid arthritis, for example, and some of the types of medication used to treat it. One should be able to describe generally the combination of methods used to diagnose rheumatic diseases and something about the medical supervision necessary to treat rheumatic disease. And finally, one should be cognizant that quackery is a 500 million dollar business that preys on sufferers of rheumatic diseases. A second aspect of education for the social worker, then, is the ability to feel comfortable giving some basic information about rheumatic disease and its treatment to the public.

The unique role of rheumatic disease education for the social worker lies in the area of adaptation to illness. In order to function at full capacity, the rheumatic disease patient must understand not only his illness, his medication, and his treatment program, but he also must be aware of the "psychological and social side effects" of living with chronic illness, and then have some resources for coping with them. A patient who is overwhelmed by the psychosocial difficulties of living with chronic illness probably will absorb very little of the other educational efforts of other staff members.

What then are the psychological and social side effects of living with chronic illness? Although there is much written on this subject (3–8), there are a few basic concepts which patients should understand. 1. Living with chronic illness can change role functioning and changes in role functioning can disrupt families and be threatening to one's self esteem. 2. Living with chronic illness means living with more unpleasant and difficult emotions. 3. Living with a chronic illness that is progressively disabling causes and requires mourning over lost functioning. 4. Living with chronic illness often puts a strain on personal relationships.

In teaching these concepts to patients, one will not be telling them anything new. If they have had any experience with their illness, they will already have experienced what one is discussing. Chances are, however, they will believe that they are unique in having to deal with these problems and may have become so overwhelmed that they have not consciously identified these problems as being connected with their illness. Furthermore, they may not yet have begun to form strategies for coping with these consequences of chronic illness.

Loss of role functioning is an area that the rheumatic disease patient feels very keenly. If one asks rheumatic disease patients how it makes them feel to live with their illness, "useless" will invariably be on the list of responses. Families, however, may not recognize the importance of helping to keep the patient functional in the roles that he defines as significant. Well-meaning families may discourage a patient from continuing to work, take care of a household, or participate in social activities. Discussing the various roles he performs and their importance may help a patient decide where energy should be concentrated. Explaining the relationship of role performance to self-esteem may help family members provide the kind of support necessary to keep the patient functional where it counts.

A second psychological symptom that rheumatic disease patients experience but may not conceptualize, is that they are having to cope with increased levels of emotional arousal. Other consistent answers to the question of how it feels to live with chronic illness are "frustrated, angry, and depressed." Frustration is a common emotion for all human beings, but for the rheumatic disease patient it can be a constant companion. Frustration is having difficulty getting out of bed, getting off the stool, brushing teeth, combing hair, lifting the coffee pot, putting on socks, buttoning clothes, cutting food, opening the car door, climbing stairs, walking, holding the phone, etc. All these moments of frustration can and do occur daily. An almost inescapable companion of frustration is anger. The rheumatic disease patient, then, is living with much higher levels of frustration and anger than he had to deal with prior to his illness. The other unpleasant companion is depression. Sad and blue feelings are to be expected when living with chronic illness but often rheumatic disease patients are unable to express the frustration and anger, thus adding to their emotional overload and contributing to their feelings of depression. Discussing these feelings with patients and families helps destroy their feelings of isolation and guilt and can help patients focus on strategies for coping with their emotions.

Not only is emotional arousal a function of situational episodes of disability, but there is often an underlying mourning process for lost functioning, identity, and self-esteem. In our society, we are what we do. We are identified and valued by our capabilities. The rheumatic disease patient who has experienced some disability has experienced some degree of death of self. It may have been the working self, the socially outgoing self, the athletic self, the independent self, or the healthy self. A psychiatrist writing on "Psychological Issues in the Management of Rheumatoid Arthritis" recently stated, "It is crucial to stress that this mourning process is not only normal but necessary if the individual is to cope with his disease." (8). Mourning takes time and if successful culminates in a readjusted individual. But the rheumatic disease patient may be experiencing a steadily worsening or periodic disability, so the grieving and adjustment process may be continual or frequently occurring. Although this sounds like a depressing subject in itself to discuss with patients, talking about mourning can give patients "permission" to express what they are feeling and, more importantly, it may help to put their feelings of loss in a more positive context.

A final side effect of living with rheumatic disease is the adverse effect it may have on personal relationships. Most rheumatic diseases are both invisible and unpredictable. Unless severely afflicted, the rheumatic disease patient "looks good" to their friends and family. Furthermore, he or she may act able one day and disabled another. An inconsistent, invisible illness is very difficult for others to understand. It is a rare rheumatic disease patient who has not gotten the feeling at one time or another that others think he is malingering. Knowing how and to whom to explain one's illness, without becoming a bore, is a crucial skill if the rheumatic disease patient is to maintain good personal relationships.

Educating the patient as to some psychosocial side effects of rheumatic disease, of course, does not prevent these problems from occurring. But foreknowledge and acknowledgement of them may lessen the impact, it may help him recognize what is happening to him, and may allow him to marshall his resources to cope with these problems when they arise.

Our responsibility for education only begins with the patient. Equally as important is educating the patient's "family" (in the broad sense of significant others). Misunderstanding by family members can hinder a patient's functioning both physically and emotionally. It is crucial for the family to understand the symptoms of the disease, it's treatment, the patient's abilities and limitations, and the psychosocial side effects with which the patient is having to deal. Furthermore, this information has more credibility to the family if delivered by a health professional. Patients are often hesitant about further discussing their illness with family members because it is already too much a part of their family's lives. And families may in fact be tired of hearing about illness. Both patients and/or families can be in a denial stage and not communicating at all about the disease. Teaching by a health professional has more authority and allows the patient and family to learn together how to understand and best manage rheumatic disease.

An employer is certainly a significant other in a working patient's life. A rheumatic disease patient's ability to continue to be economically productive may depend on his employer's attitude toward his illness and his limitations. Again, there may be more credibility when a health professional approaches an employer regarding the need for a change in a patient's duties or working conditions. The physician can supply a letter with diagnosis, prognosis, and suggested limitations, and the occupational therapist can do a job evaluation and give specific suggestions. The social worker's role here may be one of insuring that the patient desires help in approaching his employer and then coordinating the efforts of other team members.

Again the role of educator applies to the larger systems which affect patient care. Within the hospital or institution where the patient is being treated there is an opportunity to educate other staff members as to the problems, needs, and sensitivities of rheumatic disease patients. Widening the circle, we have a responsibility for educating both the lay and professional public concerning the psychosocial problems of the rheumatic disease patient. Other allied health professionals are also anxious to understand the emotional needs of the patients whom they treat and there often is a demand for social workers active in the area of rheumatic disease to speak at professional meetings. The other group who is concerned about arthritis care is the lay public who are relatives of patients or patients being treated primarily as outpatients. They eagerly attend classes or public forums concerning rheumatic disease.

The final ring of the target populations to be educated about rheumatic disease, is the public in general and politicians in particular. Not until the impact of suffering and economic loss caused by rheumatic disease is understood by the public and the lawmakers, will rheumatic disease research receive a larger share of the federal research dollar. Although this aspect of education can benefit directly from our efforts, another approach is to educate rheumatic disease patients concerning their potential or exerting political pressure. Twenty-nine million rheumatic disease patients is a very respectable potential constituency for any politician.

In summary, our efforts to educate rheumatic disease patients about the psychosocial side effects of living with chronic illness is the rock we toss into the pond. The broading rings of target populations are families, staff personnel, health professionals, the lay public already interested in rheumatic disease, the general public, public servants, and politicians. The broader we can be in defining our educational responsibility, the wider will be the understanding we foster regarding the problems and needs of the rheumatic disease patient.

Counseling

The third major area of responsibility for social workers working with rheumatic disease patients is that of counseling. This is an area which I intend to discuss more briefly because counseling skills are a part of professional social work training and would be something that a social worker would bring with him to the job. The need for counseling is usually determined during the evaluation process or in subsequent contacts with patients or families. The decision as to whether a problem is tackled through individual, marital, or family counseling has to be based on the worker's assessment and the client's desires. The worker would also have to decide whether he has the particular skills and time necessary to deal with specific problems. Many problems may be better handled through referral to a community counseling resource.

There are several roadblocks which often have to be overcome in order to successfully fulfill the counseling role. The first may be to educate physicians and other team members that you have counseling skills to offer. It often takes a while to overcome the stereotypes that social workers are welfare workers or that they do only nursing home placements. The second difficulty can lie in establishing a contract for counseling with the patient. Although one may identify individual, marital, or family problems, it is possible that at the time one sees the patient he is primarily concerned with some type of alleviation of physical problems related to his illness. At times it may be unrealistic to expect some patients who are struggling to improve their level of physical functioning, to also have the energy and motivation to deal with less concrete problems. With hospitalized patients a treatment contract may be limited to problem clarification, help with problems related to hospitalization, or community referral for future treatment. There will be other patients however, who are so uncomfortable or overwhelmed by personal difficulties that they are very anxious to commit themselves to begin working on those problems.

The final roadblock to counseling can be time itself. If one works exclusively in an inpatient setting, then one often has to operate within the confines of the hospitalization. A very short-term planned therapy approach may not only be appropriate, but a practical necessity in working with inpatients (9, 10). If one is able to follow patients on an ongoing outpatient basis, one is more likely to have the opportunity to make contracts for short- or long-term treatment.

I would like to discuss one treatment area, that of sexual counseling. As mentioned in the evaluation section, someone on the treatment team should offer the patient an opportunity to acknowledge difficulties or ask questions about their sexual functioning. However, the question then becomes how to deal with the problems uncovered. As with all areas of counseling or psychotherapy, the worker must be realistic about his/her limitation in knowledge and skills. There are, however, areas of concern regarding sexual functioning in which the worker can give useful information, suggestions, and encouragement without entering the area of sexual counseling per se. For example it is often appropriate to discuss problems of fatigue, timing, and basic positioning with patients. There are also literature and films available which can serve to provide information to staff members and facilitate communication between patient and staff or better yet between patient and spouse (11–13). If the worker has not had a specific training in sexual therapy (which most of us have not), his other responsibility is to locate referral sources in the community where patients with long standing or complicated sexual dysfunctioning problems can receive treatment.

Switching from an area of treatment to a type of treatment, I would like to advocate working with rheumatic disease patients in groups. Groups can be used both for educational and counseling purposes. A group setting can boost morale, encourage sharing, and offer an added degree of validity to ideas one is trying to communicate. Rheumatic disease patients often have a sense of isolation within their own communities, which a group experience helps to dispel. The two obvious types of groups which are being used with rheumatic disease patients are inpatient and outpatient groups. Inpatient groups of necessity are short-term, heterogeneous, and probably need to be fairly structured in order to be effective. Their purpose can be education and/or supportive therapy. Regardless of the initial purpose, they will encourage socialization among patients which is supportive especially for those patients who may be hospitalized far from families or friends. In reviewing a discussion of the curative factors in interactional group psychotherapy and then comparing it with my experience in doing arthritis patient discussion groups, I was surprised at how many of the factors I thought operated in a structured short-term group. Of the 10 factors listed, six seemed to be present in even such a limited group experience. In my opinion, patients displayed evidence of benefiting from instillation of hope, feelings of universality, imparting of information, altruism, imitative behavior, and existential factors (9, 14–16).

Outpatient groups offer limitless possibilities for membership, structure, and purpose and can be run as traditional psychotherapy groups if desired.

Looking at the counseling role within the institution, there usually is a need for supportive counseling and case consultation on an *ad hoc* basis with other staff members. If one has a staff that deals routinely with chronically ill patients, then they face the loss of omnipotence found in other areas where one can offer a cure to their patients. We all then have to face the frustration of chronicity. Patients may heighten this frustration by rebuking their care-giver's ineffectiveness. The social worker can be available either informally or on a regular basis to meet with staff members and allow them to ventilate or bring up particular problems with patients on the unit. This is not only supportive to coworkers but also can enhance their effectiveness with patients. In some hospitals, social workers or other staff members run regular nursing groups designed specifically for the above purposes.

Again broadening one's area of concern to the community, the role of counselor can be conceptualized in several ways. One cannot "counsel" the entire community but it is possible to support or create opportunities within the community for rheumatic disease patients to participate in groups or individual experiences designed to offer support or aide in personal problem solving. The creation of patient clubs, for example, offer rheumatic disease patients opportunities for socialization, education, support, and through splinter groups, group therapy. Social workers may also act as consultants to other agencies who are trying to provide services to the chronically ill or disabled.

Communication

A fourth role of the social worker is that of facilitating communication within the treatment team, both in matters concerning patient care and team functioning. Certainly all team members will be constantly communicating with each other regarding patient care. But it is inevitable that at times the comments of the patient, doctor, or staff member will be misinterpreted, orders will get lost, or suggestions forgotten. In order to insure that a good treatment plan is both formulated and carried through, someone on the treatment team has to take responsibility often for literally running or calling back and forth between the patient, doctor, nurses, and therapists. This does not sound like a particularly exciting role for a social worker but it can make the difference between haphazard care and a smoothly flowing progressive treatment program.

The other area where open communication is a necessity is among team members. Although team members share the goals of good patient care, it is not a naturally homogeneous or probably harmonious group. There are usually differences in sex, age, training, and priorities among team members. There may be distrust, misunderstanding, and disagreement about respective roles and conflict over particular issues of patient care and team policy. And yet if the team is going to be effective in planning and delivering good patient care, the divisive factors cannot be overwhelming. The primary responsibility for maintaining cohesiveness and cooperation among team members lies with the head of the team; however, it is also well within the purview of our professional training and ideals to encourage open expression of ideas, support fellow workers, and help others to work through hostile feelings so that they can address issues. The social worker's goal should always be to encourage understanding and cooperation among team members.

There is also a potential for professional benefit by assuming the latter role. A social worker who demonstrates some skills in understanding, communicating clearly, and fostering problem solving and cohesiveness with fellow workers, is in fact demonstrating his/her skills in dealing with patients. Although subtle, this display of skill cannot help but enhance the worker's image, as a therapist or counselor in the minds of his colleagues.

Discharge Planning and Community Referral

Appropriately, the last role to discuss is that of discharge planning and community referral. One of the favorite cliches of medical social work is that "good discharge planning begins the day of admission." Following the roles outlined, it would be correct to say that good discharge planning begins the day of evaluation. By the time one has completed an evaluation one should have a feeling for problem areas such as: housing, homemaking, parenting, income, marital and family relationships, and/or social isolation.

The goals of discharge planning are basically the same as the goals of rehabilitation in the hospital: those of restoring and maintaining the role functioning and, therefore, self-esteem of the patient. There may be, however, several levels of intervention in order to accomplish this basic goal. The first level of intervention is making sure that the patient's basic needs will be met once he leaves the hospital. These can be needs such as adequate nutrition, housing, income maintenance, and follow-up nursing, physical therapy, and medical care. Once one is satisfied that those needs will be met, then one can focus on the patient's role functioning and especially on those roles which he values. It is to be hoped that during the course of hospitalization the patient will have regained some of his/her abilities. If, however, the patient cannot fully return to his former level or means of functioning, then discharge planning becomes a way of augmenting the patient's abilities, providing surrogate methods of fulfilling a role, or relieving the patient of some role responsibilities so that he can use his energy and talents in an area which is more meaningful to him. For example, a single parent may feel inadequate or guilty because of his/her inability to engage in outdoor or sports activities with the children. This portion of the role of parent could perhaps be fulfilled through referral to a community resource, such as Big Brothers or Big Sisters. In another case, a homemaker might be found to fulfill the household responsibilities for a disabled mother. This surrogate homemaker, working under the direction of the disabled patient gives the patient at least a partial sense of fulfilling her role. Also, it eliminates the need for a major reorganization of household responsibilities, which can be upsetting to the entire family. A final example of relieving a patient of a role might occur when a worker helps a family find alternate child care for grandchildren who were formerly the partial responsibility of an older arthritis patient. Relieved of her baby-sitting responsibilities, a grandmother might have more time and energy for other activities which are more enjoyable and less stressful.

Discharge planning is a role that traditionally has been identified with social workers. It may be the final task in the ongoing work with the rheumatic disease patient. But even if one only is called into a case at the time of discharge planning (which has been known to happen), the successful completion of this aspect of patient care necessitates at least a brief use of the other roles. Doing discharge planning requires some assessment of the patient's functioning and priorities. One will probably have to educate the patient and other staff members as to the resources available, and one may have to do a great deal of counseling with the patient to help him accept changes in his life situation or degree of independence. Finally, the need for ongoing and productive communication with other team members is never more pressing than when one is trying to work out a complicated discharge plan.

In summary, discharge planning is an extension of the team's effort to rehabilitate the patient. The patient's progress during hospitalization is monitored and when possible, community resources are used after discharge to continue progress toward unfinished goals. When a complete return to functioning is not possible then the resources of the community are called upon to augment the patient's abilities and/or to insure maintenance of the gains that he has made.

Summary

Rehabilitation of patients with chronic illness requires a holistic approach to the problems of disease and disability. Not only must the idiosyncracies of the illness and its manifestations be understood, but there must also be consideration and understanding of the total patient with his unique personality, reactions to illness, relationships, and social support systems. The social worker by inclination and training promotes a holistic approach to rehabilitation. His tasks with rheumatic disease patients, the institution and the community are varied but can be grouped into five basic roles.

EVALUATION

The social worker does a psychosocial evaluation of the rheumatic disease patient. This evaluation focuses not only on the patient's social situation and interpersonal relationships, but also on the congruities and discrepancies between role expectation and role performance. The result of the evaluation should be that other staff members not only have a better understanding of the patient as a person, but also are cognizant of the patient's priorities for rehabilitation.

EDUCATION

The social worker has a role in evaluating and reinforcing other staff members' efforts to educate the patient and his family regarding the disease process, symptoms, and treatment. The educational responsibility which is uniquely the social worker's is to give patients and families information and skills which help them adapt to the psychological and social side effect of living with rheumatic disease.

COUNSELING

Social workers have skills in individual, marital and family counseling. They may have additional interest and expertise in group work and/or sexual counseling.

COMMUNICATION

Social workers have a role in promoting understanding between patients and staff members and in fostering open communication among the treatment team.

DISCHARGE PLANNING AND COMMUNITY REFERRAL

These two roles can become the final tasks in working with the hospitalized rheumatic disease patient. But they do not signal the end of rehabilitation. Instead discharge planning and community referral becomes the means of continuing the goals of rehabilitation and pursuit of role maintenance.

Finally, the social worker not only engages in these roles with individual patients but also applies these guidelines to the institution in which he works and the community at large. The purpose of social work in a rehabilitation setting is to facilitate the achievement of maximum functioning by the individual and to foster institutional and community responsiveness to the needs of those with rheumatic disease.

REFERENCES

1. Doremus, B. L. The four R's: social diagnosis in health care. *Health Soc. Work 1:* 120, 1976.
2. Kauffman, C., and Samuels, G. Psycho-Social Evaluation of the Patient with Chronic Disease: Arthritis. Western Pennsylvania Arthritis Project, St. Margaret Hospital, 1976.
3. Feldman, D. J. Chronic disabling illness: a holistic view. *J. Chronic Dis., 27:* 287, 1974.
4. Hyman, M. D. Social psychological factors affecting disability among ambulatory patients. *J. Chronic Dis., 28:* 199, 1975.
5. Lane, H. J. Working with problems of assault to self image and life style. *Soc. Work Health Care, 1:* 191, 1975–76.
6. Strauss, A. L. The Burden of Rheumatoid Arthritis. In *Chronic Illness and The Quality of Life.* The C. V. Mosby Company, Saint Louis, 1975, pp. 71–80.
7. Vignos, P. T. Psycho-Social Problems in Management of Chronic Arthritis. In *Total Management of the Arthritic Patient,* edited by G. E. Ehrlich. J. B. Lippincott, Philadelphia, 1973, pp. 111–117.
8. Zeitlin, D. Psychological issues in the management of rheumatoid arthritis. *Psychosomatics, 18:* 7, 1977.
9. Garvin, C. Task centered group work. *Soc. Service Rev., 48:* 494, 1974.
10. Rapoport, L. Crisis-oriented short term casework. *Social Service Rev., 41:* 31, 1967.
11. Boogs, J-A. Living and Loving with Arthritis: Information on Sex and Arthritis. The Arthritis Center of Hawaii, Honolulu, 1977 (rev 1978).
12. Ehrlich, G. E. Sexual Problems of the Arthritic Patient. In *Total Management of the Arthritic Patient,* edited by G. E. Ehrlich. J. B. Lippincott, Philadelphia, 1973, pp. 193–208.
13. Lachniet, D. and J. Onder. Sex and Arthritis and Women. Presented at the 8th Scientific Session, AHP section of ARA meetings, June 1973. Department of Social Services, University of Michigan Medical Center.
14. Erfling, J. Model for conducting arthritis patient discussion groups. *Allied Health Prof. Section Newslett. 11:* 14, 1977.
15. Sampson, E. E., and M. Marthas. *Group Process for the Health Professions.* John Wiley and Sons, New York, 1977.
16. Yalom, I. D. *The Theory and Practice of Group Psychotherapy.* New York, Basic Books, 1975.

9

Vocational Assessment, Counseling, and Training

PHILIP SPERGEL

During the 1960s much had been written about the rehabilitation of the disadvantaged and minority groups. However, in the United States, it was not until the 1970s, particularly through the Rehabilitation Act of 1973, that attention began to be focused on the physically disabled as a minority group. In 1974 the Affirmative Action Law was enacted but it was not until several years later that the law became enforced. The author had the privilege of participating in the White House Conference for the Disabled in 1977 but was discouraged to see the under-representation of arthritics as a group. Because arthritis is considered "commonplace" the general population fails to respect how formidable the arthritides are as sources of disability.

In many respects the arthritic person is an immigrant within his own country. Many are unemployed or at best underemployed and are aliens in the mainstream of society. Despite social reform, the problems seem to increase geometrically as the years increase arithmetically. Our society is abundant with paradox and promise; more specifically, the coexistence of positive factors, such as new medical and surgical advances, and negatives such as increased unemployment, marital discord, and debilitating psychological factors.

Philosophers, scientists, and novelists have long been interested in the relationship between man and his work. Psychologists have been concerned with this problem since the turn of the century and from this concern the fields of industrial psychology, vocational guidance, and rehabilitation were developed.

Following World War I large scale rehabilitation programs were first begun. There were two separate phases, one for civilians and one for veterans. The former grew modestly until World War II. The country's social values were reawakened by recognizing its obligation to returning disabled servicemen and by the successful results achieved with the application of improved restorative services in medicine and other disciplines. Almost concurrently, efforts to restore and employ civilians with disabilities quickened due to the lack of man power in an industrial environment requiring a larger labor force. There arose an increased realization of the large numbers of disabled individuals in our society as a whole and of the values of a rehabilitation approach.

Rehabilitation is a complex process and quite difficult to define. A generally accepted definition is the one formulated in 1942 by the now defunct National Council on Rehabilitation: "Rehabilitation is a restoration of the handicapped to the fullest physical, mental, social, vocational, and economical usefulness of which they are capable." Rehabilitation is a philosophy incorporating a body of knowledge from many disciplines working together as a team. A major goal is to reduce impairments as fully as modern knowledge and skills permit and to overcome the obstacles standing in the way of a full and productive life. Ideally, rehabilitation should be considered an individual process, one that is tailor-made for each disabled person. This requires a comprehensive evaluation.

Vocational Assessment

Vocational evaluation is a process that includes a survey of education, mental capacities, abilities, interests, avocational pursuits, work history, achievements, personality patterns, physical factors, social adjustment, and family relationships. In the case of the disabled it is necessary to notice special influences which infringe upon life history and to use this knowledge in making more valid assessments.

Man has continually searched for means of measuring human ability and to make valid predictions about it. In the context of massive social concern and programming for disabled individuals, deeper understanding of their behavior and potential for work is urgently needed. Considerable attention has been given to the impropriety of using present testing devices to measure the psychological characteristics of individuals who deviate from the norm because of physical, psychological, social and/or educational limitations. In the not too distant past, it was not uncommon for professionals to regard an arthritic individual as being unemployable. This attitude did not take into account the fact that work has been and will always be a fundamental organizing principle of life. People would still much rather work than be idle. All one need do is engage in conversation with an arthritic patient, or for that matter with anyone who has a disability, and one will learn of the importance of work.

The development of adequate techniques of assessment has had an important place in the rehabilitation movement. There are a number of reasons for this, not the least of which is the fact that federal and state agencies have provided considerable financial support for much of the rehabilitation effort, and thus they have a marked interest in accountability. As the rolls of the disabled increased, there was an eagerness to identify those individuals who could feasibly be rehabilitated. A major criterion for feasibility was potential to return to the labor market. The problem has been and will continue to be the manner in which one utilizes appropriate criteria to identify potential for employment. Industry and the higher educational systems have for many years been concerned with the problem of selection. Because of mass education, and our heritage of individualism, there has been a strong interest in measuring individual differences in ability and aptitude. There is a belief that the socioeconomic hierarchy reflects individual differences in capabilities and what can be said of a "normal population" can also be applied to such a disability group as the arthritic.

The United States, unlike European countries, had no hereditary labor force. It was the millions of European immigrants who arrived in the United States following the Civil War that comprised the labor market. For the most part they consisted of unskilled labor and they had to be trained and disciplined for "factory work". From this arose the development of vocational education both in the public schools and private agencies. Thus, vocational education also developed a complex structure of assessment procedures. Thus, it stands to reason that the rehabilitation movement would be quite interested in assessment techniques.

There are essentially four ways in which one can be evaluated regarding work potential. These are: 1. job analysis; 2. psychological testing; 3. work sample procedures; and 4. the situational work approach. Prior to World War II, the primary manner in which individuals were assessed regarding potential for employment was through job analysis and aptitude testing. Job analysis usually yields three kinds of information: the definition of the job; the task of the job; and the requirements which the job demands from the worker for successful performance. It was defined by the war manpower as "the process of determining by observation and study and reporting pertinent information relating to the nature of the specific job. It is the determination of the task which comprised the job and the skills, knowledge, abilities, and responsibilities required of the worker for a successful performance and which differentiates the job from all others." The compendium of jobs can be found in the Dictionary of Occupational Titles where there are approximately 25,000 job definitions which are known by over 40,000 titles. The Dictionary of Occupational Titles, commonly referred to as D.O.T., is now in its 5th edition. It is used by individuals who are involved in the selection process, counseling, and vocational rehabilitation. Job analysis is a process whereby the employment interviewer may be provided with a written statement describing the job and a statement noting the minimum hiring specifications for all jobs. It is important to recognize, however, that the job analysis only indicates what is being done on the job but says nothing about the individual performing the work.

Probably the most common method by which individuals are evaluated regarding their interests, aptitudes, achievements, and personality is through psychological testing (assuming one has a literacy level equivalent to 6th grade or better). These instruments can assess one's vocational preference, one's aptitudes (the ability to learn a particular body of knowledge with training), one's achievement (what one has attained through education), and one's personality or characterological make-up).

All of us who have worked are aware of the fact that different jobs require different levels of intelligence and responsibility. Intelligence has often been defined operationally: "as what intelligence tests measure." The movement began in Paris, France, early in the 20th Century with the development of the Binet-Simone Test of Intelligence. It was later revised in California and became known as the Stanford-Binet. During World War I the Army Alpha and Beta (nonverbal group intelligence tests) were developed. The psychometric movement has progressed by leaps and bounds since then and new tests are finding their way into the market daily. A major problem with intelligence testing is that it does not take into account deviations from the norm. Thus, individuals with educational deficits, cultural limitations, physical handicaps, sensory impairments, etc. are often placed at a disadvantage when undergoing psychological evaluation via standardized tests. For this reason it was necessary to develop other techniques, particularly work sample assessment, and situational work evaluation. The individual with arthritis who experiences morning stiffness lasting several hours could well be penalized when undergoing an examination of manual dexterity. In addition, if pain is present, this can cause distractability, creating difficulties concentrating. If these factors are not taken into account, then the individual may be rejected from a position. However, if the behavior could be observed over a period of time, one may find that as the day progresses the arthritic patient becomes more nimble and, in fact, quite productive. To do this one might have to observe the arthritic patient for several hours at a time. New problems require the development of new techniques.

Man has continually searched for means of measuring human ability so that valid predictions could be made. This must be done if we are to understand the behavior and potential for work within a handicapped population. The author was involved in seeking a solution to the problem and was instrumental in developing a series of empirically graded industrial tasks to be used as an organized method of assessing the aptitudinal factors and personality characteristics of individuals who are not amenable to standardized methods of evaluation. Over a 10-year period a systematic procedure evolved at the Philadelphia Jewish Employment and Vocational Service to enable vocational counselors to penetrate the defenses and superficial responses of hard-to-place individuals through a deeper understanding of capability, adjustability, and the irreversibility as well as of work related traits. The procedure came to be known as the J.E.V.S. Work Sample Battery.

Work samples range in complexity from very simply structured operations to difficult activities involving symbolic reasoning and abstract conceptualization. They are derived from activities performed in competitive industry and are representative of a wide variety of interrelated functions such as psychomotor coordinations, spatial relations, etc. Walter Neff has defined a work sample as a "mock-up", a close simulation of an actual industrial operation not different in its essentials from the kind of work a potential employee would be required to perform in an ordinary job. Because of this, it is less threatening and more meaningful to a population comprised of individuals with physical disabilities such as arthritis. The administration of such work samples in a vocational rehabilitation setting maximizes the usefulness of these observations.

Since these tasks are simulated job duties and do not comprise a formal test situation it is assumed that the individual being less defensive is more prone to assert his capabilities and thus will reveal his potential cognitive, connotative, and affective self-pattern. By observing the performance of an individual undergoing work sample evaluation, the vocational counselor increases his scope of information. This helps to generate more valid hypotheses about the client's employability because the counselor derives deeper insights than would be possible from a standard battery of psychometric tests. The procedure does not attempt to pinpoint specific occupational objectives but is designed to assist in the determination of one's ability for fields of work or job families. They are not selection instruments and should not be used as such. However, they are rather concrete situations that examine the degree to which the individual can adapt and perform according to a set of prescribed demands.

Further, the sustained and structured observations of selected work behaviors reveal the extent to which the individual can change or improve in particular respects thus offering a measure of adjustability along specified vocational dimensions. These dimensions are the personal and social aspects of work as well as the capabilities which are specific to the performance of various tasks.

The psychological premise upon which work sampling is based is that as functioning becomes more complex and stressful, a higher degree of personality integration is required. Simple and mechanistic behaviors may permit effective performance in the face of competing internal and external stimuli. Those behaviors involving such higher processes as discrimination, judgment, and reasoning, demand a more persuasive or global mobilization of energies which are focused on the task.

A concomitant effect of the work activity or sampling method is the response of the individual to his experience. As he engages in meaningful work he tests reality as it involves him. New cognitive and affective tones are incorporated as learnings which govern his future responses. As these become revealed to him, his work identification and motivations become formed and are part of his repertory of worker-role behaviors. In this light, work evaluation may be viewed as interacting with the work experience or treatment process; it provides a basic growth activity which may be either pivotal or supportive to counseling. The work sample approaches are reality oriented, their major virtue. They provide a close simulation of actual work demands administered in a reasonably controlled quasi-industrial setting; an unparalleled opportunity to observe basic employment behavior is provided. To be sure, it is an expensive, often time-consuming technique, that requires both an intellectual and emotional commitment to continuous revision and reconstruction, but it is, in our experience, the most effective, meaningful procedure for evaluating the vocational assets, liabilities, and potentials of the disabled population.

The situational assessment approach, like the work sample, is based on an effort to simulate actual working conditions. Work sampling attempts to assess the skills of the individual for mastering specific tasks or undergoing training for entering into a particular occupation and the situational work approach is aimed at evaluating and developing general work behavior. The situational work approach questions the potential of one to be able to work at all. The question asked is "what is it in the work situation that comprises a particular problem for the individual" (in this case the arthritic). The situational assessment attempts to assess the client's adaptability to the ordinary demand characteristics of work as a social situation. Situational assessment has its origins in the sheltered workshop movement where the objective is not so much to standardize the test situation as it is to "standardize" the observer. Observers must be trained in their judgments because the approach relies heavily on the rating scales. What is stressed here is obtaining information on the general work personality; that is, what work means to the individual; the manner in which he reacts to important other persons on the job, such as supervisors and coworkers, and those work roles that are found congenial. The situational approach is less structured than work samples since it does not really depend on the kind of work that is performed. In situational assessment, the individual is paid wages for his effort and the work is generally subcontracted, meaning that it is performed on actual commodities destined for sale. Foremen are present who set standards for quality and quantity of output and regular hours are maintained. The assessment occurs over a sustained period of hours, generally in an industrial environment. The total physical setting generally reproduces what is found in ordinary employment. Other workers are present with whom the client must interact. The activity is sustained frequently over a several week period of time so that the process of adaption can be observed and manipulated. This allows the observer to formulate hypotheses as to the particular types of problems that the arthritic person may have in adapting to work. There are several problems with this method, not the least being that it is often difficult to reproduce an industrial setting within the confines of the typical rehabilitation facility. In addition, it is not easy to duplicate the wide variety of employment that exists in the labor market and the levels of skills comprised in industry at large.

Since much arthritis, particularly osteoarthritis, is a disease of late middle-age, many patients have had an extensive work history. Because of their disability they are often unable to continue with their former level of employment. As a result, they may require a modification of their present position, a change of jobs, or in some instances an entirely new career. The psychological ramifications are great. One's role as a worker is incorporated in the self-concept. The arthritic who can no longer engage in his life's work experiences a profound sense of loss. This can be a shocking experience often followed by denial and depression. Counseling is essential in helping the individual cope with his altered body and vocational image. When a person is born with a disability, his adjustment will be influenced not only by his impairment but also by the attitudes and reactions of those important people in his environment.

Family reactions to developmental disabilities are often quite strained. Acquired disabilities, however, are frequently accompanied by a strikingly deep pain of loss, anxiety, and bewilderment as to how to restructure one's life and by disturbing uncertainty as to how to react to and deal with other people. Basic personality remains unchanged and the manner in which one reacts after a physical disability depends chiefly upon his psychological integration before the event. This means that one can predict adjustment to disease by knowing the manner in which one has reacted to stress throughout his life.

The incurrence of a severely disabling condition, such as advanced arthritis, is deeply disturbing to even well-integrated people, but the intensity is modified by such factors as previous experience with handicapped persons in and outside the family, gradual or sudden onset of the impairment, and clear or uncertain medical prognosis. This is particularly true with as whimsical a disease as arthritis. One may feel well on a given day and experience considerable pain and loss of function at another time. A disability only becomes a handicap when it prevents the individual from doing something that is important to him. For example, if one is color-blind but this impairment in no way affects his daily life activities, then it is not considered a handicap. However, if the color-blind individual has a burning desire to become an airline pilot, then the disability becomes a handicap. A major consideration is the value which society and the disabled individual place on the occasion of the disability. An injury resulting from a needless automobile accident is more difficult to reconcile than one incurred in combat or even in work. Thus the incurrence of a disability is a highly individualized personalized matter which must be considered in a social context. It is often the cause for emotional upheaval. Most individuals require a period of time to grieve. This phase must be completed before one can rebuild his self-concept in the face of new realities.

The defense mechanisms used by the disabled are similar to those of a "normal population". The individual is involved in various life roles, work being one of the more important, and thus there are many kinds of adjustments one can make. The individual must pass through the stages of shock, denial, regression, depression, and adjustment. The psychological make-up of the individual must be carefully considered. All too often researchers have attempted to correlate diagnostic categories with specific personalities and this is, in our opinion, nothing more than a myth. For example, during the late 1950s and early 1960s, the professional literature was replete with the theory that those patients diagnosed as having rheumatoid arthritis shared a distinct personality pattern. The arthritic individual was reported to be self-punitive, latently hostile, having interpersonal difficulties with parents, having less loving mothers, more authoritarian fathers, a greater tendency to divorce, and a lower income level than the normal population. A study performed at our Arthritis Center at Moss Rehabilitation Hospital refuted this theory. What appeared to be emerging was a chronic disease personality of which the arthritic patients represented only one subpopulation. The findings suggested that medical and allied health service professionals have to guard against overgeneralization. It is dangerous to consider all patients with rheumatoid arthritis as psychologically similar. Their commonality may lie in the disease process, although great variations existed even within the group. This points up the importance of viewing each arthritic patient as an individual with personalized needs and desires. To be sure, rheumatoid arthritis is a chronic disease that not only interferes with the physical life of the individual but also influences the economic and social spheres. An examination of the psychosocial factors ultimately leads to a better understanding of the disease process and to a better control of physical symptoms.

Counseling, both vocational and personal, is often as effective in the treatment of the arthritis as are the variety of pharmacological agents. The more the rehabilitation psychologist or counselor knows about the nature and specific conditions of certain impairments, such as arthritis, the better they are able to function in their own field and as team members. In seeking suitable job fields and opportunities for clients and in follow-up procedures with them, the facts about the medical examinations are crucial considerations in the counseling of these clients and their families. It is ludicrous to counsel someone for return to work when this is not a realistic possibility. Each individual has a unique set of conditions relating to impairments and to capacities and abilities. Having experience with the arthritic patient helps the counselor to understand and work through his own negative attitudes. Subtle psychological factors can impede or facilitate the patient's attitude toward himself and his disability as well as the attitude of others toward him.

Psychological Counseling as a Therapeutic Intervention

The severity and intensity of the arthritic condition significantly effects vocational outcome. The options can range anywhere from unemployment to return to former position. Arthritis is not an acute illness and because of its chronic state there is always a potential to become increasingly debilitated. Throughout the treatment process, vocational options have to be continuously assessed. The patient must be counseled regarding transferability of skills, a concept extremely important to one's vocational rehabilitation. The question raised here is what aptitudes, interests, personality characteristics, etc., can be transferred from positions requiring activities that can no longer be performed to jobs that are now within the capabilities of the individual. For example, one's general intelligence, verbal ability, numerical ability, spatial relations, and form perception can be transferred even if there is a severe involvement in all extremities. The vocational goal is similar to that of maintaining function in activities of daily living. The objective is to assist the individual in functioning as optimally as possible. Often, rehabilitation engineering can be of great assistance in developing aids and devices that can be applied to the office and business as well as home.

It has been the experience of health providers at Moss Rehabilitation Hospital that emotional stresses are frequently much more critical than physical limitations and that the extent that one's emotional feeling is affected must be taken into consideration. Interpsychic tensions and anxieties are often translated into interpersonal relationships and to coworker association. Individuals experience four stages of the disease: shock, denial, depression, and accommodation. Frequently, many patients do not progress beyond the level of denial. Although this defense mechanism can be healthy, the tendency to deny the disability is unfortunate if it interferes with realistic planning and adaptation. The goal of all team members is to minimize the effects that the arthritic condition has on one's life.

Emotional problems can be dealt with through a variety of psychological approaches. In a rehabilitation facility the psychoanalytic method is rarely used because of its extensive time and expense.

Nevertheless, behavior therapy is often introduced; particularly the teachings of deep muscle relaxation to reduce stress. This has been found to be extremely successful with almost all forms of arthritis. The advantages of the technique are that it is relatively simple, fast, and satisfying. Therapeutically, efforts are directed at teaching the patient more appropriate modes of adapting to uncomfortable situations. Group therapy and family therapy have also been extremely helpful in dealing with interpsychic and interpersonal problems.

Two primary factors interfering with the psychological and vocational rehabilitation of the arthritic patient are intensity of pain and degree of disability. Most typically, the arthritic patient experiences more pain than individuals afflicted with other chronic diseases. Pain is a significant cause of functional disability. This presents to the arthritic individual a question of motivation because of a paradoxical phenomenon. To continue with wanted activities may create exquisite pain on the one hand, but on the other to reduce pain and not be active can in fact increase loss of function. The arthritic patient often has to carry out activities of daily living, including work, with painful joints. Although mild analgesics may relieve this discomfort, potent drugs are often necessary and can create a state of lethargy. Considering all variables, it is not surprising that a number of arthritic sufferers "give up". Psychological counseling is frequently helpful in providing the support required for the arthritic to persevere.

Progressive crippling of one or more joints is rather common in arthritis. Despite good medical care, the crippling can progress and be irreversible. Surgery has been introduced to improve the disabled joint and increase mobility. Here, too, counseling is extremely important. The arthritic often looks to the future with horror expecting increasing debilitation. Although no one can guarantee that progressive crippling will not occur, permitting the patient to ventilate emotions and feelings can be therapeutic. The site of the involved joint is of major importance, particularly regarding life functions, including work. If one is a professional, such as a psychiatrist, social worker, statistician, etc., one may well continue one's life work despite crippling changes. However, if one is a laborer, craftsman, etc., a change in job may be required.

There are also important cosmetic implications with regard to arthritis. The deformities are frequently unsightly and again the patient is in need of counseling. In our program, group counseling sessions with arthritic patients and their families are held one evening a week.

An attractive middle-aged woman would come to the session with a sweater draped across her hand no matter how warm the day. Finally, at one of the meetings she was questioned about this by another patient. After several minutes of hemming and hawing, she finally admitted that she was terribly ashamed of her ulnar deviations and swan neck deformities. A lively discussion ensued and a sensitivity exercise was performed. All of the nine participants in this group session were asked to join hands with the lights off and to explore each other's hands to get some idea of what the other individual was like. When the lights were turned on and this exercise was discussed, it was interesting to note that not one comment was made about any deformities. Each person instead commented about affect or what they felt the other person was like with regard to emotionality as a result of exploring hands. The exercise had a marked effect on this woman and, in fact, increased her life space. She now felt more free to travel and she became less sensitive about the appearance of her hands. She had even begun to consider the possibility of returning to the labor market.

It is becoming more common for family members of arthritic patients to seek counseling, both personal and vocational. One must remember that relatives have been told by a physician, either insensitively or gently, of the diagnosis. By the time family members seek therapeutic assistance, the identified patient, in this case one with arthritis, has already begun to show marked limitations. Often relatives are quite ambivalent, feeling both guilty and angry at the arthritic patient. The therapist must become aware of the fact that until the family has made an adjustment to the disability, they may resist or misinterpret help of any kind.

A diagnostic family interview must include all important family members since it provides the opportunity to view the interaction of the family, with and around the arthritic member to discern attitudes, responses, and alliances. Husbands, wives, and children of the patient often provide an accurate barometer of the family cohesiveness in coping with the arthritic. It is also possible to identify the potential sources of strength and weaknesses. Family therapy may afford all members the opportunity to express negative feelings that are often aroused in the presence of slow-yielding dependency, disproportionately demanded attention, as well as expense. Family therapy can reduce both guilt and anger. Family therapy is a form of treatment that attempts to shift the balance of unhealthy interactions among the members, so that healthier forms of association can be developed. In the opinion of the author, there are two major indices to successful rehabilitation: 1. the premorbid personality structure and 2. the cohesiveness of the family. There is a consensus that the well-being of the family truly influences the degree of success with which the arthritic patient is managed. The rheumatologist must be aware of this because he can provide the family with professional support. The family can then, in turn, be supportive to the patient. Of course, if the problems in the network appear intense, the physician should refer the patient to a family agency or a family therapist.

The individual with arthritis frequently has to contend with the pain, structural deformities, loss of function, and increased dependency needs. This of course varies with the severity of the disease, environmental supports, level of medical care, and the personality of the individual. In the total rehabilitation of the individual, one must take into account the personal, social, family, and vocational aspects of life. If the psychological variables are not considered, the physical rehabilitation may be futile.

Over the years, employers have become increasingly aware of the contribution that can be made by disabled individuals, including the arthritic. The vocational rehabilitation movement is a relatively recent phenomenon and new ways of evaluating disabled individuals are being developed. In this chapter the author has discussed four major methods: psychological testing; job analysis; work samples; and the situational work experience. It is important to be cognizant of the fact that even within a diagnostic, homogeneous category such as arthritis, there are considerable individual differences.

The author has identified what he considers to be the two most important variables in the rehabilitation of the disabled: 1. strength of premorbid personality and 2. cohesiveness of the family unit. The importance of providing the patient with psychological supports has also been discussed. It should be remembered that one is not dealing with "an arthritic individual" or "an arthritic personality" but instead with an individual who has an arthritic condition that is only one aspect of the person's life. He or she bears many other roles and titles such as husband, wife, father, mother, brother, sister, lover, employee, and most of all, human being.

REFERENCES

1. Anthony, E. J. The Mutative Impact of Serious Mental and Physical Illness in a Parent on Family Life, In *The Child in His Family*, edited by E. J. Anthony. Wiley, New York, 1970.
2. Bellows R. M., and Estep, M. F. *Employment Psychology: The Interview*. Rinehart & Co., Inc., New York, 1954.
3. Borow, H. *Man in a World at Work*. Houghton Mifflin Co., Boston, 1964.
4. Boszormenyi-Nagy, I., and Framo, J. L. *Intensive Family Therapy*. Harper & Row, New York, 1965.
5. Bursten, B. Family dynamics, the sick role and medical hospital admissions. *Family Proc., 4*: 202, 1965.
6. Erickson, G. D., and Hogan, T. P. *Family Therapy–An Introduction to Theory and Technique*. Jason Aronson, Inc., New York, 1976.
7. Frampton, M. E., and Gall, E. D. *Special Education for the Exceptional*. Porter Sargent Publisher, Boston, 1960.
8. Garrett, J. F., and Levine, E. S. *Rehabilitation Practices with the Physically Disabled*. Columbia University Press, New York, 1973.
9. Goldenson, R. M., Dunham, J. R., and Dunham, C. S. *Disability and Rehabilitation Handbook*. McGraw-Hill, Inc., New York, 1978.
10. Greenblum, J. The Control of sick care functions in the hospitalization of a child: family vs. hospital. *J. Health Human Behav., 2*: 32, 1961.
11. Haley, J. *Problem-Solving Therapy*. Jossey-Bass, Washington, D.C., 1977.
12. Jackson, D. D., and Yalom, I. Family Homeostasis & Patient Change. In *Current Psychiatric Therapies*, edited by J. Masserman. Volume IV, Grune & Stratton, New York, 1964.
13. Neff, W. S. *Rehabilitation Psychology*. American Psychological Association, Inc., Washington, D.C., 1971.
14. Pattison, H. A. *The Handicapped and Their Rehabilitation*. Charles C Thomas, Springfield, 1957.
15. Spergel, P., Ehrlich, G. E., and Glass, D. D. The rheumatoid personality—A psychodiagnostic myth. *Psychosomatics, 19:*78, 1978.
16. Szasz, T. S. *The Myth of Mental Illness*. Harper & Row, New York, 1974.
17. Vroom, V. H. *Work and Motivation*. John Wiley & Sons, Inc., New York, 1964.

10

Transportation Evaluation, Counseling, and Training

MICHAEL H. BOBLITZ

Little is known about the transportation ability, needs, and problems of the approximately 3,600,000 symptomatic arthritic people in this country. In a recent study of the transportation handicapped in the United States, 44% of all arthritic people are estimated to have no mobility limitation at all, whereas 34% have some mobility difficulty (1). The researchers further estimate that an additional 13% of those with arthritis have mobility difficulties requiring the use of ambulation aids. Finally, 5% require the use of a wheelchair, and 4% are homebound. Whether these estimates are truly representative of the entire arthritic population is of little concern. The importance of the study is its implication that a large segment of the arthritic population does have transportation handicaps that affect their employment and their participation in community activities.

This chapter attempts to explore three modes of transportation—driving personal licensed vehicles, driving commercial trucks, and using public transportation—that the author has found to be of particular concern to both the arthritic population and the medicolegal and transportation professionals responsible for their safety and physical well-being. Each subsection indicates the functional requirements of a particular transportation mode and, where possible, its relationship to the clinical manifestations of rheumatic diseases. Evaluation, counseling, and training approaches that have been devised and found to be satisfactory in dealing with the specific problems confronting the patient are discussed. Also, each subsection indicates the role of respective federal agencies in resolving the transportation handicaps of the disabled (including the arthritic) population.

Personal Licensed Driving

Although the automobile is the primary mode of personalized mobility of 83% of the transportation-handicapped individuals nationally, only 32%

operate a vehicle themselves (2). This situation is primarily because a large portion of this special population does not have an operator's license. One can only guess that the reason for their not having an operator's license is because of their medical impairment.

A recent literature review indicates that there have not been any studies specifically considering the arthritic person's ability to operate a licensed vehicle, such as an automobile or van. Furthermore, it is a common practice to group patients with arthritis and those with the other rheumatic diseases together with those with musculoskeletal impairments when discussing medical impairments interfering with driving. Finally, the literature review indicates that since there is an absence of scientific data, physicians have often denied their patients an opportunity to operate an automobile on the assumption that such medical conditions as arthritis cause their patients to be hazardous drivers.

Throughout the literature review, medical clinicians and traffic specialists have found the work of Julian Waller (3) to be the cornerstone of the movement to correct this deficiency of supportive data. Waller's work suggests that the more severe the medical impairment, the higher the crash rate (3). His work estimates that as many as 20% of drivers have chronic medical impairments (other than alcoholism) severe enough to be a potential handicap to driving. His studies include cardiovascular disease, diabetes, alcoholism, and epilepsy, but he does not include studies of musculoskeletal impairments, such as arthritis. Also, Waller states that only 15–20% of the drivers with medical impairments have had crash experiences as the direct result of their impairments. His most important statement is his hypothesis that medical impairments may be a contributing factor, at a subclinical level, in many crashes. Whatever the status of a patient's medical impairment, Waller's work reminds the physician of his responsibility to understand the patient's need to operate a motor vehicle, the functional difficulties that may develop, and the potential hazards that could ensue.

EVALUATION OF DRIVING PERFORMANCE

Driving a personal licensed vehicle safely is an extremely complex psychomotor task. The driver receives information from a multifaceted driving environment. Once the driver perceives this information, he interprets it and decides upon an action. The action of the decision results in the dynamic response of the vehicle. For this sequence of events to occur safely, the driver must have a minimal level of judgmental and physical qualities.

Medicolegal and transportation professionals make no distinction between normal and disabled drivers when establishing these minimal requirement levels of driving qualities. The normal and disabled driver must possess at least the minimal judgment and physical qualities. Medical clinicians responsible for determining the presence of these qualities in the disabled driver usually evaluate the physical qualities prior to evaluating both qualities in interaction.

Evaluation of Basic Physical Driving Tasks

Due to the wide spectrum of clinical expression of the rheumatic diseases and the variable progress of these diseases in individuals, the physician should evaluate his patient's disease state and degree of ability and disability. Often, physicians delegate the monitoring of their patient's transportation problems to driver evaluation and training programs. These programs, usually hospital- or rehabilitation center-based, provide periodic patient reassessments and training activities to assist the arthritic driver in maintaining his operator's license and his safe driving skills. Most driver evaluation and training programs are supervised by an occupational therapist. These programs may operate as a section of the occupational therapy department or exist administratively as separate departments or centers.

Before admitting the disabled patient to the driver evaluation and training program, the occupational therapist requires written information from the physician. The information includes the patient's type of arthritis, present muscle strength, range of joint motion, and coordination. The physician needs to indicate any specific medical precautions that may affect the patient's driving ability. When the physician shares this kind of information in his referral, the therapist is given the background facts necessary to initiate the evaluation.

Many transportation centers use driving simulators and adaptive driving aids to assess the basic physical driving skills. A driving simulator consists of the driver's compartment of an automobile and contains a complete instrument panel and bucket type of car seat. The simulator can be equipped with a variety of driving aids to duplicate those actually used by the patient. A projector with a cinemascope lens projects full-color motion pictures depicting traffic situations on a screen in front of the room. On the screen, one sees the same thing that one would see from the driver's seat—the rear-view mirror, head of the car, and the street. The patient manipulates all of the controls and driving aids, if necessary, in response to the situation on the screen, just as though he were in an automobile.

The simulator film is marked with a binary code for performance monitoring. When a monitored error is made, a panel mounted on a simulator hood indicates the type of error: steering, braking, turn signal, speed, and accelerator position. Only one error will go on at a time, and it will remain on until either the mistake is corrected or the time elapses for that particular action. The occupational therapist records the types of errors that have occurred.

The occupational therapist gathers other pertinent information about performance besides simulation errors. The therapist must assess the manner and consistency of control of a number of basic driving tasks during the simulation exercise. For example, the therapist must determine whether steering errors are due to poor hand placement on the steering wheel or to the mild subluxation of the right wrist and the slight bilateral flexion

TABLE 10.1. *Basic Physical Driving Tasks*

Task	Evaluation Location	
	Simulator	Actual vehicle
1. Opens/closes car door		X
2. Transfers to/from seat		X
3. Opens/closes front side windows		X
4. Adjusts seat/mirrors		X
5. Fastens/unfastens seat belt and/or harness		X
6. Depresses/releases foot brake	X	
7. Releases/depresses parking brake	X	
8. Shifts gears	X	
9. Depresses/releases clutch	X	
10. Depresses/releases accelerator	X	
11. Controls steering	X	
12. Turns signals on/off	X	
13. Turns head/body upon backing/pulling out	X	
14. Turns head to observe road environment	X	

contractures of the elbow. Table 10.1 contains a list of basic driving tasks which should be evaluated during the simulation exercise. Any of the tasks that the therapist finds deficient should be resolved with or without a driving aid prior to an "on-the-road" driver evaluation. The first five tasks of Table 10.1 are best evaluated in the patient's vehicle or the center's evaluation and training vehicle.

Several major transportation centers have incorporated new evaluation tools into their basic evaluation programs. One simple and inexpensive device measures the force input capability of the severely disabled driver's upper limbs to control steering and hand-operated acceleration and braking (4). The device assists the occupational therapist in choosing the appropriate type of hand control from several variations to be prescribed. Another device for which hand controls are used allows the therapist to evaluate the major driving functions—steering, accelerating, and braking—in their interactive mode (5). This device simultaneously measures the exerted force and the force duration of the upper limbs in performing the major driving functions.

A word of caution needs to be made about static evaluation tests, such as those involving turning a steering wheel to the left and to the right a specific number of degrees. Recent research on electromyographic studies of the function of muscles of the upper limb in car driving has shown that there are marked differences between the function of the muscles during controlled static movements of steering and those during simulated driving (6). The researchers state that one reason for this difference is that the study's subjects are not allowed to change their hand positions during static steering, whereas no such instructions are given to them during the simulated driving experience. This performance difference could become apparent when the occupational therapist finds the patient's steering ability poor during the on-the-road evaluation and not during the static steering test.

As soon as the basic driving skills have satisfactorily been demonstrated in the simulator and any needed aids, an on-the-road driver evaluation by a state-approved driving instructor is given. Currently, simulation is not a replacement for on-the-road driving experiences because it cannot duplicate the degree of danger with respect to the capabilities of the arthritic driver and the ever-changing roadway and traffic conditions.

Evaluation of on-the-Road Driving Performance

Measuring driver performance in a vehicle on the highway is an important part of the evaluation process. Since most arthritic patients are predominantly in the wage-earning age (7), those that are referred for evaluation already possess an operator's license. Many states do not legally require the arthritic driver to report any change in his medical status until license renewal. This permits the program's state-approved driving instructor to conduct the on-the-road evaluation.

Most driving instructors, often occupational therapists, have the patient operate the program's dual-control vehicle equipped with the necessary driving aids. Usually, the evaluation is at least an hour in length and includes a variety of traffic situations on highways, urban streets, and secondary roads.

The usefulness of the information gained about the arthritic patient from the on-the-road evaluation is dependent upon the evaluative skill and experience of the driving instructor. Presently, there is no standardized approach to driver performance evaluation. Most driving instructors rely on the performance criteria used at the state's license examining stations since the patient is going to have to meet the state's established minimal performance competency to maintain his license.

A Study of Driver Evaluation: Rheumatoid Arthritis

During 1975, this author had an opportunity to evaluate 22 rheumatoid arthritic drivers in s simulated driving situation and to observe their performance on the road with a state-approved driving instructor. The author conducted these evaluations while serving as Coordinator of the Transportation Evaluation and Training Center at Moss Rehabilitation Hospital, Philadelphia, Pennsylvania. The study group consisted of 17 men and 5 women. They had been diagnosed as having classic or definite rheumatoid arthritis by the rheumatologists at the Albert Einstein Medical Center's Arthritis Center. All of the drivers were in stages II and III, as defined by the American Rheumatism Association. Their ages ranged from 37–62 years of age, with a mean age of 57. These drivers were referred to the Transportation Center because of driving problems that the physicians of the Arthritis Center documented at the time of admission.

TABLE 10.2. *Range of Joint Motion/Pain Profile of 22 Rheumatoid Arthritic Licensed Lrivers at Admission*

Joint Location	Males																	Females				
	A	B	C	D	E	F	G	H	I	J	K	L	M	N	O	P	Q	R	S	T	U	V
Upper limbs																						
Shoulder	3/3*	0/0	0/0	2/0	2/0	3/3	1/1	0/0	1/0	1/1	1/1	1/1	3/3	3/3	0/0	0/0	0/0	1/2	2/2	1/3	3/3	1/1
Elbow	0/3	0/0	3/2	3/1	2/0	0/0	0/0	3/2	0/0	1/1	1/1	0/0	0/2	0/0	0/0	0/0	3/0	1/1	3/3	0/0	1/1	0/0
Wrist and hand	3/3	0/0	2/0	3/3	0/0	3/3	3/3	3/1	1/1	1/1	3/3	3/3	1/3	3/3	0/0	1/1	3/3	1/1	0/0	2/2	2/2	2/2
Lower limbs																						
Hip	0/0	2†/2	0/0	0/0	0/0	0/0	2/2	0/0	3/1	1/1	1/1	2/2†	2/2	3/3	1/1	0/0	0/0	2†/3	3/3	0/0	0/0	0/0
Knee	0/0	1/0	2/3	0/3	0/0	0/0	1/1	1/0	0/0	1/1	3/1	2/2	1/1	0/3	1/1	3/3	3/3	3/1	3/3	1/1	1/1	3‡/2
Foot and ankle	0/0	0/0	1/1	0/0	1/1	0/0	0/0	0/0	1/1	1/1	1/1	0/0	1/1	3/3	1/1	1/1	1/3	1/1	3/1	1/1	1/3	1/3
Spine																						
Cervical	0	0	0	0	0	0	2	0	0	1	1	3	3	0	0	0	0	1	0	0	1	0
Lumbar	0	1	0	0	0	0	0	0	0	0	0	3	2	0	1	1	0	0	0	1	0	0

* Right and left side, respectively. Key: 0 = pain and range of motion limitation absent; 1 = pain present but range of motion limitation absent; 2 = pain absent but range of motion limitation present; 3 = pain and range of motion limitation present.

† Total hip replacement arthroplasty.

‡ Knee arthroplasty.

Each patient's range of joint motion, pain status, and the existence of surgical intervention was documented. Table 10.2 contains the summary profile of the 22 rheumatoid arthritic drivers at the time of their admission. None of the patients had other medical impairments that were contraindications for driving. Four patients had experienced surgical intervention for their arthritis prior to their admission to the Arthritis Center. Patients B and R had undergone right total hip replacement arthroplasties, whereas patient L had had a left total hip replacement arthroplasty. Patient V had experienced a right knee arthroplasty. Finally, patients J and R wore Philadelphia cervical collars because of their atlantoaxial joint subluxation.

Each simulation session began with an orientation period. During this period, the limitations, whether due to pain, restricted movement, or surgical intervention, were determined. The patient was given an explanation of the driver simulator and an opportunity to try out various appropriate driving aids. The author suggested vehicle modifications that the patient might find helpful in making his driving experience possible or easier. Each was then evaluated driving in the simulator, using a driving aid if needed. The simulator offered the patient experience in rural, multilane expressway, and city driving. Table 10.3 summarizes the driving aids and vehicle modifications recommended to the 22 patients at the time of this initial driving task evaluation.

Nine patients were found to need vehicle modification. In other words, 9 patients prior to admission were driving automobiles that potentially could have aggravated their arthritis and decreased their safe driving. Patients J, P, R, and T were found to need such a number of vehicle modifications that they probably needed to purchase new automobiles before their on-the-road performance would prove to be acceptable. Power steering and automatic transmission were the most common vehicle features needed.

Two patients, M and R, needed the benefits provided by hand controls. The most common needed driver aids were additional mirrors and steering aids.

Since simulation driving is not a standardized evaluative test, the patients were scheduled for an on-the-road driving evaluation by a state-approved driving instructor. The in-car evaluations took place 2 or 3 weeks after hospital admission. Some of these patients had been discharged and were outpatients by the time of the on-the-road evaluation. The automobile used contained all of the vehicle modifications in Table 10.3 with the exception of lever-type car door openers, power seat, and power windows. The automobile was equipped for only the push-pull style of hand controls and not the push-right angle-pull style. After a 10-min review of the operation of the automobile used, each arthritic patient was evaluated on his performance during a 40-min driving experience. All of the evaluations occurred over the same type of streets in afternoon traffic conditions.

As a result of the on-the-road evaluation, the state-approved driving

TABLE 10.3. *Driving Aids and Vehicle Modifications Recommended as a Result of Basic Driving Task Evaluation*

Aids and Modifications	Males																	Females				
	A	B	C	D	E	F	G	H	I	J	K	L	M	N	O	P	Q	R	S	T	U	V
Key lever	X					X											X	X				
Car door opening aids	X					X											X	X				
Side mirrors on fenders							X			X	X	X	X					X			X	
Full-view rear mirrors							X			X	X	X	X					X			X	
Steering knob			X^R	X^L		X^R		X^L					X^R					X^R	X^L	X^R		
Quad-type steering cuff	X^R																					
Right-side directional signal	X																					
Left-side gear shift lever	X																					
Complete hand controls (push-right angle-pull)													$?^L$					$?^L$	X^R			
Hand-operated brake pedal														X	X^R							
Hand dimmer switch		X	X										$?^L$					$?^L$	X^R			
Horn extension													$?^L$					$?^L$	X^R			
Left-foot gas pedal		X							X													X
Automatic transmission		X								X						X				X		
Power steering	X					X				X			X			X		X		X	X	
Power brakes		X								X						X		X		X		
Power seats										X						X		X				
Two-door sedan										X						X						
Power windows	X									X						X		X		X		
Lever-type car door opener										X						X		X				

^{R} Recommended for right limb.
^{L} Recommended for left limb.
? = questionable driving aid.

TABLE 10.4. *Driving Status as a Result of on-the-Road Evaluation*

Driving Status	Males																	Females				
	A	B	C	D	E	F	G	H	I	J	K	L	M	N	O	P	Q	R	S	T	U	V
Satisfactory		X	X	X		X		X	X		X				X	X					X	X
Unsatisfactory																						
Needs training with aids	X						X							X						X		
Needs training with performance skills					X												X					
Needs both aid and performance skill training										X		X										
Aids not satisfactory													X						X			
Arthritis believed too severe																		X				

instructor found 50% of the drivers had satisfactory driving skills (Table 10.4). Four arthritic drivers had potential to drive provided they would have additional training with the required driving aids. Two drivers needed training to improve their performance skills. Another two arthritic drivers needed both aid and performance skill training to operate a vehicle safely. Drivers M and S were not able to be evaluated effectively because their recommended aids were not available on the vehicle and they were not able to operate the push-pull type of hand controls satisfactorily. Finally, driver R's stage of rheumatoid arthritis was found to be too severe to permit her to operate a vehicle safely.

Although this evaluation study of rheumatoid arthritic drivers was based on a small sample and need not be representative, it does offer an approach that may be used in evaluating driver performance and in determining vehicle aids and modifications. Also, the study indicates that conventional driving aids, like hand controls, which were designed for the severely disabled patient seemed to be inappropriate for the severely disabled arthritic. Finally, the study indicates the importance of additional training on the road since 8 drivers had potential to drive if they had further training.

VEHICLE, VEHICLE MODIFICATIONS, AND DRIVING AIDS

Various automotive features are commercially available when an individual purchases a vehicle. On some automobiles, these features are considered standard, and they are included whether the purchaser wants them or not. Usually, the more expensive vehicle contains several automotive features that are considered luxury items. Unfortunately, the arthritic patient who purchases a new personal licensed vehicle finds these luxuries are, in reality, necessities.

The automobile of choice is an intermediate or full-sized, 2-door vehicle. The doors on a 2-door car are wider and allow entrance into and exit from the vehicle more easily. Automatic transmission, power steering, and power brakes are almost always necessary features since they help conserve energy expenditure. The availability of cruise control could be a great energy saver for long-distance driving. The arthritic driver could also benefit from auxiliary power features, such as power windows, power door locks, and power seats. In parts of the country where snow and freezing rain are experienced, a rear window defroster is desirable. A tilting and telescoping steering wheel and a pivot seat provide for more comfortable positioning. Finally, the arthritic driver whose hands are painful and deformed should purchase an automobile that has lever door openers. The author knows too many arthritic patients who have had to stand in inclement weather because they were physically unable to open a frozen car door that had push-button openers.

Several foreign manufacturers have exceptionally well-designed vehicles available in this country. For example, the Volvo has been designed with several features appropriate for the arthritic driver. A key feature is the Volvo's front orthopedic-designed reclining seats with adjustable lumbar support. Volvo conducted and sponsored medical research which demonstrated that a firm lower-back support, along with a properly reclining backrest, can greatly reduce forces on the lumbar spine (8). This concept has been incorporated into their automobile and could be an outstanding feature for those with low back pain.

For those arthritic drivers who have difficulty ambulating and require the aid of a manual or powered wheelchair, a van may be able to meet their mobility needs. The use of the van with hand controls, powered steering and braking boosters, and a powered lift can permit driving from a wheelchair if transfer to a modified vehicle seat is impossible. Obviously the van must be modified with additional features so that the operation of the lift can be controlled both inside and outside the vehicle, and the wheelchair secured in the van.

On occasion, modification of the vehicle is easier and less costly than purchase of a new model. For example, if the arthritic driver has automatic transmission and needs power steering, he can retrofit his vehicle with this needed modification. Two new vehicle modifications for those who need to reduce further their steering and braking effort are the Saginaw steering valve and the Bendix aviation brake-assist booster. The Saginaw steering valve can be installed in General Motors and Ford vehicles to reduce the effort necessary to turn the steering wheel further than that offered by factory power steering. The Bendix aviation booster is designed to assist stopping the vehicle when normal braking systems are unsatisfactory.

In addition to vehicle modifications, driving aids also can be retrofitted to a vehicle to make it more barrier free. One important example is the need for additional mirrors on both front fenders. Since many arthritic drivers cannot turn their heads and often their upper torsos a total of 150° they have difficulty in backing up the vehicle and observing oncoming cars when pulling out into traffic. The additional fender mirrors, if properly positioned, can provide this important visual ability.

Conventional mechanical brake-accelerator hand control systems are aids which often have not been found satisfactory for severely disabled arthritics who are unable to brake safely and accelerate their vehicle. The problem is not the required right-angle pull toward the driver's lap to actuate the accelerator; but the push effort to actuate the brake lever often causes considerable discomfort and pain at their wrist. The recent limited availability of the CCI Harden Servo Control has shown that the servo system may eliminate this problem. This servo-control system is designed to provide acceleration and braking power amplification for those drivers who lack the strength to operate the conventional hand controls. Vehicle acceleration and braking is controlled by the displacement of a control handle. The servo-control handle unit is usually attached to the driver's door in front of the armrest. This system uses engine vacuum for its power source. The brake and accelerator have their own vacuum reservoir. The brake system reservoir has enough vacuum supply to make several complete high-speed stops if the vehicle engine stalls.

In the future, there may be a single servo control that operates the brake, the accelerator, and the vehicle's steering. This servo control system operates like the proportional "joy stick" control of an electric wheelchair. Displacing the joy stick forward and reverse controls the braking and acceleration of the vehicle. Moving the joy stick to the left or right from its neutral position controls the vehicle's steering. This special system is currently experimental and is undergoing further development and testing by the Veterans Administration Prosthetics Center (VAPC).

TRAINING AND COUNSELING

The objective of driver training and counseling is to maintain or obtain a state operator's license for everyone enrolled in the training phase. The driving instructor repetitively works with each patient until consistent performance has been demonstrated in the areas found deficient during driver evaluation. This phase of the transportation program is almost always conducted in the program's dual control vehicle. If the driver training requires the use of the candidate's own vehicle because of special driving aids and modifications, a temporary training dual brake may be installed on front passenger's side of the vehicle for about $60. The driving instructor can only conduct the training in the candidate's vehicle if the program's insurance permits. The in-car training should always begin with the patient becoming familiar with the training vehicle on a driving range or an out-of-the-way area. As the candidate obtains skill proficiency, the driving instructor will increase the degree of traffic difficulty. The driving instructor should not overlook reviewing techniques of parallel parking and emergency driving situations.

Successful completion of the training phase does not guarantee that the arthritic is now a safe driver, because the transportation program does not have the legal responsibility to make such a decision. The arthritic driver should be counseled to have his driving performance reevaluated voluntarily by the state licensing agency. I have found that if the disabled driver reports his medical status and is reevaluated and his performance is found satisfactory, the driver's disability will not be prejudical in a future accident. Otherwise, a future accident may lead to cancellation of his vehicle insurance and forfeiture of his operator's license

PHYSICIAN REPORTING OF DRIVING IMPAIRMENT

Recent legal decisions in California (Tarasoff v. Regents of the University of California, 118 Cal. Rptr. 129, 1974) and in Iowa (Freese v. Lemmon, Iowa N.W. 2d 576, 1973) have established that the physician is liable if he fails to warn the patient who has a driver impairment of the potential danger of continuing to operate a motor vehicle (9). This new physician responsibility has created controversy among physicians. Many physicians fear becoming a part of the policing apparatus of licensing jurisdictions, and they also fear that their patients will conceal information and fail to seek any medical treatment in an effort to avoid a revoked operator's license (10).

The possible solution to this controversial issue may be to establish medical advisory boards in each state's licensing agency to develop impairment criteria. Each state medical society could then recommend a course of action to the state advisory board that seems ethically satisfying and medically sound regarding a particular physical impairment like arthritis. It is to be hoped that rheumatologists, orthopedic surgeons, and physiatrists will become involved in this issue since they are professionally oriented toward human performance.

ROLE OF CONCERNED FEDERAL AGENCIES

Recent federal interagency cooperation between the Veterans Administration (VA), the Department of Education, and the Department of Transportation has led to significant progress in permitting the disabled to operate a personal licensed vehicle. These agencies routinely exchange research findings and, where possible, jointly share in the cost of funding research, demonstration, evaluation, and research utilization.

The enactment of Public Law 91-666, entitled "Disabled Veterans' and Servicemen's Automobile Assistance Act of 1970," in June 1971 mandated the VA to address the disabled veterans' driving problems. The public law, in addition to making adaptive driving aids or devices available to disabled veterans, required the VA to establish safety and quality standards for adaptive driving equipment. Since May 1971, the VAPC in New York City has been testing hand control systems and van lifts. This testing effort has led to equipment standards which have been accepted by all of the concerned federal and state agencies. The VA, in collaboration with Texas A & M University, has been studying modified vans to develop prescription indications, safety requirements, and acceptable standards of function and comfort. Recently, Texas A & M University, under a VA contract, has evaluated several experimental servo-control systems which may lead to revolutionary new approaches in resolving the driving barrier for the more severely disabled.

The United States Department of Transportation's National Highway Traffic Safety Administration (NHTSA) has begun research and development projects to provide data on the disabled driver's performance, with or without adaptive controls and driving aids, and to develop education and licensing programs which can improve the disabled driver's performance. Recently, NHTSA and the Department of Education's Bureau of Education for the Handicapped conducted a joint project concerning the impact of motor vehicle driving on public roadways by "special populations."

In addition to the Department of Education's involvement with NHTSA, the Department's National Institute of Handicapped Research (NIHR) has established a Rehabilitation Engineering Center at the University of Michigan to investigate vehicle systems for the severely disabled. This Rehabilitation Engineering Center has established an effective liaison with the automobile industry, and this relationship has begun to generate a greater concern for vehicle redesign and vehicle barrier removal.

Commercial Truck Driving

Arthritis and clinical manifestations associated with rheumatic diseases are prevalent among qualified commercial truck drivers. In 1976, the Bureau of Motor Carrier Safety (BMCS) of the United States Department of Transportation conducted an in-depth study of 4699 qualified commercial drivers to consider the relationships between commercial vehicle accident involvement and the medical fitness of the drivers at fault (11). The study, although not significant, did document the 58 most commonly diagnosed specific health impairments of its subjects. Ten medical conditions were specifically related to arthritis and the clinical manifestations of rheumatic diseases (Table 10.5)!

Skeletal integrity, muscular strength, and joint mobility and stability are necessary physical qualities for effective performance of the commercial driver's driving activities and his related manual tasks. Drivers with rheumatoid arthritis and osteoarthritis are usually disqualified by medical examiners in very early stages of the diseases because of the clinical findings of joint limitation and joint pain when these are reported as detected! A major problem confronting both the physician and the driver is deciding

TABLE 10.5. *Arthritis and Clinical Manifestations of Rheumatic Diseases Found among Commercial Truck Drivers*

Medical Conditions	ICDA Codes*
Arthritis (unspecified)	715
Vertebrogenic pain syndrome	728
Diseases of the knee or operations	729.8, 80.6, 86.5
Pain in joint	787.3
Diseases of bone or operations	720–723, 80.4
Diseases of joint or operations	724–729, 87
Diseases of muscle, tendon, or fascia or operations	730–732, 734, 88–89
Fractures or operations	805–829, 80–84
Dislocations	830–839
Sprains	840–849

* International Classification of Diseases adapted code.

when operating a commercial vehicle has become a hazard to the driver's well-being. For an examining physician to certify or disqualify the driver, he must be familiar with the demands and the environmental stresses involved.

CHARACTERISTICS OF COMMERCIAL DRIVING

Work Patterns and Vehicle Types

Approximately 70% of the nation's commercial drivers are straight-truck drivers. A straight-truck driver operates a truck with various truck body configurations which may have up to 5 axles and 16 wheels. He frequently begins work before 5 AM, loading his truck and arriving at a delivery stop by the time the place of business opens. His work day often exceeds 9 hr, spending much of this time climbing in and out of his truck to load and unload his cargo.

The remaining commercial truck drivers are long-haul or over-the-road drivers. These drivers operate tractor trailer trucks which are comprised of a tractor or front unit and one or two back units called a "semitrailer." There are four types of long-haul drivers: short-relay, long-relay, straight-through, and sleeper.

The short-relay driver leaves his home terminal at a regular time and drives 4–5 hr. At a predetermined place and time, he meets another driver, exchanges trucks, and drives it to his home terminal.

The long-relay driver travels about twice as far as the short-relay driver from his home terminal, accumulating about 10 hr of driving. Upon arrival at the turnaround point, this driver takes an 8-hr rest and subsequently drives another vehicle to his terminal.

The straight-through driver may take several days to reach his final destination. This driver works 10 hr and then sleeps 8 hr in a motel. He repeats this process until he reaches his destination. At the destination, the straight-through driver may or may not have a chance to reload the truck.

His new cargo destination may or may not coincide with his home terminal. Several weeks of "moving on" may occur before he receives a cargo destined for his home terminal which will reunite him with his family.

Like the straight-through driver, the sleeper driver operates his truck in a straight-through fashion except that the tractor is always equipped with a sleeping bunk. The sleeper driver shares the driving and related tasks with his "codriver." Usually, one driver is sleeping or resting in the bunk while the other driver is operating the truck. Sleeper drivers usually follow a rigid "4-hr driving" and "4-hr resting"schedule. At their destination, they may uncouple the trailer or unload their cargo. They may have to divert to another terminal to take on a new cargo or trailer for transport to a new destination. Sleeper drivers are away from home for several weeks at a time.

The tractors that the long-haul drivers operate are custom-built. The owner-operator, a driver who owns his own tractor, often has the tractor built to his specific needs. The fleet motor carrier orders a large volume of tractors at a time, often with little regard to the specific needs of its hired drivers. With the recent Teamster national contract, the cost of driver wages and fringe benefits have often led the motor carrier to hire owner-operators to move the freight since the owner-operators are not bound to Teamster rules and wages.

Environmental Stresses

The truck driver is exposed to both physical and psychosocial stresses that can affect the driver's susceptibility to accidents. Vibration and excessive noise are the prevailing physical stresses, whereas monotony, negative life situations, and lack of social support are the psychosocial stresses. The physical stresses are often overlooked and misunderstood by both the examining physician and the driver.

The source of the vibration is the running truck engine. Truck vibrations are in the 0–15-Hz frequency range, and they are usually applied in the vertical direction via the seat, the floor, and the steering wheel. Vertical axis vibration in the frequency range of 4–6 Hz will produce whole-body resonance or vibration of the seated driver. Research has shown that the driver's performance capacity is affected by frequencies in this range (12). Whole-body vibration in this vicinity can interfere with the driver's ability to maintain his upright posture while driving or his use of his limbs upon exiting the cab. During prolonged driving, the driver uses his body musculature to dampen the strain associated with vibration-induced, internal-pressure oscillations. Unfortunately, the effectiveness of muscle activity as a dampening technique is gradually lowered in relation to driving time, and fatigue occurs. The occurrence of whole-body resonance for some drivers has led to their having experienced chest pain and decreased respiratory function (13). Also, whole-body vibration has been linked with a higher-than-expected prevalence of certain spinal and supportive-structure disorders among truck drivers (14).

In addition to the stress of vibration, truck drivers frequently are exposed to stressful noise levels in excess of 90 db from the roar of the diesel engine. Continued exposure to the meaningless engine and exhaust noises may interfere with the hearing and the health of the driver. Research has shown that noise levels in excess of 75 db can produce cardiovascular alterations and may cause cardiovascular disorders (15). Fatigue, altered thought processes, and nausea also have been reported as disturbances from noise in the range of 75–90 db (15).

Although a few laboratory studies have described the physiological effects and the performance degradation of individual environmental stresses found in the operation of a vehicle, these stresses are rarely experienced as a single stress. Under normal circumstances, the truck driver is exposed to an intricate interplay of environmental stresses while performing several critical tasks during operation of the vehicle. No literature is currently available on combined stress interactions of operating a commercial truck.

Critical Components of Operating a Commercial Truck

Twenty-seven routine and emergency tasks have been identified to be highly critical for a driver with arthritis or any other structural defect to operate a commercial vehicle safely (16). The task descriptions are written in their present form in Tables 10.6 and 10.7 to reflect the current terminology used by truck drivers. Table 10.6 contains those tasks that are performed by the upper left and right limbs. Table 10.7 contains those tasks that are performed by the lower left and right limbs. Some of the tasks are found on both tables because they require both upper and lower limb or limbs to complete these tasks safely.

In addition to the tasks involving the upper and lower limbs, the mobility of the neck is also of considerable importance in permitting the driver to complete critical visual monitoring tasks. While scanning the road ahead, the driver must continuously monitor a sophisticated dashboard of instruments providing information concerning the vehicle's operational status. He also must scan an elaborate system of rear-view mirrors for traffic and such signs of vehicle malfunction as loose cargo covers or burning tires.

Although the critical components or tasks are listed individually, many are completed in combination with each other. Steering, gear shifting, and clutching are often performed by the driver in unison. The driver steers with his left hand and arm while he shifts through as many as 24 gears that require considerable clutching with his left foot and leg. The steering is controlled by an oversized steering wheel of 20–26 inch in diameter requiring, in emergency situations, 70–80 ft lb of force by the driver to maintain vehicle control. Gear shifting, itself, requires moderate strength and timely coordination. Truck engineering has recently incorporated both the main and

TABLE 10.6. *Critical Tasks Involving the Upper Limbs*

Critical Task	Limbs or Limbs Involved			
	Left	Right	Both	Either
Enters/leaves cab			X	
Gets up/down to hook/unhook			X	
Hooks/unhooks electrical cables/air hoses			X	
Fastens/unfastens seat beat			X	
Turns engine on/off (key with push-button starter)			X	
Operates switches (i.e., headlight)				X
Sounds horn				
Air (with lanyard)	X			
Electric (center of wheel)		X		
Shifts gears				
One gear box, single-speed rear axle		X		
One gear box, 2 or more speed rear axle, axle control on shift lever or dashboard		X		
Two gear boxes, 1 shift lever, range control on shift lever		X		
Two gear boxes, 2 shift levers			X	
Perform emergency downshifting		X		
Control steering			X	
Pumps off air brake pressure until "emergency conditions"; depresses 3rd-tank air supply control button and tractor parking brake control button and holds down simultaneously			X	
Operates independent trailer brake		X		
Releases 5th-wheel locking device				X
Operates signals				
"Stalk" turn signal	X			
Push-button type	X			
Emergency flashers			X	
Raises/lowers landing gear assembly			X	
Operates emergency equipment (i.e., fire extinguisher)			X	
Inspects engine compartment				
Conventional cab			X	
Short nose cab			X	
Cab over (hydraulic hand pump)			X	
Applies/releases (hand) parking brake	X			

auxilary transmission into one shift lever eliminating the need for a shift lever for each transmission, in most tractors. For example, the driver operating a 2-range transmission would begin to accelerate and shift the lever in an "H"-shaped pattern, 1-2-3-4-5. While in the 5th speed, he would pull a range button up to move the lever to the 6th speed (Fig. 10.1). The driver would then shift progressively through to the 10th speed. Throughout this process, the driver is engaging and disengaging the truck's power train through the clutch pedal as he shifts transmission gears in response to the rpm reading of the tachometer and the speed of the vehicle.

TABLE 10.7. *Critical Tasks Involving the Lower Limbs*

Critical Task	Limbs or Limbs Involved			
	Left	Right	Both	Either
Enters/leaves cab			X	
Gets up/down to hook/unhook and maintains balance			X	
Inspects 5th wheel			X	
Checks wheels, tires, brakes, and suspension system			X	
Applies (foot) parking brake	X			
Applies brakes				
Applies deep initial pressure on foot brake; as vehicle decelerates, gradually reduces pressure to initiate stop (air)		X		
Applies light initial pressure on foot brake; as vehicle decelerates, gradually increases pressure to initiate stop (hydraulic)		X		
Depresses brakes and clutch simultaneously			X	
Drags brakes while accelerating to dry wet brakes			X	
Operates floor dimmer switch	X			
Operates windshield-washer pump				X

Some of the critical tasks involve nondriving duties, such as coupling and uncoupling the tractor to one or two trailers (Fig. 10.2), and the inspection of the vehicle's mechanical system (Fig. 10.3). These activities demand driver agility as he bends and crawls under the vehicle to evaluate the condition of the brakes, suspension system, tires, and the 5th-wheel engagement (tractor trailer hookup). The driver's physical strength is required in releasing the 5th-wheel locking device, raising and lowering the trailer's landing gear (Fig. 10.4), and inspecting the tractor's engine compartment. Finally, the driver's ability to climb and balance himself is critical in coupling and uncoupling the trailer electrical cables and air hoses (Fig. 10.5). These nondriving tasks are as critical as those involved in driving the vehicle. Some drivers with clinical manifestations of rheumatic diseases have been disqualified because they were unable to perform these work-related duties safely, even though they were fit to drive. Unfortunately, for these drivers, there are few simplifications or vehicle modifications available to simplify or eliminate these nondriving tasks.

TRACTOR MODIFICATIONS FOR THE ARTHRITIC DRIVER

There are only a few tractor modifications available to the arthritic driver. Although these modifications are costly, they can greatly improve the arthritic driver's comfort and safety, as well as decrease the physical effort required in performing some of the critical driving tasks. The availability of these modifications are dependent on whether the driver can afford them as an owner-operator or, as a company driver, acquire them from his motor carrier.

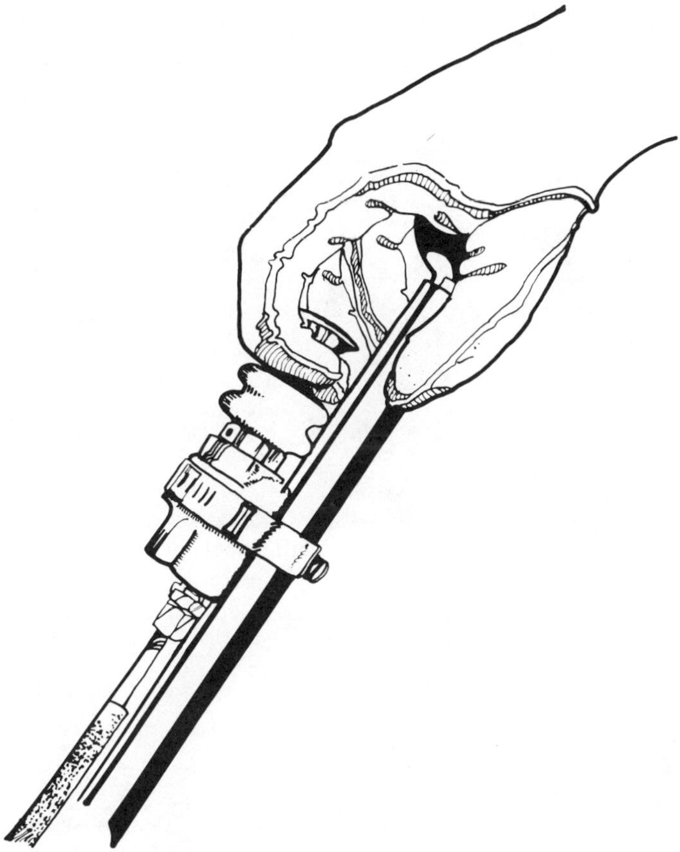

Fig. 10.1. Pulling up on the range selector button to shift into the higher range.

The fully automatic transmission recently has arrived as an important modification in the commercial truck field. Proper shifting and clutching with a commercial truck manual transmission is a complex physical skill that requires a great deal of experience. A gearbox that provides automated shifting eliminates the use of the clutch in driving and automatically provides the shifting of gears for efficient truck operation. The extra cost of the automatic transmission has, of course, been a major roadblock. The additional cost of a heavy-duty fully automatic transmission is at least $5000! The automatic transmission permits an arthritic driver to reduce trip time, decrease bodily fatigue, and increase highway safety because the driver can concentrate on the traffic and keep both hands on the steering wheel.

Power steering, hydraulic and air-powered, is another item that can greatly aid the arthritic driver. Today, with the pressure of crowded streets

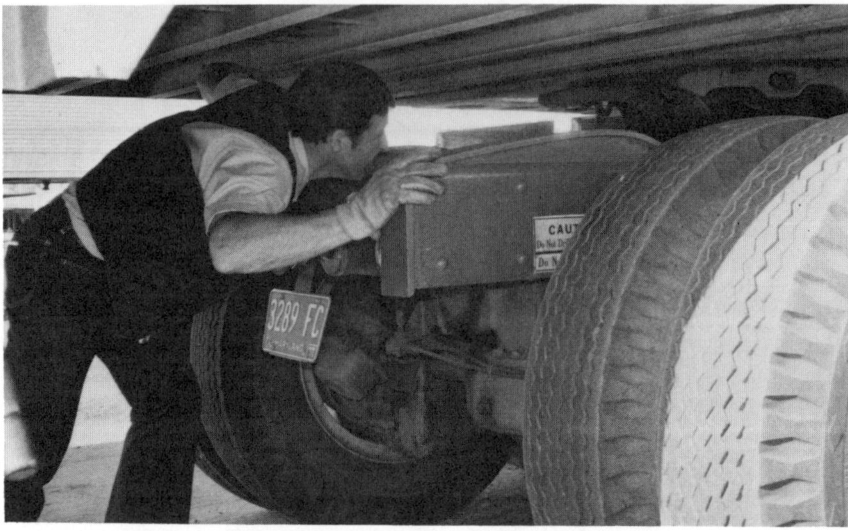

Fig. 10.2. Inspecting the 5th-wheel engagement.

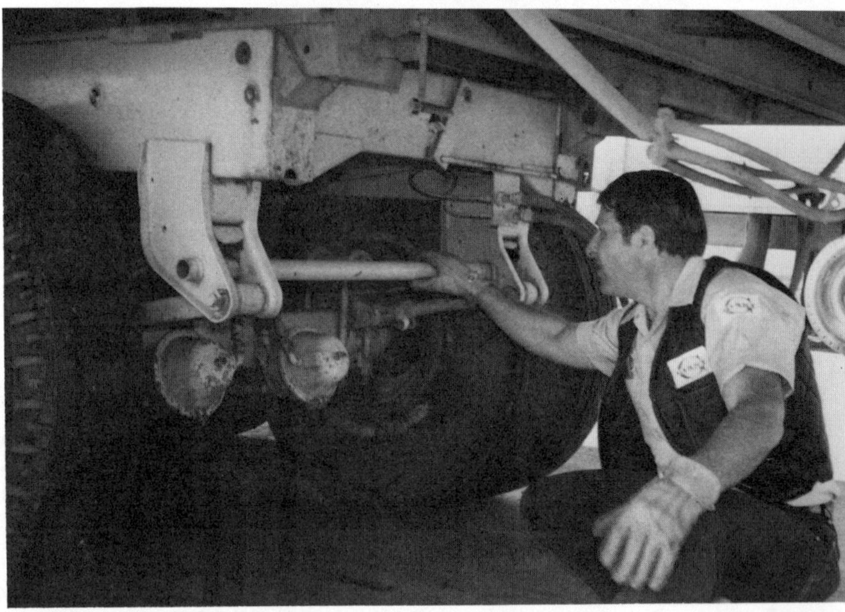

Fig. 10.3. Inspecting the vehicle's suspension system, tires, and braking system.

and highways, with greater emphasis being placed on the dangers of driver fatigue, power steering is getting a second look by truck drivers. Hydraulic power steering has been around for a number of years, but because it cannot be readily installed after the tractor has been built to manual-steering

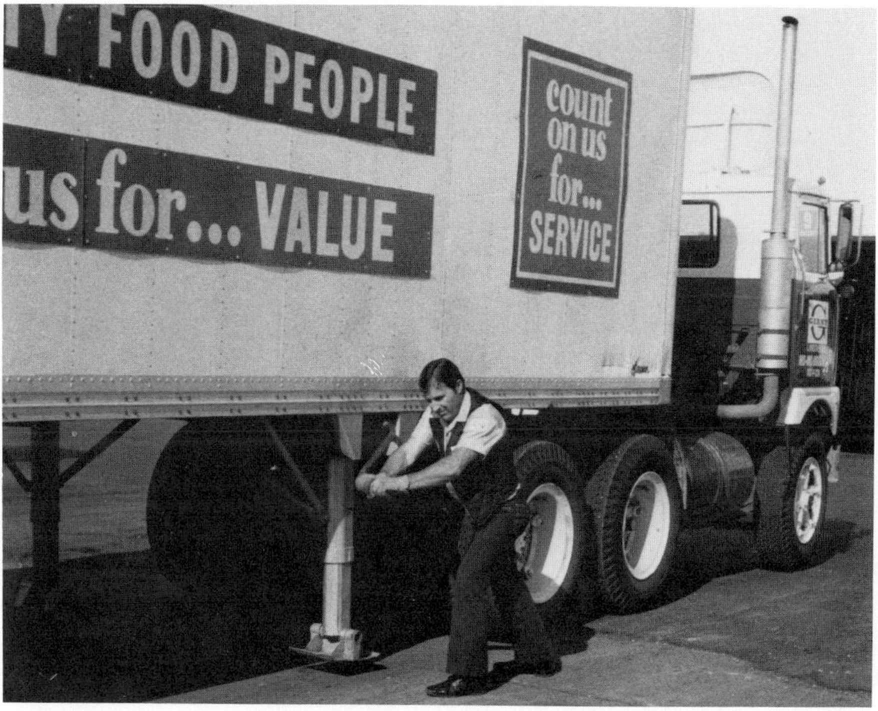

Fig. 10.4. Raising the trailer's landing gear.

specifications, it did not succeed in the trucking industry. Air-actuated power steering, on the other hand, can be installed on any truck without being limited by the geometry of the front end or the ratio of the steering box. One overriding reason for choosing power steering on a truck is the safety benefits it offers. Normally, if a driver were to let his right front wheel drop into a deep shoulder area off the road pavement, it could spell disaster. A manually steered unit will normally whip the steering wheel around in the driver's hand grip enough to cause him physical pain and, in some cases, tear the wheel loose from his hands. Power steering will absorb the shock in this type of situation and, in effect, set up a reverse steering element action as the front wheels try to follow the road edge. When the truck has decelerated to less than 5 mph, the driver can return the wheels to the road.

The deluxe air-ride seat is another vehicle modification which can greatly improve the arthritic driver's comfort and back support. Many standard vehicle driver seats, especially those found in a short-wheelbase tractors are uncomfortable because they vibrate and cause the back of the seat to "backslap" the driver repeatedly in the lumbar spine area. The deluxe seat, suspended on a cushion of air, can be height-adjusted, much like a barber's chair. Also, the deluxe seat has an adjustable lumbar support. A key feature of this seat is that the driver can "dial" his weight into the seat so that it

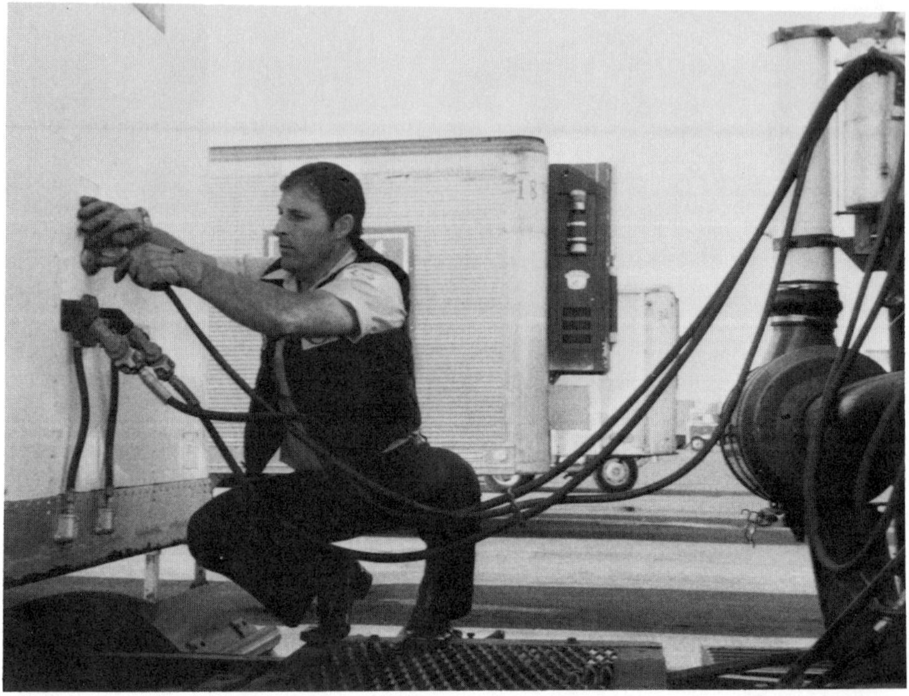

Fig. 10.5. Balancing while coupling the trailer electrical cables and air hoses.

can smooth out the road bumps and vehicle vibrations. The cost of the deluxe seat is between $250 and $350.

The three recommended modifications together could cost the arthritic driver approximately $8000. If the driver is an owner-operator and is still paying for his $50,000 tractor trailer, he may be reluctant to consider any additional expense, even with the need to prevent further clinical manifestations of his rheumatic disease. This is also true of the company driver who fears the loss of his job if he makes his financial demand of the motor carrier. In either situation, the driver needs counseling and professional support if his needs are to be met.

ROLE OF BMCS

The BMCS of the United States Department of Transportation is responsible for establishing adequate medical standards and ensuring that only those persons who are physically and mentally fit drive in interstate commerce. The Bureau relies mainly on the medical profession and the safety investigation cadre of the United States Department of Transportation in discharging these responsibilities.

The established medical fitness standards are subject to the interpretation of the examining physician. Under existing regulations, any licensed physician may medically certify any of the 4–5 million full- and part-time interstate drivers. This regulation is currently being considered for modification. Medical specialists, orthopedic surgeons, and physiatrists are being considered for exclusive certification of all drivers with diseases of the musculoskeletal system and connective tissue. The physician must understand and interpret the established medical fitness standards, be familiar with the applicant's job demands and stresses, and determine the driver's medical fitness in relation to specific work-load factors. The examining physician may incur professional liability through medically certifying a commercial driver who has had a known disqualifying condition if that driver were to use that certificate to drive and were to become involved in a major commercial vehicle accident.

The safety investigator, one of approximately 125 nationwide, can be called upon to evaluate the driver who has clinical manifestations of a rheumatic disease or diseases. The safety investigator can individually examine each case by actually accompanying and determining the arthritic driver's performance of operating a tractor trailer on the highway. Because he is often in contact with motor carrier fleet operators, he may be of assistance to the driver in resolving a disagreement that might lead to the driver's loss of certification. If the arthritic driver's performance is questionable but felt by the safety investigator to be correctable with the use of vehicle modifications, the safety investigator may require that the arthritic driver apply to the Bureau for a waiver under Sections 391.41 and 391.49 of the Motor Carrier Safety Regulations. This waiver, if approved, permits the driver to operate a vehicle (other than a vehicle that transports hazardous materials) in interstate commerce but only if the vehicle is equipped with the required modifications. The waiver application must be submitted jointly by the person who seeks the waiver and by the motor carrier that intends to employ him. The owner-operator can file a waiver application by himself since he at least owns his tractor unless he leases himself to a regulated motor carrier. The Director of the Bureau (Department of Transportation, 400 South 7th Street S.W., Washington, D.C.) has the sole responsibility at the current time to approve or disapprove the waiver application. Should the arthritic driver's performance be unsatisfactory or his waiver be disapproved, the safety investigator can refer the arthritic driver to a vocational rehabilitation counselor for assistance in finding a new vocation if the driver desires.

Use of Public Transportation

The arthritic patient's inability to use pubic transportation to travel to his physician's office or to an arthritis clinic has been a major factor interfering with his ability to secure appropriate medical care for his arthritis (17). A recent study by the United States Department of Transportation supports this statement. Public transportation, in areas served by mass transit, is a critical mode of transportation for the disabled and elderly in securing medical care and therapy (2). Seventy percent of transportation-handicapped people 16 years of age and older depend on public transportation to travel to medical or therapy settings!

Among the many problems confronting the disabled arthritic patient's use of public transportation is the variety of design and travel barriers found on the system that he uses. The travel barriers fall into two categories: those barriers in which the individual acts on the system, and those barriers in which the system acts on the individual (18). The first category refers to the individual's psychosocial and attitudinal barriers as well as his physical disability status. The second category comprises those difficulties encountered by the individual in using the transit vehicles and the terminal facilities. Response to transportation barriers is a highly individual matter. Individuals react differently to the different kinds of barriers. Some elements in the transportation environment which pose serious obstacles for some individuals affect others little or not at all. Both categories of travel barriers can be improved and, in some cases, eliminated through training, but it is quite clear that permanent elimination of the major architectural barriers lies at the heart of any effective or realistic solution for the disabled passenger.

DESIGN OF THE CURRENT PUBLIC BUS AND ITS OPERATION

Of all vehicles used in urban mass transit 80% are buses, and 75% of all urban mass transit riders take buses. The current public bus is usually a 51-passenger vehicle without any provisions for wheelchairs. The bus has a 34-inch floor height with the front door first step approximately 15-inch from the street. The distance of the last rear door step to the street is approximately 16 inch. The two interior steps at both the front and rear door are approximately 9½ inch high. The Flxible Transit Coach, the most common transit bus in urban cities, like Philadelphia, is equipped with two distinct types of doors. The front door, for boarding and alighting, is totally controlled by the vehicle operator. The rear door is an electrically operated touch-type door which is used for exiting only. When the bus operator places the door control lever in position, a green light above the rear door illuminates to tell the passenger that he can disembark. The passenger needs only to touch either door handle to open the door. The rear door will close automatically when the passenger has descended onto the street and is no longer in contact with the door handle.

The interior of the current public bus has a narrow aisle with occasional stainless-steel stanchions and overhead grab bars that run the length of the bus. The seats of the bus are not padded and vibrate when the vehicle's engine is running. The two-bench style seats at the front of the vehicle, located over the wheel well, have been exclusively reserved for disabled and elderly passengers. The cord to signal the operator of a pending exit is located above each seat window.

Because of the pressure from the disabled and elderly population to eliminate the design barriers of the current public bus and the recent federal legislation to implement such an action, a new public bus is now available for purchase by the transit industry. This "interim" vehicle is primarily the General Motors' RTS-II bus, which it began to develop in late 1973. Although this bus can be equipped with a factory-built wheelchair lift, it has not been found to be the answer by the disabled and elderly in meeting their needs and in solving their travel problems. Although the bus floor is 33 inch high and similar in height to the current model, the bus is equipped with a special "kneeling" feature which can lower the floor 9 inch. The kneeling feature can bring the 1st step at the front bus entrance in line with the top of the curb when passengers are boarding. Although this bus can accommodate wheelchair passengers and "kneel" for its ambulatory passengers, the bus still is equipped with the significant interior barriers found in the current model.

The vehicle operator plays an important role in improving or eliminating some of the travel barriers that those disabled experience while traveling on either the current or interim design of public bus. For example, when the vehicle operator pulls the bus up to the curb instead of stopping in the street, the passenger's distance required to climb onto the bus is reduced. This operator courtesy decreases the disabled passenger's potential for physical harm while boarding the bus. With the expanded responsibility of transit agencies to serve passengers with transportation handicaps, disabled passengers are now requiring the operator's physical assistance as well as his courtesy. This new request has presented both the operator and his employer with some grave safety concerns. For example, there is the question of whether a vehicle operator should lift a passenger into or out of the step-entry bus. Potential danger exists for both the person lifted and the person lifting; yet this assistance is, at times, requested and provided. In the best interest of transit operators and their passengers, transit agency management is continually reviewing employee policies and responsibilities, making sure that vehicle operators are aware of their expected roles and are properly trained to carry out these roles.

FUNCTIONAL ACTIVITIES REQUIRED IN PUBLIC BUS USE

The design of the current public bus requires the rider to follow a characteristic profile of functional activities. Due to local conditions or vehicle design, there may be some variations in the profile among passengers. The passenger's functional activity profile begins with walking at least two blocks, often carrying packages weighing up to 10 lb, locating the bus stop, and then waiting until the bus arrives. The passenger frequently stands for more than 10 min in the outdoors during all kinds of weather. Once the desired bus has arrived, he must climb the bus steps, deposit his fare and possibly obtain a bus transfer, and locate a seat—all while maintaining his balance as the bus proceeds to the next stop. If a seat is available, he has to negotiate the often crowded aisle to be able to sit down. If all the seats are occupied, he must ride standing, holding onto a vertical stanchion or overhead grab bar to support himself. As the passenger approaches his destination, he has to be able to locate his stop, pull the signal cord, and exit down either the front or rear door steps. Once the passenger has disembarked and has safely moved away from the vehicle as it departs, he often walks at least 2 or 3 blocks to his destination. In some cases, the passenger has to repeat this process as he transfers from one bus to another before reaching his final destination.

Twenty-four specific functions or activities are listed in Table 10.8 in a sequence most often followed by passengers using the current public bus as

TABLE 10.8. *Categorical Functional Activities Required by Ambulatory Passengers in Public Bus Use*

Activities	Critical Activities	Potential Operator-assisted Activities
1. Walks 2 blocks to bus stop carrying 10 lb	X	
2. Stands waiting at least 10 min	X	
3. Identifies correct bus	X	
4. Ascends front bus steps from curb	X	
5. Ascends front bus steps from street	X	
6. Places change in coin box/shows reduced fare card/ obtains transfer		X
7. Walks to seat while bus is stationary	*	*
8. Walks to seat while bus is moving		X
9. Transfers to seat while bus is stationary	X	
10. Transfers to seat while bus is moving		X
11. Sits and maintains balance while bus is moving	X	
12. Stands and maintains balance while bus is moving		X
13. Stands up from seat while bus is stationary	X	
14. Stands up from seat while bus is moving		X
15. Pulls signal cord		X
16. Walks to front exit while bus is stationary	*	*
17. Walks to front exit while bus is moving		X
18. Walks to back exit while bus is stationary	*	*
19. Walks to back exit while bus is moving		X
20. Descends front bus steps to curb	X	
21. Descends front bus steps to street	X	
22. Descends back bus steps to street		X
23. Walks 2 blocks to destination carrying 10 lb	X	
24. Stands waiting at least 10 min to transfer to another bus	*	*

* Neither critical nor potential operator-assisted activities.

their transportation mode. A passenger may not perform all of the activities found on the list at one time because the person making the trip may not desire to carry out certain activities, or he may be forced to perform others because of unplanned situational factors. Ten activities are designated critical activities that all passengers must be able to perform to use the current designed bus safely. Nine activities are designated potential operator-assisted activities. These nine activities do not preclude a passenger from traveling safely and independently because the vehicle operator can and does, in cities like Philadelphia, routinely assist the passenger in these activities. For example, the vehicle operator, if asked, can maintain the bus stationary until the passenger is safely seated. This operator courtesy eliminates the passenger's need for physical assistance in getting to a seat while the bus is in motion.

BUS USE BY THOSE DISABLED BY ARTHRITIS

In January 1975, the Moss Rehabilitation Hospital in Philadelphia expanded its Transportation Evaluation and Training Center to investigate the effects of public bus transportation on people with physical disabilities and to train them in its use. One area that was studied was the assessment of the ability of 25 rheumatoid arthritic patients to use the current public bus found in Philadelphia (19). This study developed from the combined efforts of the Transportation Center, the Southeastern Pennsylvania Transportation Authority (SEPTA), and the 24-bed Arthritis Center of Moss Rehabilitation Hospital-Albert Einstein Medical Center. The study utilized the 19 functional activities (activities 4–22) found in Table 10.8.

Twenty-five patients (20 women and five men) with rheumatoid arthritis, with a mean age of 61 years, took part in this study. All of the patients were diagnosed as having classic or definite rheumatoid arthritis, as defined by the American Rheumatism Association. All of them were in stages II and III with the exception of one 69-year-old man and one 67-year-old woman classified as in stage I. Forty-four percent (10 women and one man) stated that they used the current public bus as their primary mode of transportation prior to admission to the Arthritis Center.

The functional assessment tool consisted of a 4-point scoring system describing performance of the 19 functional activities. The individual's performance of each activity was scored as independent, requires supervision, requires assistance, and not feasible/a hazard. Upon the individual's completion of all 19 activities, he was graded functionally as to his ability to use public bus transportation. The four possible scores were: travels independently, travels with supervision, needs training, and travel not feasible. An individual was functionally scored "travels independently" if he received a score of "independent" in all 19 activities or in combination with those activities scored "required assistance," as found in Table 10.8 under the column entitled "potential operator-assisted activities." These nine activities did not preclude a subject from traveling independently because of vehicle operator courtesy. If any of the critical activities found in Table 10.8 among the 19 activities were scored "not feasible/a hazard," the subject was graded functionally "not feasible" in traveling by public bus. The investigators believed that these seven critical activities, if performed unsuccessfully, designated a significant hazard to the patient's safety in traveling by public bus.

Of the 11 rheumatoid arthritis subjects who stated that they used the public bus prior to admission, only four subjects (three women and one man) were found to be able to use the public bus independently at the time of the evaluation. The investigators stated three possible reasons for this discrepancy in the subject's performance. The reasons were: reduced physical performance from disease exacerbation during the current hospital admission, denial of the limitations of rheumatoid arthritis, and the necessity to use the public bus, irrespective of one's physical state, just to meet basic personal needs.

EVALUATION, COUNSELING, AND TRAINING IN PUBLIC BUS USE

During February 1975, the Moss Rehabilitation Hospital Transportation Center and SEPTA mutually agreed to an exchange of services, initially for 1 year, so that the center could expand its program to provide public bus evaluation and training for its ambulatory patients. A major obstacle in reaching agreement on the exchange of services with SEPTA was the question of liability for patient injury. The issue was resolved by the hospital agreeing to self-insure the program. The Transportation Center agreed to provide an audiovisual employee training package for SEPTA in return for the use of a SEPTA current-designed public bus once a week during a weekday off-peak period. At that time, the center decided to charter a SEPTA bus for a 2nd weekday each week to provide continuity for the training portion of the Center's activities.

Since that time, a SEPTA bus has been used on each Tuesday and Thursday between the hours of 12:30 PM and 2:30 PM. This period of time is divided into two 1-hr sessions. The 1st session is primarily used for outpatients, and the 2nd session is primarily used for inpatients. Each hourly session is further divided into smaller blocks of time. The first 20 min of the session are devoted to a series of stationary activities, with the next 30 min used for the moving activities. The moving portion involves a 6-mile bus ride. The bus travels over various road conditions, with heavy to light traffic, with turns, and with frequent starts and stops. The moving portion of the session is always over the same fixed route at the same time of day. Upon the bus's return to the hospital, the remaining time is spent on ascending and descending the front door as well as on descending the back exit to the street.

Each arthritic candidate accepted for the public transportation program spends at least 1 hourly session being evaluated. He is observed performing the 24 bus activities (see Table 10.8) by an occupational therapist. The performance is evaluated in both the stationary and moving activities by using the 4-point scoring system previously described. If the patient is found to have potential for independent use of the public bus but still requires training, a minimum of two sessions are spent with the therapist to resolve problems and reinforce techniques.

A considerable effort has been made in the public bus program to consider and incorporate training of pedestrian activity. The arthritic must be able to walk several blocks before and after taking the public bus if he is going to be completely independent in this mode of transportation. Instruction includes gait training with the proper use of ambulation aids. Techniques for handling intersections, choice of pedestrian routings, and approaches to long waits and crowds are taught.

With the proper identification of the arthritic patient's public bus transportation difficulties by the rehabilitation team, the patient will be able to be trained, with or without adaptive methods, so that he can safely travel on public transportation with minimal physical trauma and maximal energy conservation. For those patients found not to be able to travel by public bus safely, the rehabilitation team should assist in finding an alternative mode of public transportation and counsel them in the hazards of continuing to use the public bus.

ALTERNATIVE AND FUTURE PUBLIC TRANSPORTATION

Many urban mass-transit agencies throughout this country have assisted a number of private nonprofit agencies in their local service areas to apply for funding to purchase equipment for transportation services under Section 16 (b) (2) of the Urban Mass Transportation Act of 1964, as amended. The purpose of these capital grants was to assist these private nonprofit agencies in the provision of transportation to the elderly and disabled where mass transit services for this special population were unavailable, insufficient, or inappropriate. Two distinct types of specialized transit services have been developed as a result of Section 16 (b) (2): door-to-door and door-through-door services.

Door-to-door service, with lift-equipped vehicles, can provide travel for elderly and disabled people who are uneasy about travel on regular transit vehicles or are unable to use regular vehicles because of their disabilities. The vehicles used by this service are often vans or small buses designed to make getting on and off and riding easy and comfortably. The passenger is picked up at his door and is provided with necessary assistance by a trained driver. The passenger is taken to his destination in a reasonable length of time, with several other passengers boarding and exiting while the vehicle is in route. Once the passenger has reached this destination, he is again given necessary assistance by the driver to exit the vehicle. It may be necessary to request this service 24 hr in advance. The cost to use this service would be at least three times the cost of the current public transportation fare or approximately less than half the cost of a taxi fare for the same distance.

Door-through-door service is a highly specialized service utilizing on-vehicle escorts or multiduty drivers to provide passenger assistance. The escort would provide such assistance as helping the passenger into his home, carrying his packages, and providing social service information. This type of service is particularly health- and welfare-oriented, serving disabled persons who are not independently mobile. The cost for this service often approaches that of a taxi fare. Recently, several private profit-making systems have been established throughout this country on a franchised basis to provide door-through-door service. These private systems are expensive and usually beyond the income of most of those disabled.

Both types of specialized transit service can and do provide true mobility to the user whether he is infirm and elderly or disabled by arthritis and wheelchair-bound. Several major urban transit systems have developed a complementary specialized service that is flexibly routed, with vehicles designed for but not limited to the nonambulatory disabled. This complementary service links with the regular fixed route system at selected barrier-free surface routes.

In the next 10 years, specialized transit services will become integrated with the conventional fixed transit system in major urban areas. Also, many small towns and rural settings will develop new rural transportation systems which will be both barrier-free and specialized from the outset. By 1984, many major transit systems, like SEPTA in Philadelphia, would have begun to receive the Transbus, a radically different intracity bus designed specifically to meet the needs of the disabled and elderly and to replace the interim bus. The Transbus or "low-floor bus" was to have its floor only 22 inch above the ground. Also, the vehicle was to have the capability to "kneel" down to 18 inch. A retractable ramp or a lift and a 44-inch-wide door would have permitted those confined to wheelchairs to use the buses. Unfortunately, the Transbus has been discontinued because of bureaucratic red tape, engineering design problems, and manufacturer unavailability. It can be hoped that a bus like the Transbus will be available to the elderly and disabled in the near future.

ROLE OF URBAN MASS TRANSPORTATION ADMINISTRATION (UMTA)

UMTA of the United States Department of Transportation is an outgrowth of federal legislation passed in 1964. This was a start in recognizing public transit, whether by bus or by rail, as a necessary public service in urbanized areas. UMTA has been working to remove the travel barriers confronting the elderly and disabled since the late 1960's. The agency's elderly and disabled transit activities initially centered around its administrative initiatives, its research, and its demonstrations. Recently, the agency's efforts have been mostly administrative through its regulatory process. Because of UMTA-sponsored programs, public transit systems in the United States have been responding to the needs of the elderly and disabled in three ways: reduced fares or special fare systems, specialized transportation services, and accessible vehicle and facility design (18).

In the National Mass Transportation Assistance Act of 1974, Section 5 amended, Congress provided UMTA with a new formula grant program for operating and capital assistance to urbanized public transit systems. In this act, Congress included an obligatory half-fare for elderly and disabled riders during the off-peak period of transit use. Most of the transit systems have been operating this program on a simple cash-paid reduction basis, once the disabled or elderly riders have shown some form of identification attesting to their eligibility.

During 1973, the Urban Mass Transportation Act was amended by adding Section 16 (b) (2). Section 16 (b) (2), as previously stated, provided capital grants to private nonprofit corporations for the provisions of specialized transportation to the elderly and disabled where mass transit services for this population were unavailable, insufficient, or inappropriate.

Since 1970, the national mass transit policy, as encompassed in Section 16 (a) of the Urban Mass Transportation Act and more recently in Section 504 of the Rehabilitation Act of 1973, has mandated that publicly funded mass transportation vehicles and facilities be accessible to the elderly and disabled. The progress of "mass transit accessibility" has been very slow and almost always negotiated under the pressure of litigation. Both the question of cost for implementing accessibility and the question of the need for fully accessible transit systems have caused the delay. Recently, UMTA has proposed new regulations that state that existing bus systems must have, within 6 years of the regulation's implementation, a level of "accessible" regular service equal to half of the peak-hour service and all of the off-peak service. Also, all interim buses ordered prior to the availability of a "Transbus" must be fully accessible if it is technically feasible. Obviously, the existence of a barrier-free and personalized public transportation system in urban areas is at least 20 years away for both the UMTA and the disabled and elderly.

Conclusion

For arthritic individuals, transportation is the "life line" which permits them to maintain or obtain employment, transact personal business, enjoy the social and recreational opportunities which are available to the able-bodied, and obtain appropriate medical care (for arthritis, dental, and eye corrections) we take for granted. Until recently, however, research has not addressed the special transportation requirements and needs of those who have arthritis. Most of the research effort in transportation modes—personal licensed driving, commercial driving, and use of public transportation—has centered around the questions of what the transportation requirements are for each mode, and what the evaluation and training goals should be for the normal population in each mode. Researchers have believed that until this information is known, as it now is, it is difficult to specify what deviations or changes are necessary for a special population.

This chapter has attempted to inform both the physician and therapist of the state of the art of each of the three transportation modes and of each mode's relationship to the clinical manifestations of the rheumatic diseases where possible. It is hoped that each health professional will utilize this information to better evaluate, counsel, and train his arthritic patient in the safe and appropriate use of a transportation mode.

REFERENCES

1. Michaels, R. M., and Weiler, N. S. *Transportation Needs of the Mobility-Limited.* The Northeastern Illinois Planning Commission, Evanston, Illinois: Transportation Center, Northwestern University, 1974.
2. United States Department of Transportation, Urban Mass Transportation Administration. *Summary Report of Data from National Survey of Transportation Handicapped People.* Washington, D. C., June 1978.
3. Waller, J. A. Medical impairment and highway crashes. *J.A.M.A., 208:* 2293, 1969.
4. Koppa, R. J., McDermott, M., Leavitt, L. A., and Zuniga, E. N. Handicapped driver controls operability: A device for clinical evaluation of patients. *Arch. Phys. Med. Rehab., 59:* 227, 1978.
5. Reger, S. I., Law, D. F., McGloin, A. T., and Spence, R. E. Development of a Driver Evaluation-Trainer Aid for the Handicapped. In *Proceedings of the 5th Annual Conference of Systems and Devices for the Disabled.* Baylor College of Medicine and Texas Institute for Rehabilitation and Research, Houston, Texas, 1978, pp. 106–108.
6. Jonsson, S., and Jonsson, B. Function of the muscles of the upper limb in car driving. V. The supraspinatus, infraspinatus, teres minor and teres major muscles. *Ergonomics, 19:* 711, 1976.
7. Duff, I. F., Carpenter, J. O., and Neukom, J. E. Comprehensive management of patients with rheumatoid arthritis. Some results of the regional arthritis control program in Michigan. *Arthritis Rheumat., 17:* 635, 1974.
8. Andersson, B. J., Örtengren, R., Nachemson, A., and Elfström, G. Lumbar disc pressure and myoelectric back muscle activity during sitting. IV. studies on a car driver's seat. *Scand. J. Rehab. Med. 6:* 128, 1974.
9. Jacobs, S. Reporting the handicapped driver. *Arch. Phys. Med. Rehab. 59:* 387, 1978.
10. Hames, L. N. Physician reporting of driver impairment; searching for answers. *J.A.M.A., 234:* 1027, 1975.
11. Gruber, G. J., Calvert, E. K., and Bernet, J. M. *The Role of Chronic Medical Conditions in Commercial Vehicle Accidents.* Bureau of Motor Carrier Safety, United States Department of Transportation, Contract no.: DOT-FH-11-8274B, Washington, D.C., 1976.
12. Hornick, R. J. Vibration. In *Bioastronautics Data Book,* Ed. 2, edited by J. F. Parker and V. R. West. NASA SP-3006, United States Government Printing Office, Washington, D.C., 1973.

13. RAMEY, J. I. Occupational Vibration. In *Occupational Medicine Principles and Practical Applications,* edited by C. Zenz. Year Book Medical Publishers, Inc., Chicago, pp. 553–562, 1975.
14. FISHBEIN, W. I., & SALTER, L. C. The relationship between truck and tractor driving and disorders of the spine and supporting structures. *Indust. Med. Surg. 19:* 444, 1950.
15. HODGE, D. C., AND GARINTHER, G. R. Noise and blast. In *Bioastronautics Data Book,* Ed. 2, edited by J. F. Parker and V. R. West. NASA SP-3006, United States Government Printing Office, Washington, D.C., 1973.
16. WILSON, A. B., AND BOBLITZ, M. H. *Limb Prosthetics for the Bureau of Motor Carrier Safety.* Bureau of Motor Carrier Safety, United States Department of Transportation, Control no. DOT-FH-11-9047, Washington, D.C., 1977.
17. EHRLICH, G. E. *Total Management of the Arthritic Patient.* J. B. Lippincott, Philadelphia, 1973.
18. REVIS, J. S., AND REVIS, B. D. *Transportation and the Disabled: an Overview of Problems and Prospects.* United States Department of Health, Education, and Welfare, Office of the Assistant Secretary for Planning and Evaluation. Washington, D.C., October, 1976.
19. ROSENTHAL, D., BOBLITZ, M. H., AND RAO, V. D. Bus use by disabled arthritics: functional requirements. *Arch. Phys. Med. Rehab., 58:* 220, 1977.

11

Joint Conservation and Protection

EVELYN ROSSKY

Joint conservation has increasingly become accepted as the most important program that occupational therapists can offer the patient. Most chronic inflammation, the most chronic disease of the joints, does not destroy the joint completely. Inhibitions and alterations in function may occur as a result of connective tissue disease, and these can often be overcome by intelligently conceived programs of exercise and functional use, especially when initiated at the inception of the disease.

Written instructions have been developed in our Arthritis Center to supplement individual and group training *and* concrete experiences—behavior is *not* changed by a lecture. The following pages are adapted and elaborated from this manual, and are presented as if addressed to the patient, in language intended to persuade. The references and their bibliographies represent the growing support in the literature; they provide the health professional with a current index to the body of knowledge fundamental to the understanding essential for preparation of an informed patient capable of participating in his own care.

Why Joint Protection?

For you with joint disease, a major purpose of treatments prescribed by our doctors—drugs, injections into your joints, splints, or surgery—is to keep *your body* functioning. This booklet is your Owner's Manual.

If you have rheumatoid arthritis, you know that it affects your whole body, *including* your joints. This manual is for you, most of all.

For you with degenerative joint disease alone or other problems related to connective tissue disease, your therapist will point out specific sections.

Techniques that can save energy, reduce stress and pain, are worth learning. You're not an athlete in training; you are eager to do what needs doing when you can and to find pleasure where you can; knowing the best ways can free you for both.

Remember: when rheumatoid arthritis is active, you need added REST (1, 2). This is the time for *isometric* exercises—muscle tightening without joint movement—so that there's no pain (3, 4). Count out loud as you hold the muscle contraction (this keeps you from holding your breath) for about 6 sec (5), and your lungs will be ready to fill again when you let go.

All joints should be gently taken through their *pain-free range* of motion; even once a day can prevent stiffening and loss of use (6, 7). When moving the weight of your arm is more than the shoulder muscles can sustain, a family member can be taught to help you, or you can use stronger muscles to help the weak ones (8). You may need splints to relieve pain and provide local rest for your joints in good position (9–12). Simple devices and special techniques can help you care for yourself: a sponge instead of a washcloth lets you press the water out. A buttoning device protects tender, painful joints and fingertips. A dressing stick will ease clothes off tight, hard-to-move shoulders and arms, pull a drawer open, or move a shoe closer.

When arthritis is not acute, regular activity, using all joints to their fullest range, is very important—but in the right way. Your home exercise program planned for you by your therapists, for stretching and for strengthening, should be built into your daily routine where it fits best. Be sure you know one or two easy exercises for each joint so that you never skip a day (e.g., moving limbs while lying in bed so that gravity is eliminated (13)). Add the activities that are a necessary part of your day—and an important part of that is play—and you should be able to plan for a total that permits the highest level of satisfying function for you, without leaving you exhausted. Staying mobile is part of your personal responsibility (14).

You know that you have good days and bad days. We know that if you consistently get some rest on your good days (as tempting as it is to try to "get everything done"), the bad days will not be as bad or as frequent.

Remember: joints that have been affected by inflammation, that have been or are swollen, can be damaged more easily than normal joints. They are vulnerable because they don't "fit" as perfectly as they once did. Pressures from outside and inside can contribute to deformity. You'll be learning new ways of doing the things that are part of your typical day—not only to avoid pain, but to *protect your joints.* You will be changing some old habits—not *you,* just your habits.

Consider: each person with arthritis has different interests, desires, and problems. The principles of joint protection that follow are important to all, and their value will become evident as you talk with your therapist and as you begin to apply them. If you don't understand any part as you read, or how it relates to you, you *must ask.*

BE AWARE OF BODY POSITIONING

A position of flexion (bent knees, hips, elbows, fingers) can lead to deformity if held for long periods, so: lie face down, if possible, for 10 or 15 min or more twice a day, *with your feet over the end of the bed* for total muscle relaxation. Your body weight helps to straighten hips and knees. This is called "proning," and balances time spent in a chair with hips and knees bent. If you cannot lie on your stomach, even with a pillow under your chest to protect tightened shoulder muscles, lie on your back or side and s-t-r-e-t-c-h with your heel toward the foot of the bed—first with one leg, and then with the other (15). But do it daily without exceptions.

You know that a pillow under the knees eases the knees and the low back, *but* if you have rheumatoid arthritis, you must choose instead the positioning and stretching just described.

If propping your face on your hand is a comforting habit, uncurl fingers and straighten them against your cheek, chin in palm.

Sitting for long periods leaning on bent elbows? Relax your arms into your lap; and if your hands are puffy, rest them at a comfortable height on a table or on a fat, light pillow (16, 17); or pinch back your shoulders as you cross your arms on your chest, thumbs down, fingers up (18). Notice that the curves of your fingers fit the curves of your arms, gently stretching each joint without stressing other joints. Breathe in, then out, filling and emptying the lungs fully just twice—a simple mini-tension-reliever you'll find useful.

You can see that extension (opening out) of all joints is being emphasized along with support in good position and reduced muscle tension to ease pain and improve motion: BE AWARE.

THINK GRAVITY: BECOME AN EXPERT IN BODY MECHANICS

You have seen weightless spacewalkers on television, but *we* have to move our arms, legs, bodies, and other objects against—or *with*—the forces of gravity. A tall ladder standing perfectly upright can be easily held in that position. But it takes power to hold a ladder that has begun to fall. This concept also applies to your body. Your body is balanced if, as you walk, you hang your shoulders under your ears, with your knees, hips, and back in good alignment. When you begin to slump all of your muscles have to work harder to keep you "upright" against gravity (19). In this position you'll tire more quickly, and weak or damaged supports around your joints are challenged (20).

Good sitting posture also insures that your arms are in the best functional position, and that your lungs have room to fill when you breathe. You'll tire less quickly, feel better, and *look* better.

Learn the most efficient way to get up from a chair: slide your buttocks forward, knees together, your feet (flat on the floor) back under the chair, then lean forward so that you are looking down at your shoes. Now, with palms on the chair arms, push off as you push up with hips and knees. With your center of gravity brought forward in this way, you're using good body mechanics, with all muscles working together. Choose to sit in the chair with arms but if this is not possible, turn sideways and with one arm on the chair back, the other on a table top, push up.

Remember: you've got to keep at it. When you're taking a shower, when you're brushing your teeth, when you're walking to work or around the house (put up extra mirrors), when you're sitting at the table, at your desk, or in your car—THINK GRAVITY.

THINK CHANGE: DON'T OVERWORK MUSCLE GROUPS OR JOINTS

Tired muscles cannot share in protecting your joints and the work is left to ligaments and other supporting structures. The abnormal tensions and pressures affect joint surfaces as well as circulation (21–23).

Stand if you can, for some of your work, but sit *before* your legs are too tired. Any sturdy stool that is higher than an ordinary chair makes getting up and sitting down easier. To shift weight or to relieve a tired back, put one foot up on a small stool, or up on the floor of your opened sink cabinet or work table.

If you are talking to a friend at the market, support your back against a wall or support your arms on a shopping cart. Lean against the sink if you're doing the dishes—it "unweights" the hip and knee joints.

If your responsibilities include vacuuming, cleaning windows, or waxing the family car or silver with repeated, tiring movements (often against gravity) as well as gripping (often a heavy object), break the job down into small parts, change the way you do it, or get help in getting it done.

The static grasp of handwriting is eased by a foam cylinder (from a curler) by a felt-tipped pen—or use an electric typewriter if you can. Knitting and crocheting are not therapeutic because these activities involve holding more than moving. But if they mean joy to you, stop approximately every 10 min to stretch and rest. A fat, lightweight pillow in the lap cradles the arms and holds the work high. THINK CHANGE.

THINK POWER: USE BIGGEST MUSCLES, STRONGEST JOINTS

Our chewing muscles are among the strongest in the body. Rest your fingers on each cheek in front of the ear as you clamp your teeth and feel those muscles tighten (now take a second to let your jaw hang loose and feel those muscles "let go"—it's good practice for learning to release muscle tension). The jaw is a powerful lever that lifts and positions the teeth, providing the force for grinding food. When a tooth is lost, that same power becomes an abnormal force that tilts strongly rooted teeth into the empty space, causing joint pain (24).

Now look into the palm of your open hand. Curl the fingers in, then out, then spread them apart. Your "knuckles" are very mobile joints, and each *finger* is *jointed* so that you can pick up a grape, a lemon, an orange, a grapefruit—or pat a child's head (25, 26). Each joint is constructed for a lifetime of "normal" use, but the repeated swelling and inflammation of rheumatoid arthritis (27) as well as the repeated stresses of some jobs (28–31) can change joint construction. New ways of doing things can protect unstable joints from deforming forces.

Your fingers, then, are not for weight-bearing, so push up on your palms, or use forearms on a firm table. To move about in bed, try a portable trapeze, and consider slippery, satiny sheets. To get out of bed, try a portable bed-rail or a straight chair backed to the bedside.

Use body weight to move an object: close a drawer with your buttocks or move a chair with your hips.

The power for lifting comes from the muscles of your legs, not your back, so do not bend over without bending the knees. THINK POWER.

THINK PRECISION: USE YOUR HANDS THOUGHTFULLY

The special way your *thumb* works with your fingers makes the hand a precision tool—an engineer's "impossible dream." Your fingertips "see" to button up under the chin or to tie an apron behind your back (32). In order to ease stress on fingers lubricate dials and knobs and locks. Use needlenose pliers for power-pinch (33–35). Use a gadget to open your car door, an adaptation for the car-key, and never a thumb for a thumbtack. Hooking replaces pinching when you attach cotton tape loops where needed: a long loop stitched into each side seam of your slacks (if you do not have belt-loops) and you can "hook" them on with your palms; a loop on each end of washcloths and towels, and you can not only reach to bathe and dry back or feet but you can hang the cloth by its own loop to drip dry.

For you with rheumatoid arthritis, almost from the beginning *gripping* has been sometimes painful, sometimes impossible. If you make a fist and look at it in the mirror, you can see that your knuckles slope down from index to little finger. The bones of the hand are shaped and attached to each other to allow the small and ring fingers to hold while the middle and index fingers work with the thumb to do precision tasks—like knot-tying. In the hand with chronic synovitis (inflammation of the joint lining), that built-in sloping contributes to deforming forces (36, 37), and gripping (making a fist) can tear at damaged pulley systems of the tendons in the palm (38–41). Therefore, choose workshop and kitchen tools with fat handles and light weight. Wrap foam on handles of tools you use often to fatten and soften the gripping surface.

As loops spare and protect small muscles, so do levers, with more efficient use of available power from large muscles, protect your hands from twisting forces. Use offset screwdrivers and long-handled wrenches. Consider an oven-spade as a lever to lift mattress corners while making a bed. Find lever-type doorknobs and sink faucets, or change round ones to levers with adaptations. Allow handwash to drip dry; don't wring it. Use lightweight handwipes or sponges and *press* out moisture instead of twisting.

Stop and think: whether you are holding a golf club or a steering wheel, you can do it with less tension without losing good control (42), saving energy as well as practicing good joint protection. PAY ATTENTION.

WATCH YOUR HANDS

During your usual way of doing some familiar activities, you'll see that the fingers are being pushed against each other, as when you hold a knife to cut, rather than supporting each other in good alignment, as when you hold a knife like a dagger. Therefore, hold your razor-sharp, thick-handled steak knife like an ice pick (or a dagger), and use a pulling action to cut. Your joints are more stable in this position and you get more power per pull.

Slide, don't lift (gravity again). If you must lift, slip palms of both hands *under* plates, bowls, or pans. Do not grip edges. Use oven mitts for removing hot dishes from the oven.

Dishwashing in hot water feels good. Use your hands as you've learned to, and wear your wrist splints under large lined rubber gloves.

Open screw-top jars by leaning your palm on the lid and using shoulder motion. Place the jar on the sink bottom (low for leverage), a sponge-cloth under and on top for stability and traction. NO FINGERS. Remind the family not to tighten them again.

Never hold a cup by its handle (look at your fingers!). Use a thermal cup and hold it palm to palm. The comfortable heat feels good.

LOOK AT YOUR FINGERS

In the small jobs your fingers do again and again, day after day, individual finger joints can be placed under abnormal pressures that can cause pain and even dislocation over time. In activities such as button-pushing or dialing: slip a foam curler over a pencil, hold it like an ice pick, and use the eraser end as a fingertip—or ask your occupational therapist for a device to help you (43).

For opening cans: use a wall-mounted (low, of course), crank-operated opener, or an electric opener with good leverage.

For using scissors: try several electric models at the store for weight, comfort in the hand, and ease in using the on/off button—as with any appliance. Long handles with short blades improve leverage, sharpening and lubrication improve efficiency and both reduce joint stress.

RESPECT PAIN

The body usually gives the danger signal of pain if joints are placed under harmful stress. Be alert for stiffness that lasts more than an hour after an activity (not passing discomfort). Stop and think about the cause of the discomfort so that you can change the method or the time. Apply the same rules to your exercise program; *more is NOT better.*

Remember, skill that you acquire in relieving muscle tension (44, 45), whether by positioning, breathing, partying, listening (to music, a talk show, or a friend) helps you to ease your own pain (46).

PLAN FOR A BALANCE OF REST AND ACTIVITY

In addition to your medications, you need 8–10 hr of sleep at night, and a rest period during the day. Teach yourself to do part of a job, then stop *before* you are tired. Alternate hard and easy jobs, remembering that working with your arms can be tough even if you're sitting (47).

Have at least one chair that really fits you, comfortably supporting your arms, back, and head. To remove the pressure of a chair edge from your thighs, make a simple support to elevate your feet slightly (e.g., using a slab of styrofoam or a phone book). Consciously relax your body in a position of good alignment—neck to toes.

CONSERVE YOUR ENERGY

Re-plan your work areas to save yourself, on the job, in the workshop, and around the house.

Use wheeled tables or carts to move food, laundry, and projects (more than one is even better).

A cutting board placed across an open kitchen drawer makes a high work area to pull up a stool.

Use convenience foods in simple nutritious menus (48, 49).

Check out the supermarket freezer for tempting, balanced frozen meals to keep your body fueled. Prepare in a tabletop oven, if energy or mobility are limited.

When your shoulders are painful—or if those muscles just can't lift the weight of your arms against gravity: put nose or eye drops in while still in bed; support your elbows on a table (or washbasin) while combing your hair or shaving; or prop your arm against the wall to don a shirt. You'll use less power, control the pain, and keep your shoulders mobile.

PLANNING

Not buying impulsively, not moving unthinkingly, not waking up to an unplotted day does not mean an end to spontaneity. But planned purchases reduce frustration, and planned motion reduces muscle tension; rushing against time wastes energy and invites the pain of a surprised joint.

The quality of attention and awareness you would give for expected guests is appropriate and rewarding when planning for time spent with your mate, with your family, or for an hour alone. DO IT!

Adaptations and devices make life easier (50). *Consider*: clothing made of stretchy fabric, with front openings and easy-on-the-fingers fastenings (51); a free-standing dustpan to be used to bring the floor up to you; a 2-inch slice of broomstick slit to fit over the end of a knife blade making it a 2-handed chopper; three yards of nylon net cut in half the long way with a loop knotted into each end to make one foot-scrubber and one back-scratcher; a wooden back scratcher as a dressing stick.

You have problems to solve and solutions to share. Make notes, *ask questions*. START NOW.

REFERENCES

1. Smith, R. D., and Polley, H. F. Rest therapy for rheumatoid arthritis. *Mayo Clin. Proceed., 53:* 141, 1978.
2. Ditunno, J., and Ehrlich, G. E. Care and training of elderly patients with rheumatoid arthritis. *Geriatrics, 25:* 168, 1970.
3. Muller, E. A. Influence of training and inactivity on muscle strength. *Arch. Phys. Med. Rehabil., 51:* 449, 1970.
4. Magness, J. L., Lillegard, C., Sorenson, S., and Winkowski, P. Isometric strengthening of hip muscles using a belt. *Arch. Phys. Med. Rehabil., 52:* 158, 1971.
5. Nutter, D. O., Schlant, R. C., and Hurst, J. W. Isometric exercise and the cardiovascular system. *Mod. Concepts Cardiovasc. Dis., 41:* 3, 1972.
6. Lowman, E. W. *Arthritis.* Little, Brown and Co., Boston, 1959. p. 182.
7. Flatt, A. *Care of the Rheumatoid Hand,* Ed. 3. C. V. Mosby Company, St. Louis, 1974, p. 37.
8. Wilson, C. H. Exercise for Arthritis. In *Therapeutic Exercise,* Ed. 2, edited by J. V. Basmajian. Williams & Wilkins Co., Baltimore, 1978. pp.514–530.
9. Thomas, H. O. *Diseases of the hip, Knee and Ankle Joints,* Ed. 2, 1876, with supplement *A Review of the Past and Present Treatment of Inflamed Joints.* Little, Brown & Co., Boston, 1962, pp. 141–147.
10. Partridge, R. E. H., and Duthie, J. Controlled trial of the effect of complete immobilization of the joints in rheumatoid arthritis. *Ann. Rheum. Dis., 22:* 91, 1963.
11. Mills, J. A., Pinals, R. S., Ropes, M. W., Short, C. L., and Sutcliffe, J. Value of bed rest in patients with rheumatoid arthritis. *N. Engl. J. Med., 284:* 453, 1971.
12. Ehrlich, G. E. Rest and Splinting. In *Total Management of the Arthritic Patient.* J. B. Lippincott Company, Philadelphia, 1973, pp. 47.
13. Swezey, R. L. Exercises with a beachball for increasing range of motion. *Arch. Phys. Med. Rehabil., 48:* 253, 1967.
14. Cailliet, R. Chronic pain: is it necessary? *Arch. Phys. Med. Rehabil., 60:* 4, 1979.
15. Baier, R. E., Shafrin, E. G., and Zisman, W. A. Adhesions: mechanisms that assist or impede it. *Science, 162:* 1360, 1968.
16. Plewes, L. W., and Owen, J. The swollen hand. *Physiotherapy, 45:* 59, 1959.
17. Weeks, P. M., and Wray, R. C. In *Management of Acute Hand Injuries.* C. V. Mosby Company, St. Louis, 1973, pp. 119–120.
18. Hollis L. I. Splint substitutes. *Am. J. Occup. Ther., 21:* 139, 1967.
19. Williams, M., and Lissner, H. R. *Biomechanics of Human Motion.* W. B. Saunders Co., Philadelphia, 1962, p. 40.
20. Radin, E. L., Paul, I. L., Rose, R. M., Simon, S. R. The Mechanics of Joints as it Relates to their Degeneration. In *Symposium on Osteoarthritis, American Academy of Orthopedic Surgeons.* C. V. Mosby Company, St. Louis, 1976, pp. 38–39.
21. Thomas, H. O. *Diseases of the Hip, Knee and Ankle Joints,* Ed. 2, 1876, with supplement *A Review of the Past and Present Treatment of Inflamed Joints.* Little, Brown & Co., Boston, 1962, pp. 172–173.
22. Goldthwait, J. Rheumatic diseases: pathological considerations. *Am. J. Occup. Ther., 19:* 127, 1965.
23. Basmajian, J. V. *Muscles Alive,* Ed. 4. Williams & Wilkins, Baltimore, 1978, pp. 178–179.
24. Marbach, J. J. Arthritis of the temporomandibular joints and facial pain. *Bull. Rheumat. Dis., 27:* 919, 1977.
25. Landsmeer, J. M. F. *Anatomical and Functional Investigations of the Articulation of the Human Fingers.* S. Karger, New York, 1955. p. 64.
26. Napier, J. Evolution of the hand. *Sci. Am., 207:* 56, 1962.
27. Brewerton, D. A., and Lettin, A. W. F. The Rheumatoid Hand and its Management. In *Rehabilitation of the Hand,* Ed. 2, edited by C. B. Wynn Parry. Butterworth and Co., London, 1973, p. 298.

28. Backhouse, K. M. Mechanical factors influencing normal and rheumatoid metacarpophalangeal joints. *Ann. Rheumat. Dis., 28 (Suppl.):* 15, 1969.
29. Swanson, A. B., and Swanson, G. deG. Disabling Osteoarthritis in the Hand and its Treatment. In *Symposium on Osteoarthritis.* C. V. Mosby Co., St. Louis, 1976, pp. 199–200.
30. Hadler, N. M., Gillings, D. B., Imbus, H., Levitin, P. N., Makuc, D., Utzinger, P., Yount, W., Slusser, D., and Moskovitz, N. Hand structure and function in an industrial setting. *Arth. Rheumat., 21:* 210, 1978.
31. Howell, D. S., Woessner, J., Jimenez, S., Seda, H., and Schumacher, H. A view on the pathogenesis of osteoarthritis. *Bull. Rheum. Dis., 29:* 996–1000, 1979.
32. Moberg, E. Methods for Examining Sensibility of the Hand. In *Hand Surgery,* Ed. 2, edited by T. Flynn. Williams & Wilkins Co., Baltimore, 1975, p. 295.
33. Cooney, W. P., and Chao, E. Y. Biomechanical analysis of static forces in the thumb during hand function. *J. Bone Jt. Surg., 59A:* 36, 1977.
34. Linscheid, R. L. Demonstration of subluxing forces at the metacarpotrapezial joint. *Clin. Ortho., 123:* 87, 1977.
35. McGrath, M. H., and Watson, H. K. Arthroplasty of carpometacarpal joint of the thumb in arthritis. *Ortho. Rev., 8:* 127, 1979.
36. Hakstian, R. W., and Tubiana, R. Ulnar deviation of the fingers. *J. Bone Jt. Surg., 49A:* 299, 1967.
37. Swezey, R. L., and Fiegenberg, D. S. Inappropriate intrinsic muscle action in the rheumatoid hand. *Ann. Rheum. Dis., 30:* 619, 1971.
38. Smith, E., Juvinall, R., Bender, L., and Pearson, J. Role of the finger flexors in the rheumatoid deformities of the metacarpophalangeal joints. *Arth. Rheum., 7:* 467, 1964.
39. Wise, K. S. The anatomy of the metacarpophalangeal joints with observations of the aetiology of ulnar drift. *J. Bone Jt. Surg., 57B:* 485, 1975.
40. Herbison, G. J. Finger Motion Related to Rehabilitation. In *Symposium on Reconstructive Hand Surgery,* edited by J. W. Littler, L. M. Cramer, and J. W. Smith. C. V. Mosby Co., St. Louis, 1974, pp. 246–262.
41. Bywaters, E. G. L. Jaccoud's syndrome—a sequel to the joint involvement of systemic lupus erythematosus. *Clin. Rheum. Dis., 1:* 147, 1975.
42. Basmajian, J. V. Motor learning and control. *Arch. Phys. Med. Rehabil., 58:* 40, 1977.
43. Making Adaptive Equipment with Polyform (Bull. 2-128-R1). Roylan Medical Products, Menomonee Falls, Wisconsin.
44. Heep, R. B. Effects of Biofeedback Assisted Muscle Relaxation on State Anxiety Levels and Cognitive Processes in an Anxious Physically Disabled Population. Doctoral Dissertation for Temple University, Philadelphia, 1977, p. 15.
45. Green, E. E., Green, A. M., and Walters, E. D. Verbal Procedure Used in Developing Voluntary Control of Internal States in Autogenic Feedback Training. In *Stress and the Art of Biofeedback,* edited by B. B. Brown, Bantam Books, New York, 1978, p. 257.
46. Melzak, R. *Puzzle of Pain.* Basic Books, New York, 1973, pp. 31, 201.
47. Semmler, C., and Semmler, M. Counseling the coronary patient. *Am. J. Occup. Ther., 28:* 611–612, 1974.
48. *Mealtime Manual,* Ed. 2. Campbell Soup Co., New Jersey, 1978.
49. Parrish, L. *Cooking as Therapy.* Avon Books (Arbor House), New York, 1975.
50. *Self Help Manual for Arthritis Patients.* Arthritis Foundation, Atlanta, Georgia.
51. Kernaleguen, A. *Clothing Designs for the Handicapped.* University of Alberta Press, Alberta, Canada, 1978.

12

Splinting in the Rheumatic Diseases

HANNA GRUEN

Splinting for the patient with rheumatic disease continues as a primary treatment modality used by occupational therapists. It is important to comment, however, that the efficacy of this practice remains, in *most* instances highly subjective and controversial. This is by no means to imply that it should be discarded: only that we are made aware of the need to study and validate our procedures.

Even basic splinting terminology remains variable among centers and authors. For purposes of this chapter let us simply label splints relative to the function they are expected to perform. 1. Static or resting—those used exclusively for rest. They may be placed on various parts of the extremities with the wrist and hand in combination (Fig. 12.1) and the knee being the most common. 2. Functional—those which in any way assist functional ability. The traditional wrist cock-up (Fig. 12.2) is used to stabilize a subluxed wrist or to support a painful wrist in order that hand function may be enhanced by decreasing pain. 3. Dynamic—those providing force or energy. The classic Swanson postoperative splint serves as a good example.

In the case of metacarpophalangeal (MCP) synovitis a functional splint may include immobilization of that joint and, though not allowing for power grasp, it may allow for fine pinch activity with decreased pain and decreased stress to the inflamed joint. This splint may be used solely as a rest splint. The metacarpal ulnar deviation splint is one of several antiulnar deviation devices used when there is little or no wrist involvement (Fig. 12.3). It is believed by many that these offer good MCP alignment in the presence of moderate ulnar deviation of the digits (this splint was devised in and has been widely used in the United Kingdom). The Quest-Cordery splint is a similar splint used to enhance function by alleviating ulnar deviation and restricting MCP flexion while the hand is actively in use.

There are a number of small individual finger splints using a three point pressure principle to assist in the reduction of swan neck and boutonierre

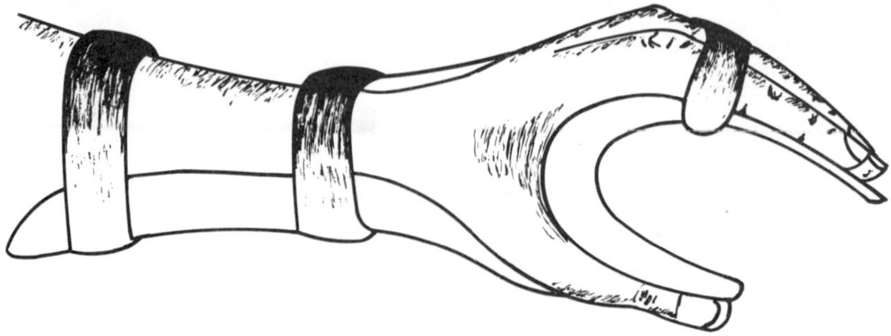

Fig. 12.1. Resting wrists, hands, and fingers type of splint. This is used to immobilize, *rest* joint during acute inflammatory painful episode to decrease pain.

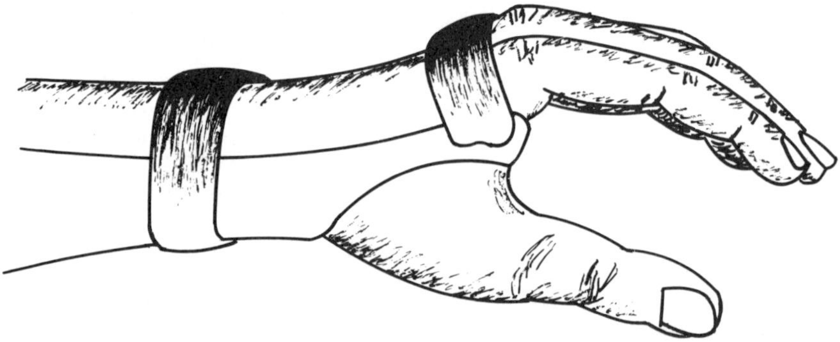

Fig. 12.2. Wrist cock-up splint. (*A*) Stabilize subluxed wrist mechanically, increase hand *function.* (*B*) immobilize wrist to allow for pain-free hand *function.*

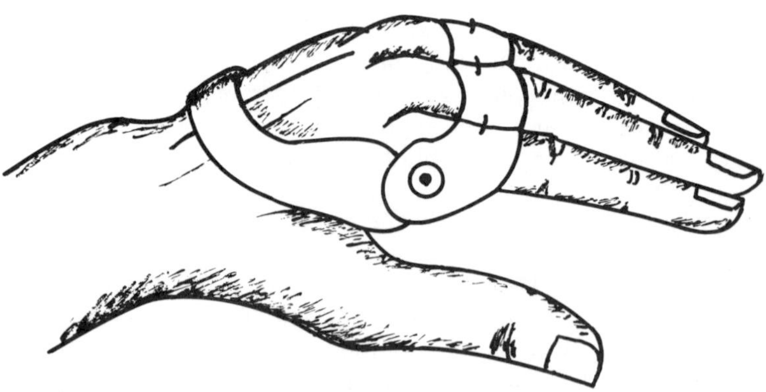

Fig. 12.3. Antiulnar deviation splint. Align MCP and restrict MCP flexion in presence of ulnar drift to increase *function*.

deformities commonly referred to as ring splints. Miniature knuckle bender splints offer dynamic force and are used by some in effort to release contracture.

Thumb splints have received more attention lately. They are functional splints that either include the carpometacarpal (CMC) and proximal thumb joints or are used correctively to gain better function in the case of a boutonniere or hyperextended distal thumb joint.

Probably the most frequently used postoperative splint is either the Swanson or some facsimile of it designed to maintain postoperative alignment and position of the MCPs after synovectomy or replacement arthroplasty—the wrist is maintained statically in functional position and the outrigger or extensor assist reduces possible extensor lag and minimizes ulnar deviation. Sometimes flexor assists are added when that motion is problematic. These assists may be used along with flexor straps or flexion gloves for stretching intrinsics with early tightening.

The next question is—do they work? Let us look at splinting for the purpose of providing the hot, inflamed joint with rest. The fact that this will produce favorable results is well documented. Gault and Spyker (1) splinted one side of their experimental group (that side which was most involved) and allowed the patient to be his own control. Plaster of Paris resting splints were used for a period of 3 weeks and were removed briefly for heat application and gentle exercise after which they were reapplied. The nonsplinted side was used for all functional activity. Participating patients did not have advanced disease. Swelling was decreased in wrists and fingers and, though joints did flare during the period of immobilization, no flares were noted in those joints that had been immobilized. At the end of the study, the nonsplinted extremity was found to have more active disease than the side which had been splinted. Partridge and Duthie (2) also substantiated decreased inflammation directly related to rest. Numerous other studies in which hands, wrists, and knees have been splinted bear out the thesis that rest through immobilization does indeed reduce swelling and pain, thus offering one source of control to the inflammatory process. Smith and Polley (3) used the Mayo Clinic Proceedings to advance their thesis that "rest therapy for rheumatoid arthritis" is beneficial. The paper is a strong advocate of articular and systemic rest during the acute phase of inflammatory disease. In their concluding paragraph they state: "Until more specific therapy for rheumatoid arthritis becomes available, the balance between exercise and systemic and articular rest should be the cornerstone, if not the keystone, of all other therapy." Thus we have substantial evidence that splinting during the acute stages of the disease is indeed indicated and valid!

It seems appropriate at this point to mention the use of stretch gloves which might, with some stretch of the imagination, be considered a form of resting splint! Ehrlich (4) in 1971 wrote of the use of stretch gloves for night resting for a group of 44 women complaining primarily of morning stiffness and or night time pain and tingling as a result of interphalangeal osteoarthritis primarily. Disease activity was varied initially. After 2 weeks, the great majority of patients reported relief of symptoms. Similar results were obtained in some instances of rheumatoid arthritis and of scleroderma, and later confirmed by Moskowitz.

While discussing the use of splinting in acute, painful conditions it should be stated that there are conditions, often rheumatic disease related, for which splinting is also a valid consideration. Those that come to mind are DeQuervain's Disease, acute tenosynovitis of the long abductor and short extensor tendons of the thumb, occurring over the radial styloid, and the often painful flexor tenosynovitis with median nerve entrapment known as carpal tunnel syndrome. Both present as acute wrist problems with subsequent influence on hand function. It has also been documented, however, that in the case of the latter, surgical intervention, even if delayed, in most cases will eventually take place.

Lest we get too excited, it must also be stated that these studies are relatively short term and do not speak of recurring bouts of inflammation over the time span that one is affected by the disease.

Let us now look at the wrist cock-up splint used to improve hand function by eliminating or diminishing wrist pain and/or by stabilizing the wrist to mechanically enhance function of the hand. Remember, Adrian Flatt (5) long ago said that "the wrist is the key to hand function as it influences extrinsic muscle balance." Chaplin et al. (6) have espoused this theory relative to juvenile arthritis, and Fried, in Licht's book on arthritis in 1969, said "A painful wrist interferes with function" in an experimental study in a nonstructured clinic setting in Pittsburgh, 54 patients were splinted at the wrist and instructed to use them for activities of daily living and night resting. When they were recalled within the year, most reported "good wrist support and relief of pain." They did wear them for heavier activity but reported them cumbersome for fine coordinated movements. Documentation validating this type of splinting is difficult to find. Subjectively, there is little question that patients using it do report relief of discomfort while working with it on. Patients with painful wrists report liking it while lifting and carrying because of stress reduction on the weakened, painful joint. Again, we must look at the practical side of this issue. Occasionally, patients have adapted to using the hand in a poor mechanical position to such an extent, that function is actually decreased by the application of such a splint. Another unfortunate but realistic consideration is the negative attitude of employers, insurance companies, and unions whose policies prohibit the use of such devices on the job. Therefore, the evaluation for splint use must be composed of more than anatomical consideration and may often be a matter of trial and error.

Other antideformity splints are highly controversial and there is to date no substantial evidence that they have value. In the case of the MCP flexion contracture with or without ulnar deviation, an anticontracture splint, if you are able to fit it, may be of great help in maintaining hygiene of palm and avoiding maceration of the skin. In the presence of ulnar drift, maintaining the hand in a more functional position has been known, subjectively to decrease pain and enhance function—if that be the case, splinting would appear to be appropriate. However, again, many patients find these splints awkward and believe that they actually decrease their functional ability, in which case you may be sure the splints will be unused!

Personally, I have had little experience with anti-swan neck (Figs. 12.4 and 12.5) and boutonniere splints. I have on several occasions placed a small lightweight ring splint on a patient with early and correctable swan neck deformity of the index finger (Fig. 12.5) and it did appear to enhance pinch; I cannot, however, report on length of compliance! Others have become interested in this type of splint and are using it, again, very subjectively, reporting short-term positive results. Very few seem to advocate stretch of boutonniere deformity via splint as there is no evidence that it is effective. In fact, this type of dynamic splinting is viewed by some with disdain. Convery et al. (3) believed that dynamic splinting neither enhanced function while applied nor attained deformity correction. Further they believed that deformity progression was not prevented and, in fact, frequently there was greater limitation of motion after a period of splinting. Swezey (7) has stated "since the deformities are dynamically induced, immobilization of the hand

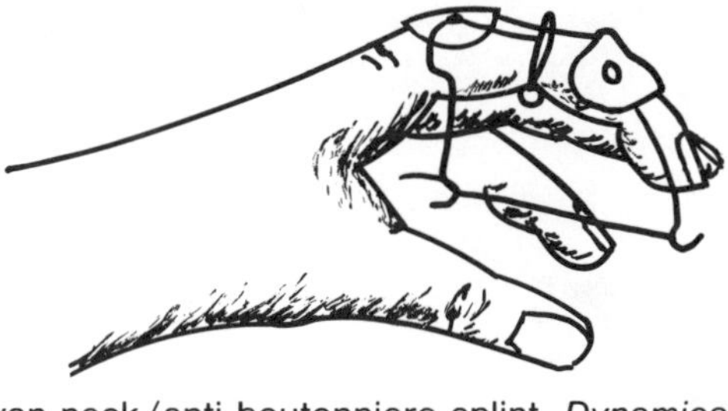

Fig. 12.4. Anti-swan neck/anti-boutonniere splint. *Dynamically* stretch contractures.

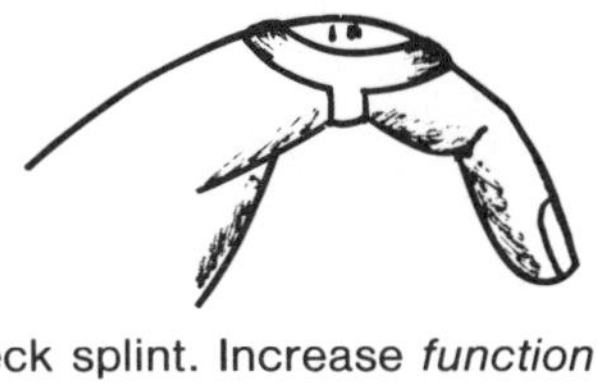

Fig. 12.5. Anti-swan neck splint. Increase *function* by splinting actively correctable deformity.

to protect it against the deforming forces is impractical as this would preclude use of the hand for protracted periods of time."

Much of the literature regarding thumbs relates to surgical stabilization of either the proximal or distal joints (8–16). However, there are instances in which splinting does help by either repositioning the distal thumb into slight flexion to allow for pinch (e.g., thumb boutonierre) (Fig. 12.6) or in the case of the painful CMC and/or proximal joint in osteoarthritis. My experience with this splint has been positive. Patients whom I have fitted with such a splint have worn them when they had pain resulting in a problem with function. Two examples stand out in my mind—one, a butcher with involvement of the carpometacarpal joint of his dominant hand, the other, a real estate saleswomen, also with dominant CMC involvement—her problem involved unlocking and opening doors in both cars and the homes she was showing.

Let us momentarily backtrack to the wrist—remember, again its importance to hand function. Early wrist contracture is worth trying to ameliorate via serial splinting. I have not found the literature helpful in substantiating this finding: or can I offer more than minimal experiential evidence of its effectiveness. I have used this for both juvenile and adult patients.

Results on postoperative dynamic splinting are less well substantiated. It seems that authors on the subject concur on early postsurgical hand mobilization for which a splint is usually most appropriate (Fig. 12.7). In a 1977 publication by Madden et al. (8) the final sentence of their abstract reads: "although this study does not compare various post-surgical schemes in a controlled experiment, we believe that the early motion and prolonged splinting program outlined is a major factor responsible for increased range of motion." In an unpublished study by McDowell et al. (9) the following is

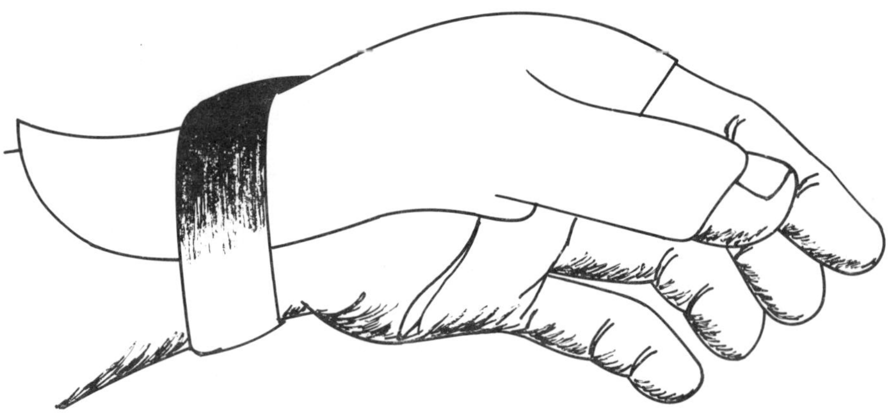

Fig. 12.6. Thumb splint. (*A*) Increase *function* by offering decreased pain to CMC and/or proximal joint. (*B*) Increase *function* by correcting actively correctable boutonniere.

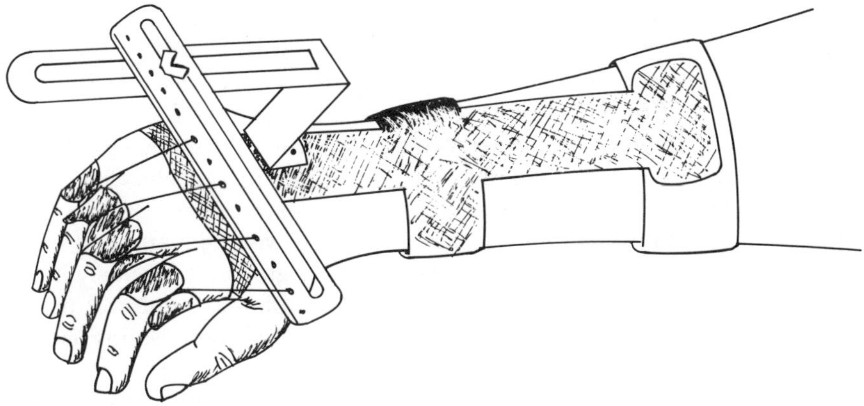

Fig. 12.7. Postoperative splints. *Dynamic* assist to maintain surgical correction during healing process.

stated: "while our data do not exactly define the contribution of dynamic splinting to the results of silastic replacement it is clear that it is of major importance." The group in the former study has advocated probably one of the most aggressive postoperative hand programs of which I am aware. Early passive range of motion (5 days postoperative) together with 6 weeks of continuous dynamic splinting was done routinely. Most splints were individually made to accomodate various hand deformities of nonoperated joints. The 4th and 5th digits were taped together to ensure active MCP flexion of the 5th digit. Flexion bands were in some cases applied by the 4th postoperative week and used initially for 2 hr with gradual increase to overnight use. Daytime splinting was discontinued after 6 weeks and patients were encouraged to use their hands for light activity. After 8 weeks all activity was encouraged without any restriction whatsoever. The study followed patients for no less than 6 months, and some for over 2 years, with apparently good results.

Of late, patient education has become a favorite modality. There is no doubt that patients need to know how to use their splint, that is how to apply and remove it, how to care for it, frequency of use, potential problems (pressure) and, most of all, the rationale for use. Many patients do not understand why they have been fitted with a splint; frequently they report awkwardness, inability to function with it on, to say nothing of the bill they have received for an appliance which they see as valueless.

Some of the inexpensive commercially made splints may be of value under certain circumstances. When it can be well fitted without causing discomfort or dysfunction, it often serves as a test splint prior to making a more costly one. Families should also be instructed in splint usage; their understanding and support may increase patient adherence.

Now that we have waded through the controversies and hypotheses—how does one make the decision "to splint or not to splint"? What are the indications and guidelines? Relief of inflammation, is one unquestionable indication. Relief of pain, subjective though it may be, is always a worthy consideration. Beyond this there are no definitive answers. However, Dr. Maria Musur of Warsaw, Poland offers a simple little guide. She classifies hands into three categories with subsequent treatment goals; the splinting application portion is as follows. 1. Hands with swelling, pain, and minimal to no deformity night resting splints or isotoner gloves. 2. Hands with early deformities (ulnar deviation, swan neck, boutonniere, thumb) all passively correctable—patient may or may not be able to maintain. Splint useful for: maintaining position; decreasing inflammation; stretching intrinsics; supporting of arches (support of MCP may allow PIP flexion in Swan neck). 3. Hands with noncorrectable, fixed deformity splinting of little value except to provide comfort for dislocated wrist.

It is clear that the majority of contemporary splints are made for the hands and wrists to enhance function and to reduce inflammation (11–13). Long leg splints to assist knees in extension still have an important place. They may well hinder the development of flexion contractures. The knee, as the wrist, may also benefit from serial plaster casting especially in the presence of early soft tissue contracture (14, 15).

Ankle, foot orthoses, especially the fitted plastic variety, can help improve continued active arthritis in the ankle, especially if pronation-eversion deformities are present (15, 16). Not to be forgotten is an important supportive foot splint, namely a properly fitting shoe! Extra depth shoes made of soft leathers and having few seams often enhance patient mobility.

Collars and spinal corsets and braces also help special problems. A well-fitted collar may help the patient with early atlantoaxial subluxation. It certainly serves as a reminder to the patient to avoid extremes of neck motion which are contraindicated and pain producing in the presence of cervical involvement.

Various types of splinting materials are now available. The low temperature products that can be molded directly on the patients have added much to the efficiency of splint application. There are also a few ready made lightweight splints which work very effectively but they must be used judiciously as they do not properly fit all clients.

It is known that splinting is effective for short-term pain relief, and in some instances long-term relief. That is the aim of all splinting and functional enhancement represents an additional bonus.

REFERENCES

1. Gault, S. J., and Spyker, J. M. Beneficial effect of immobilization of joints in rheumatoid and related arthritides: a splint study using sequential analysis. *Arth. Rheumat., 12:* 1, 1969.
2. Partridge, R. E. H., and Duthie, J. J. R. Controlled trial of the effect of complete immobilization of the joints in rheumatoid arthritis. *Ann. Rheumat. Dis., 22:* 91, 1963.

3. CONVERY, F. R., CONATY, J. P., AND NICKEL, V. L. Dynamic splinting of the rheumatoid hand. *Orthot. Prosthet., 22:* 41, 1968.
4. EHRLICH, G. Stretch gloves: nocturnal use to ameliorate morning stiffness in arthritic hands. *Arch. Phys. Med. Rehabil., 52:* 479–480, 1971.
5. FLATT, A. The Care of the Rheumatoid Hand, Ed. 3. C. V. Mosby Co., St. Louis, 1974.
6. CHAPLIN, D., PULKKI, T., SAARIMAA, A., AND VAINIO, K. Wrist and finger deformities in juvenile rheumatoid arthritis. *Acta Rheum. Scand., 15:* 223, 1969.
7. SWEZEY, R. L. Dynamic factors in deformity of the rheumatoid arthritic hand. *Bull. Rheumat. Dis., 22*: 1 and 2, 1971–72.
8. MADDEN, J. W., DEVORE, G., AND AREM, A. J. A rational postoperative management program for metacarpophalangeal joint implant arthroplasty. *J. Hand Surg., 2:* 358, 1977.
9. McDOWELL, J., GRUEN, H., WINGERT, B., AND KAPPAKAS, G. Silastic replacement of rheumatoid metacarpophalangeal joints: four year average follow up. Unpublished 1978.
10. MUSUR, M. Personal communication.
11. MALICK, M. Manual on Static Hand Splinting. Harmarville Rehabilitation Center, Pittsburgh, 1976.
12. NICHOLAS, J. J., GRUEN, H., WEINER, G., CRAWSHAW, C., AND TAYLOR, F. Do patients really wear splints? Unpublished data, 1978.
13. BARR, N. R. *The Hand: Principles and Techniques of Simple Splint Making and Rehabilitation.* Butterworth and Co., Boston, 1975.
14. MELVIN, J. *Rheumatic Disease: Occupational Therapy and Rehabilitation.* F. A. Davis Co., Philadelphia, 1977.
15. SMITH, R. D., AND POLLEY, H. F. Rest therapy for rheumatoid arthritis. *Mayo Clin. Proc., 53:* 141, 1978.
16. WINGERT, B. Lecture notes and personal communication.

13

The Role of the Physiotherapist in a Multidisciplinary Arthritis Program

PAULINE NEUBAUER

This discussion of the role of the physiotherapist is based on the background of a multidisciplinary setting within an Arthritis Centre. In this situation the various team members (Fig. 13.1) including the physiotherapist, occupational therapist, social worker, nurse, physician, orthopaedic surgeon, and bioengineer, work closely together, and the physiotherapist may work with some or all disciplines at any one time. In addition, at times other specialized services such as ophthalmology or dermatology may be required for the care of the patient.

Within a multidisciplinary setting the role of the physiotherapist is a rewarding and complementary one. The therapist provides the appropriate physical treatment to the patient, based on careful assessment, recognizing that most of the patient's other needs can be handled by the various other team members. The therapist thus avoids the frustration brought about by patient's needs which cannot be met.

To function most effectively in this environment the physiotherapist should develop a good working understanding of the roles of the other members of the team with a responsibility to maintain good communication and good relationships. There is a stimulating and satisfying climate that comes through close communication of the team members who are working toward common goals. This is of benefit to everyone involved and subsequently and more importantly, to the patient.

The broad role of the physiotherapist in this type of program can be divided into the areas of treatment, research, and education.

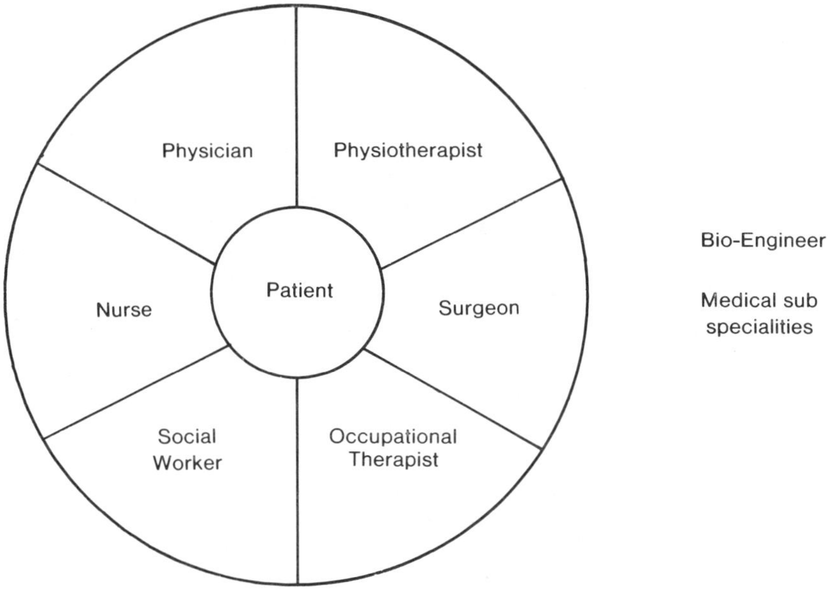

Fig. 13.1. The team in an arthritis control program.

Treatment

While pain and loss of function are the main reasons that prompt the patient to see the doctor, and relief of pain may be the patient's primary objective, in the long-term problem such as rheumatoid arthritis, the physiotherapist must take the longer range point of view.

The referred patient comes to physiotherapy basically to learn more about the physical aspect of the arthritis, and to learn how to handle the disease in the home setting. He is anxious about what it might do to his lifestyle, and wonders what can be done for his problem. Physiotherapy treatments should therefore be geared toward education of the patient including the specifics of the home program while at the same time supporting the patient by the use of specific techniques in pain relief and restoration of range of motion and muscle strength during the scheduled treatment times. The patient should take an active part in treatment, thus avoiding becoming dependent on the continuing treatment as a sort of psychological crutch or support. The patient may, however, be given further support by means of regular interval follow-up after discharge.

Assessment

In our ambulatory treatment setting the newly referred patient is assessed by the physiotherapist.

There are various basic history and assessment forms that are suitable for this purpose.

In the case of an inflammatory type of arthritis with involvement of many joints, the therapist takes a basic brief pertinent history of the events leading up to the referral. Assessment of all the joints of the body is then carried out. Any discrepancy in range of motion is noted in degrees. Muscle power is evaluated and muscle strength graded on a scale of 0 to 5. Pain, heat, and swelling of joints are also noted, together with any ligamentous laxity. Structural abnormalities, such as scoliosis or leg length discrepancy, are recorded together with any observations about the patient's gait pattern. The patient is then asked about any functional deficits relating to his ability to walk, stand, and negotiate steps, and about function in the working environment, kitchen, or bathroom area. The therapist also notes the patient's disposition and attitude toward treatment.

Based on the assessment, an appropriate treatment plan is then drawn up, which would be suited to the patient's specific requirements. This usually includes some pain relieving modality such as ice or heat for painful and/or swollen joints, to be applied prior to exercise. Other specific methods are used to increase joint range of motion and improve muscle strength. Hydrotherapy is a useful adjunct in many cases, particularly if the patient is very stiff, has many joints that have lost range of motion, or is very apprehensive. In the case of the juvenile patient, it is also especially useful as children are often less prepared to do more formal types of exercise.

Patient Education

Patient education is a most important part of treatment today. Compliance with the home program and with instructions about the type of activities to be encouraged or avoided is considerably improved by better understanding on the part of the patient.

The patient education program used in our centre is based on the assumption that the patient needs to know and understand the structure and function of a normal joint, what it is made up of, how it moves, and also to learn and understand some of the terminology that is used by medical personnel. Words such as flexion and extension can be confusing to the patients but are easily understood once explained. The patients also need to know what can happen to joints with the onset of arthritis, why it is important to follow the home program of exercises, and why it is important to avoid stressful activities. They need to learn the importance of rest periods, how to pace themselves, and the use of appropriate aids to conserve energy and avoid stress on joint structures.

Patient education may be carried out with other members of the team in a group situation, or may be done on an individual basis, therapist to patient. The group situation has the advantage that it allows for patient interaction, using a question and answer format. This opens up the possibility of going into greater depth and the voicing of concerns which might otherwise not come up in the standard treatment format, therapist to individual patient. The group situation also lends itself to the use of audiovisual techniques, such as films or slide tape presentations, which further enhance the teaching skills of the therapist. This technique provides some standardization in information given to the patient and does not rely on the individual disposition of the therapist. For this purpose we use a standardized slide tape presentation in five sessions (3). Each session takes 13 min covering subjects of anatomy, pathology, medication, energy conservation, joint stress reduction, and exercise programs. Used in this manner it is a tool to assist the therapist, providing the basis for patient questions and further discussion.

Home Program

The individual home program should not only be specific to the patient's requirements, but should be short and simple. Lengthy complicated home programs are usually short lived. The program should include the application of pain relieving methods, which the patient can easily do at home, appropriate exercises, and additional written instructions helpful to the patient which he can follow at home on a daily basis. The program for a rheumatic patient will often embody exercises to be carried out for short periods such as 5 or 10 min, two or three times a day.

Follow-up after Discharge

The physician-approved follow-up after discharge from physiotherapy treatments provides a very useful adjunct to the treatment and monitors the patient's physical condition over the long term. It provides the therapist with the opportunity to suggest to the family physician reinstitution of physiotherapy treatments or appropriate referral to another discipline, according to the patient's need, based on the findings at the time of the follow-up appointment.

Follow-up after discharge is most useful in patients with continuous inflammatory types of arthritis and most particularly, rheumatoid arthritis. Rheumatoid arthritis produces progressive problems that for the most part respond well to treatment. Many developing deformities and consequent loss of function can be prevented by the proper institution of a suitable physical program at the right time. The follow-up provides continuous support for the patient and also a useful review of a home program which may need to be amended. It may also uncover other needs, such as a need for occupational therapy or social work help or, for example, the need for further exposure to education programs. This type of follow-up program is also a valuable support to the family physician in the management of his patient. Occasional medication problems or other medical problems such as redness and soreness of eyes, skin ulcers, or other unusual complaints may come to light at the time of the physiotherapy follow-up appointment and these, the therapist can quickly bring to the doctor's attention. The follow-up interval time might be every 3 months, 6 months or a year, depending on the patient and the judgment of the therapist and physician.

Research

A research component in any physiotherapy program is a most valuable asset, but particularly so in a multidisciplinary program. Some research projects can be done with two or more disciplines jointly, such as physiotherapy and occupational therapy, physiotherapy-occupational therapy-physician, physiotherapy-occupational therapy-surgeon. As an example, in our program a physiotherapist, engineer, orthopaedic surgeon and rheumatologist collaborated in a study of the gait in patients receiving total knee replacements (1). In our experience, exposure of all the team members to the process of such research projects assists the team members in understanding each others expertise as well as providing a very stimulating climate and an attitude of continuous questioning and learning. Studies being conducted in the treatment setting are essential if a specialized program such as a multidisciplinary arthritis program is to continue to develop and refine treatment methods in the specialty. Reasonably simple on-going studies should be done to reevaluate current standard methods of treatment being used in the program. For example, a reexamination of the value of cervical traction in the treatment of cervical spondylosis was recently conducted by the physiotherapist in our setting (2). This together with review of current literature enables the researching therapist to determine current thinking and this information can quickly spread to all interested staff.

In order for effective research to be done, a specific research therapist should be designated and funded, with definite time allotted for the purpose of research. Ideally, this therapist's role in the program is to do research, so that there is no conflicting priority. To tell treatment staff that they should be doing research does not work in most settings as treatment demands always take precedence, with the result that the research does not get done. The research therapist should, however, conduct the research as part of the whole treatment program and not something separate from it.

It is important that the researcher also have an education role, so that the physiotherapy staff are informed of studies being done and of the results emanating from them. These changes can be incorporated into practice as a result of this.

Education

The physiotherapist has an education role in a multidisciplinary arthritis program. This is a specialized program and like any area of physiotherapy service, has its share of new and rotating staff, from time to time. There are also students to be handled as well as visiting professionals, whether these are physicians, nurses, physiotherapists, occupational therapists, or social workers. To keep therapists actively informed, regular in-service education sessions for the staff on this service are held, specific to the arthritis program. A working climate of continued interest in up-grading, and a thirst for knowledge in the subject are ideal if they can be fostered and this may be possible in a specific program such as this, where the interests and concerns of the therapists are not watered down by a general service concerning the whole gamut of diseases and conditions.

The addition of undergraduate students to such a program is not only beneficial to the student but also to the staff, who, in teaching and in responding to questions, develop inquiring minds about the treatment procedures rather than continuing methods from habit. The climate is, therefore, set for the development of a resource group of physiotherapists who might be called upon at any time to impart information to other members of the team, to visiting professionals, to the unit, or through courses which may be put on by the hospital or professional associations.

Summary

To summarize, the physiotherapist in a multidisciplinary arthritis program has a treatment, research, and education role. This not only provides effective treatment to the patient but lends itself to the evaluation of current methods of treatment and to educating other members of the team or other professionals on an undergraduate or graduate basis. Good communication with an understanding of the role of other members of the team is necessary to provide the best possible patient care. The aims of such a program seem to be best met in a specialized setting which allows energies and interests to be focused on the special challenges of the arthritis patient.

REFERENCES

1. McGraw, R., Foort, J., Robinson, H., Gillies, J., and R. Hannah. Multi-joint electrogoniometric assessment of patients receiving knee implants. National Health and Welfare Canada, Vancouver, B.C., project 610-1128-Y, August 1979.
2. Galbraith, M. A study of the value of cervical traction in the treatment of cervical spondylosis. Personal communication.
3. Patient Education. Rheumatoid arthritis slide/tape program. Available from the Arthritis Society B.C. Division, 895, West 10th Ave., Vancouver B.C. V52 1L7 Canada.

14

The Role of the Podiatrist in the Rheumatology Team Approach

RICHARD D. ROTH

The rheumatology team approach was established in order to centralize services of physicians and allied health personnel available to the arthritic patient. This centralization optimizes available services, facilitates research, encourages intra- and interprofessional communication and education, and reduces the overall costs involved. Any medical or surgical specialty capable of offering unique and beneficial services to a significant number of arthritic patients should be represented on the team. Such representation increases the scope and quality of care, promotes research and education, broadens team perspectives, and further reduces the overall cost of patient care.

One of the primary goals of the rheumatology team is to afford each patient maximal ambulatory ability with the least possible discomfort. To attain this goal the team must include members able to diagnose, evaluate, and treat factors known to limit the arthritic patient's ambulatory potential. The team must also encourage and support related research, communication, and education.

The foot is the structural foundation of erect ambulation. Pain, instability, and deformity involving the foot are factors that can significantly detract from an arthritic patient's ambulatory potential. The foot is frequently the initial site of symptoms in arthritic patients. A large number of arthritic patients initially presenting no symptoms in the foot later go on to develop pedal symptoms. In some of these patients pedal symptoms represent a constant annoyance, while in others they may progress to marked deformity, instability, and severe pain on any attempted ambulation.

Deformity, instability, and pain in any foot can be the result of a wide variety of traumatic, biomechanical, inflammatory, infectious, neoplastic, genetic, or developmental etiologies. Whether related or unrelated to a patient's arthritic disease, afflictions of the foot can significantly impair ambulatory ability, predispose to arthritic involvement in the foot and other areas, and exacerbate on-going symptoms in areas within, adjacent to, or even remote from the foot.

Many arthritic patients have significantly impaired ability to reach their feet and maintain the manual dexterity necessary for proper foot care. A large portion of the arthritic patient population presents with compromised peripheral vascular status or neurological deficits in the lower extremities. Others present with decreased or absent visual acuity. These findings may be related to arthritic disease, other medical etiologies, side effects of current or previous medications, or other causes. Improper nail care, neglect of the feet, poorly fitting shoes, and side effects of medications can predispose these patients to ulcerations, infections, and even gangrene. Subsequent amputations and even death may result. Insufficient evaluation or inadequate care of these patients' feet can predispose to similar sequelae.

Arthritic patients frequently have impaired inflammatory responses or reduced immunological competence due to their disease processes, antiinflammatory medication, or cytotoxic medication. Irritations, inflammations, tissue defects, and infections that would pose little threat to most individuals' feet can have disastrous sequelae in many arthritic patients' feet.

Extensive review of current orthopaedic and rheumatological literature revealed that the majority of treatment described for foot problems in arthritic patients consisted of measures aimed at relief of pain and accommodation of deformity. Frequently mentioned therapeutic measures included use of orthopaedic shoes, arch supports, shoe inserts, internal and external shoe modifications, braces, and surgical procedures. Descriptions of those aberrations of normal foot architecture or function found in the arthritic patient that predispose to deformity, progression of deformity, abnormal stress patterns during gait, and progressive pain were conspicuously absent throughout relevant literature. DuVries' text (1) was the only source presenting biomechanical considerations in foot structure and function.

Available information regarding the functional biomechanics in normal and deformed hands has helped to elucidate the mechanisms that may predispose to progressive deformity in the hand of the rheumatoid arthritic patient. Application of this biomechanical knowledge in modifying wrist splints has proven valuable in attempts to slow progression or even prevent rheumatoid hand deformities (2). Similar application of biomechanical principles in the foot would appear to have significant potential for amelioration, slowing progression, or even prevention of many etiologies of foot pain, instability, and deformity in the arthritic patient.

Functional biomechanics of the foot has been the subject of extensive study over the past few decades. Information derived from such research appears valuable in elucidating many of the mechanisms that predispose a foot to excessive internal stress, transmission of excessive stress, arthritic involvement, instability, functional impairment, and deformity. Consideration of these biomechanical mechanisms appears to have significant potential for improving palliative, preventive, remedial, and surgical therapeutic approaches to the foot problems of the arthritic patient.

The podiatrist is a specialist trained and experienced in the medical and surgical treatment of disorders of the foot. His training, with rare exceptions, includes 4 years of undergraduate college studies followed by 4 years of study at an approved college of podiatric medicine. Many have additional training in 1 year hospital-based residency programs or preceptorships. Some have completed 2 years of postgraduate residency training. After completion of formal training most podiatrists enter a private practice which includes care of a wide variety of foot disorders. A few choose to limit the scope of their practices to such subspecialty areas as podopediatrics (care of foot disorders in children), podogeriatrics (care of foot problems in elderly patients), or surgery. The podiatrist with extensive postgraduate training and/or extensive experience in a practice encompassing a wide variety of foot disorders offers the greatest potential benefit to the rheumatology team approach.

Over the past 20 years the profession of podiatry has developed expertise in the diagnosis, evaluation, and treatment of foot disorders. The inclusion of such expertise in the rheumatology team approach insures each patient optimal preventive, palliative, and therapeutic care of foot disorders. The role of the podiatrist within the rheumatology team includes a wide variety of highly beneficial and necessary patient care services.

Many arthritic patients have disorders of the feet that are unrelated to arthritic disease processes. The arthritic diseases of these patients frequently limit their ambulatory potential. Unrelated foot disorders often further limit that potential. Some of the more common disorders that may be found in any patient's foot include ingrown toenails, painful skin lesions, local infections, ulcerations, soft tissue tumors, nerve entrapments, sprains, strains, fractures, dislocations, functional abnormalities, and structural deformities. The team podiatrist, through his special interest, is uniquely helpful in differentiating these conditions from those other causes of foot pain and instability directly associated with an arthritic patient's disease processes. He can determine and evaluate the relationship of these disorders to the patient's arthritic disease. He can also determine effective treatment alternatives and render the therapy of choice to each individual patient.

The podiatrist can prevent recurrence of ingrown toenails through initial treatment followed by patient education in proper nail cutting techniques or by surgical excision of the offending nail or nail border and chemical destruction or excision of associated nail matrices. Discomfort associated with tender hyperkeratotic skin lesions can be temporarily alleviated by local débridement and padding around the involved area to prevent excessive pressure. More permanent relief can be obtained through fabrication of removable devices designed to alleviate pressure on involved areas or through various surgical procedures. A variety of other disturbing skin lesions that commonly present on the feet can be diagnosed and treated with various dermatological preparations or regimens under the podiatrist's supervision. Local infections can be treated by appropriate antiseptic soaks, incision and drainage, and/or local or systemic antibiotic use. Ulcerations are managed through removal of offending pressure on the involved area, surgical débridement, enzymatic débridement, methods of increasing circulation to the area, and/or decreasing fluid stasis in the involved area, use of grafting material or plastic surgical techniques, application of various nutrient preparations, and appropriate preventive long-term relief of pressure from the area.

The podiatrist's knowledge of the anatomy of the foot is invaluable to the team charged with the need to diagnose and treat local lesions through conservative methods such as aspiration, injection therapy, and removal of offending external irritation and pressure or through surgical excision. He can diagnose various nerve entrapments in the foot and provide relief in most cases either through injection therapy or surgical release.

Minor sprains and strains in the foot are commonly encountered in podiatric practice. They are usually treated effectively with antiinflammatory agents, and flexible or semirigid immobilization. More severe strains and sprains may require biomechanical and radiographic evaluations combined with splinting or casting. The treatment of joint dislocations and fractures varies according to the degree of injury and the area involved. Treatments for these conditions may include closed or open reduction, internal or external fixation, flexible or semirigid immobilization, or cautious observation.

Discomfort associated with digital deformities can be alleviated through alterations in footgear, construction of removable padding devices, or surgical intervention. Discomfort arising from other foot deformities or functional abnormalities in the foot can be ameliorated or even eliminated through alterations in footgear, addition of modifications to existing or prescribed shoes, use of various orthotic devices, identification and treatment of relevant proximal factors, and surgical intervention.

The team podiatrist offers essential services to those arthritic patients with compromised peripheral vascular circulation. Patients with previously diagnosed diabetes mellitus or peripheral vascular disease and those with significant findings of decreased peripheral blood flow, venous stasis, edema, or vasculitis should be considered in this category. Decreased tissue viability and compromised defense mechanisms in the feet predispose these patients to significant problems following even the most minor trauma. Those patients receiving prolonged courses of steroid therapy or immunosuppressive drugs should also be considered here due to their compromised defense mechanisms. Improper care of toenails, inadequate care of skin lesions, poor foot hygiene, and failure to recognize and treat areas of excess stress can lead to tissue breakdown, infection, gangrene, and even amputation in these patients.

Many arthritic patients are unable to render adequate or proper care to their feet. These patients may be limited in their mobility, dexterity, or visual acuity. The podiatrist can render initial foot care to these patients and instruct those responsible for their follow-up care in proper methods of nail and hygienic care of their feet.

Other arthritic patients are confined to bed for prolonged periods of time due to their arthritic disease, other medical problems, or postoperative convalescent periods. The podiatrist can be of assistance in maintaining proper foot care for these patients. His care can help in preventing tissue breakdown over the heels or other areas of the feet. Should such breakdown occur the podiatrist can be of assistance in providing the best possible treatment to these areas while the patient is bedridden. He can modify footgear to prevent irritation to the involved areas after ambulatory status is regained. The team podiatrist can also prescribe additional modifications in footgear and provide any necessary follow-up evaluations or care that recurrences of ulcerations may necessitate.

The foot of the arthritic patient presents painful and limiting deformities or imbalances similar, if not identical, to those seen in the foot of the nonarthritic patient, but optimal care of the arthritic patient's foot must include consideration of how its deformities or imbalances can progress to greater deformity and imbalance, adversely affect arthritic or as yet normal joints, and lead to progressive ambulatory dysfunction. Recognition of these factors presupposes a thorough knowledge of the biomechanical function of the normal and abnormal foot. The podiatrist is well-educated in this area of biomechanics. Through use of a biomechanical examination and interpretation of its findings, the team podiatrist is able to undertake preventive therapeutic measures. Preventive measures can be directed against minor structural or functional abnormalities that have the potential to induce significant discomfort and progression of joint disease. Orthotic splints and devices can be constructed from molds taken directly from the foot of an individual patient. They can be adjusted to accommodate structural and functional deformities and to help prevent progression of such problems or their sequelae. Special exercise and gait training programs can be designed with the physical and occupational therapy departments to assist in overcoming several functional abnormalities or imbalances. Such preventive measures hold great promise in attempts to prevent progressive deformity and functional limitation in the arthritic patient's foot.

Many arthritic patients present with advanced painful and limiting foot deformities. In these patients accommodative orthoses, prescription molded shoes, or surgical intervention may provide significant relief and marked improvement of ambulatory potential. The team podiatrist should evaluate each such case and determine the potential benefits offered by each treatment alternative.

A significant percentage of arthritic patients present with active arthritic disease in the feet and considerable pain on ambulation. Often symptomatic or remittive systemic therapy reduces foot pain but does not eliminate it. In these patients and in those whose initial arthritic symptoms present in the feet, a complete biomechanical evaluation of foot structure and function is warranted. Findings of such a survey will often reveal abnormal structural, functional, and stress relationships in involved feet. Podiatric treatment of these imbalances may provide significant symptomatic relief and may serve to slow or even prevent future arthritic involvement.

The team podiatrist is a highly qualified and valuable addition to the rheumatology team approach to total care for the arthritic patient. His responsibilities include the diagnosis and evaluation of foot disorders in the arthritic patient population. He determines various therapeutic, remedial, and palliative alternatives for each patient's foot problems, and he selects appropriate regimens of care for each patient based on the diagnosed disorder, the patient's status and prognosis, the overall team evaluation of the patient, and goals set for the patient.

The rheumatology team has two potential methods of obtaining a team podiatrist. The first is to utilize one or more podiatrists in the capacity of consultants. This involves requesting individual consultations for specific patients from podiatrists whose main responsibilities are to their individual private practices. Due to limitations in private practitioners' available time, the team consultant podiatrist will usually spend most of his time dealing with nonarthritic private patients. The time that he is able to devote to team functions such as special team conferences and charting rounds will be limited, and the time that such a consultant will have available for relevant research will likewise be limited.

The second method of obtaining a team podiatrist involves recruitment of a practitioner who is willing and able to devote the majority of his time to the team's arthritic patients. In such instances the team facility will have to be of sufficient size to provide an adequate patient load for the team podiatrist. Additionally, team members and other practitioners in the team facility will have to be receptive to granting the team podiatrist overall delineation of privileges consistent with his training, ability, and scope of licensure. Where such staff privileges are granted, the team podiatrist will be capable of utilizing the team facility to the maximum of his ability.

REFERENCES

1. INMAN, V.T., AND MANN, R. A. Biomechanics of the Foot and Ankle. In *DuVries Surgery of the Foot*, Ed. 4, edited by R. A. Mann. St. Louis, C. V. Mosby, 1978, pp. 3–21.
2. EHRLICH, G. E. Rest and Splinting, Functional Wrist Splint. In *Total Management of the Arthritic Patient*, edited by G. E. Ehrlich. Philadelphia, J. B. Lippincott, 1973, pp. 47–54.

15

Organization of Community Resources

WARREN L. BENSON

In the beginning, there was only the physician. If he was the Indian medicine man, he played the drum, did sand paintings, sang healing chants, ground the herbs, and applied the poultices. Then, gradually, he trained others to assist.

Not infrequently, the present day healer must either train others or encourage the formation of organizations that will furnish the modalities a patient needs.

This chapter will deal with existing organizations, private and public, that provide services to the arthritis patient. Reference will be made to organizing agency resources that do not presently exist in an effort to meet unmet needs. Some space will be devoted to necessary segments within these agencies. Obviously, these comments cannot be all inclusive but, rather, are intended to touch on the various areas to which health professionals can turn for assistance in meeting the total need of patient and public.

Because of rapid growth in the numbers of agencies now serving patients, the health professional will likely need help in finding the best sources of services. Some ideas are formulated here for simplifying the process.

Community Resources

Community organizations can play an advocate role by cutting through governmental red tape. An example is having government service applications on hand, thereby eliminating a visit to pick up a required form. If a physician refers a patient for help in obtaining special license tags or parking decals, the process can be expedited by a referral letter detailing the need. Many cities have special bus rates for handicapped or elderly patients, and the doctor's office can refer clients to a social agency that will assist in the application process.

Clients may frequently be referred to community agencies. Community agency personnel must remember that overall control of the patient's treatment remains in the hands of the referring physician, and not with the agency except for the particular services for which the patient was referred. Should agency personnel perceive additional treatment needs, this perception must be shared with the referring physician who may then take whatever action is deemed necessary. The agency would be acting unethically to take it upon itself to suggest a course of action to the patient. An agency wishing to receive referrals must observe accepted practices and procedures.

Where needed services have not been established in a community, a Junior League or Women's Club may propose funding of projects that fill the gap. Arthritis Foundation Auxiliaries have frequently been founded by rheumatologists' wives, and still other auxiliaries have been strongly supported and staffed by volunteers familiar with the valuable services such organizations can provide.

During the last 10 years, federal and state government aid to the handicapped has exploded into many areas. Regulations governing many programs are constantly being revised and very few organizations indirectly affected keep abreast of all the changes, so staff must maintain communication pipelines to the various departments. If an agency has an ongoing relationship with knowledgeable employees in various governmental departments, this can mean easier access for the patient who seeks services.

Social Security disability benefits can be obtained if the eligible client is made aware of applicable programs. Currently about 350,000 men and women disabled by arthritis are receiving monthly payments under Social Security. The programs cover disabled workers under 65 and their families if the person has worked long enough and recently enough in a job covered by Social Security. If a parent covered under Social Security retires, becomes disabled, or dies, the child who is disabled before age 22 is eligible for payments. One need not be totally disabled to receive benefits, since Supplemental Security Insurance makes payments to disabled people who have limited incomes and resources.

Services offered by just one of the federal and state agencies, Vocational Rehabilitation, include the following.

1. Physical examinations to determine the extent of disability, work capacity and possibilities for improvement.
2. Counseling and guidance to aid the client in personal and social adjustment.
3. Vocational evaluation to aid in the selection of a suitable vocational objective.
4. Medical, surgical, and hospital services to reduce the disability as much as possible.
5. Artificial appliances, such as braces, needed to increase work capacity.
6. Vocational training to provide the education and skills necessary for suitable employment.

TABLE 15.1. *Governmental Organizations with Services Applicable to Arthritis Patients*

State	Municipal and County	Federal
Welfare	Area councils	Rural Health Federation
Food stamps	Senior recreation centers	Champus
Employment	School districts	Diagnostic and Technical Assistance Center
Vocational rehabilitation	City health centers	Health Systems Agency
Civil rights division	Health departments	Indian Health Center
Schools for deaf and blind	Hospitals	Social Security Administration
Cooperative extension services		Talking Book Program
Economic protection division		Veterans Administration Hospital
Rehabilitation facilities		
Crippled children's programs		

7. Needed tools and occupational equipment, including licenses, in order for an individual to enter the employment for which trained.

These services may be dependent upon the state of the agency's finances when the client applies.

Here we have mentioned just a few of the services covered by federal departments. The list of governmental agencies with arthritis related programs is long (Table 15.1).

Where federal programs are involved, information can be secured from any Federal Information Center. This is simply a phone number, located in any large or midsize community from which information can be gained. The service will locate the branch of the Federal Government which has programs dealing with whatever problem the caller is concerned about.

Any community will have private social agencies providing services. The number and scope will vary according to the size and social awareness of the city. The list in Table 15.2 represents just a few of the agencies in one community which furnish services helpful to arthritis patients. Although an agency's name may be different, the function will still be there in other areas.

A physician may not be thoroughly acquainted with available agency services, because it is difficult for health personnel to keep abreast of changing staff and facilities in the community. Establishing a relationship with a community-wide organization can be a productive method of matching needy clients with community services.

The Organization

Each organization should have a board, staff, standing committees, and community relations component. Every organization relies on a great deal

TABLE 15.2. *Community Agencies Helpful to Arthritis Patients*

Agency	Services
Easter Seal Society	Transportation, speech therapy, and home modification.
Volunteer Bureau	Transportation—office help.
City Transportation Service	Handicapped transport.
Red Cross	Convalescent sitters.
Children's Hospital	Braces, surgery, eye exam, drugs.
Information and Referral	Individual assistance for problems.
Lutheran Social Ministries	Transportation.
Neighborhood Health Center	Patient care for other than arthritis.
St. Elizabeth's of Hungary Out-Patient Clinic	Patient care for other than arthritis.
Homemaker's	Homemaker services.
Visiting Nurse Association	Nursing, physical therapy, and occupational therapy.
Meals on Wheels	Mobile meals.
Sick Room Loan Chest	Adaptive equipment.
Senior Now	Make adaptive aids.
Arthritis Foundation	Information, education, treatment modalities, legislative advocacy, transporation, physician referral, self-help devices, quackery information.

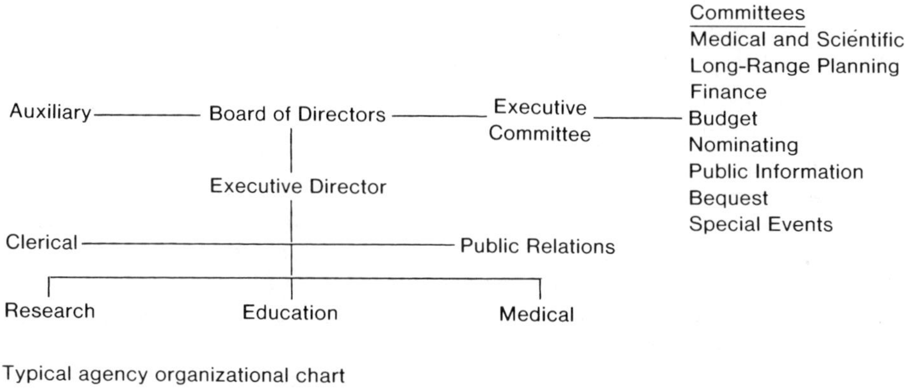

Fig. 15.1. Typical agency organizational chart.

of internal interactions (Fig. 15.1). When starting a community organization to meet a need not presently being met, planning is a necessity for best results. Various committees working together will produce planning. Cross fertilization of ideas can multiply results. A committee that does not seek input from other volunteers and from staff is not utilizing its resources to the fullest extent possible.

BOARD AND EXECUTIVE

Every organization needs a governing group with a variety of skills. This group is usually known as the Board of Directors, and is ultimately responsible for the organization's success. The Board must be concerned with planning, budgeting and setting policy. The program is implemented by staff and volunteers within the parameters established by the Board. Volunteers generally operate through committees which deal with specific segments of the organization's activities.

Although the entire Board of Directors is, and must be, responsible for the activities and actions of the group, it is frequently expedient to delegate responsibility for day-to-day decisions to an executive committee and/or staff. Requiring that every decision come from the Board can stifle initiative and reduce opportunities. An executive committee composed of officers and committee chairpersons can easily make lower echelon decisions.

All actions taken in executive session should be reviewed by the total Board at their regular meetings, and it is a good idea to make regular mailings to the Board if they meet less than once a month. These mailings provide members with summaries of actions taken. On receipt of these, Board members may want to note them for discussion at the next meeting, or if the matter is of extreme concern, can ask to be present at the next executive committee meeting to express opinions.

If the matter is of utmost importance, any Board member should be able to request a special meeting of the entire Board. Care should be taken not to overuse this privilege or, as the boy who cried wolf discovered, eventually no one may respond to a legitimate emergency meeting.

STANDING COMMITTEES

Composition of standing committees must be given serious consideration in the primary stages of group organization. Avoid an authoritative whirlwind leader who dominates decision making, fund raising, and budget planning. Should this dynamic person move, become interested in a new project, or become disenchanted with coworkers, the organization that relied on him (or her) can founder.

It is considered a good idea to include nonboard members on standing committees. These should be people with an interest in the organization, and they should have expertise and experience in the area the committee is concerned with. This serves two purposes. First, community expertise is utilized. Second, the committee chairperson is able to evaluate the volunteer's possible value as a future board member.

Although standing committees usually do not take unilateral action, a situation may arise where the Executive Committee authorizes such a procedure. Generally, the standing committee makes a recommendation to the Executive Committee, which in turn may take action or report to the Board of Directors. Reports are accompanied with a recommendation based on the information obtained. This is very helpful to the Board, many of whose members may not feel informed enough to make decisions of far-reaching impact.

Over the years, the use of standing committees allows the Board to accumulate knowledge and expertise which can be brought to bear on matters that concern a particular committee. For example, the Finance Committee may research a variety of methods for insuring the availability of on-going funding for a segment of the program, existing or planned. The committee may investigate how similar groups have instigated a successful bequest program, memorial giving, or membership drive. Other committees will be involved in various aspects of the organization, including recruitment of new Board members.

Boards have often expected great things from a new Board member, only to be disappointed. This might not have occurred if the prospect had been given an opportunity to test his or her interests and abilities via committee membership and assignments. *Nominating Committees* can be established to continually seek new board material by carefully screening volunteers and committee members.

A *Personnel Committee* can prepare and regularly review policies governing employee hiring, working conditions, salary and benefit standards, and severance. Personnel policies should be reviewed and revised at least once every 5 years. Members of this committee should personally interview every employee annually, and recommend salary and fringe benefit revisions to the budget committee.

The success of a particular agency may depend in large part on its ability to project true estimations of its fund-raising potential. An improperly prepared budget may survive 1 year, but continued unorthodox budgeting procedures can precipitate an exodus of board members, and eventual fiscal disaster. Glorious dreams of magnificent programs must be tempered by the reality of available dollars. Program people can make proposals to the budget group, but they should be based on a realistic assessment of available funding. The *Budget Committee* must work closely with the Finance and Long-Range Planning Committees.

Responsibility for setting fund-raising goals lies with the *Finance Committee*. This group must examine the agency's past history and current capabilities to determine where changes might be made to increase income. A continuing examination of all options will uncover new areas to explore. A special event, or other types of income producing programs that did not work a few years ago may be feasible today. It is particularly critical that the Finance Committee chairperson not allow one loudly expressed opinion to shut off discussion and cause a hasty decision. The Finance Committee must look at short-term and long-term agency programs, as well as events sponsored by outside groups. This committee can bring tremendous rewards to its members as they see the organization grow due to its endeavors.

An organization may be very successful over a period of time, but unless its course is charted over a long term, events may suddenly crop up that present programs cannot cope with. The organization may be plunged into chaos if it is not ready to shift its emphasis to other service roles in the community. *Long-Range Planning Committees* should keep up-to-date on legislative planning as well as activities of other agencies which may impact on future program needs. This committee may recommend to the Finance Committee certain areas in which funding should be sought to anticipate future demands.

Staff members are generally responsible for carrying out the day-to-day Public Information and Public Relations programs. A *Public Information Committee* can augment the thinking of staff and offer new approaches as well as establishing guidelines for disseminating information to the community.

Every health organization should have adequate representation of physicians and allied health personnel to guide decisions on matters relating directly to treatment and research. Representation of a variety of skills will help broaden the outlook of the *Medical and Scientific Committee.* A good committee will reflect a balance of University-based or research physicians with private physicians. Members should be sought from other agencies such as the Veterans Administration and County Health Department. A representative group of Nurses, Therapists, and other Allied Health Personnel are essential.

The deliberations of this committee, as with all committees, should be reported to the Executive Committee with recommendations for future action. These are then acted upon, or passed along to the Board of Directors for consideration if changes of philosophy or policy are involved.

Standing committees perform many useful functions in an organization. Care should be taken to utilize committees for the function for which they were formed. This enables the organization to establish tested criteria for the selection of committee members.

VOLUNTEERS

It is important not to take a volunteer's length of service for granted. A person who signs up for a 3-year term may be given a company promotion to a position in another city. Do not wait until that happens to train a successor, since the volunteer will be too busy moving to assist in training.

Potentially valuable volunteers will be lost if they are ignored, or given nothing meaningful to do. A feeling of accomplishment or sense of a job well done will secure the loyalty of the volunteer, as well as the staff. Be sure to publicly recognize a job well done. A pat on the back from the Board chairperson is nice, but it becomes even more meaningful if it is given at an annual meeting. A plaque, certificate, or some other material expression of appreciation can generate continued interest and support, as well as attract new support.

COMMUNITY RELATIONS

Since no community organization operates in a vacuum, thought must be given to publicizing the concerns of the group, its activities, and its need for volunteers. Everyone can be involved in the publicity effort. A radio station manager who sports a certificate of commendation on the wall is constantly reminded of the agency, and will refer to the agency with positive statements. If board and committee members have been well-oriented, motivated, and educated, they can generate significant support by just telling a case history of a need they know exists. A Publicity and Information Committee can take responsibility for the educational aspects of the agency, and most health agencies believe education to be an important, vital aspect of the program. Special events, if given adequate exposure and adequate planning, can be very effective community relations tools.

GRIEVANCE PROCEDURES

Volunteers and staff must realize that all your constituents will not be pleased all the time. Yet the organization must attempt to carefully examine any and all complaints. Even though the organization means well, someone is bound to be annoyed in the course of a year's operation. It is usually a good idea to have a neutral party (board member) take a look at the problem. Occasionally, some members of the public may be unreasonable in their expectations, but at other times complaints may lead to necessary changes in operating policies.

ORGANIZING

Here are some steps a health practitioner wishing to assume a leadership role might take: document the need; discuss the need with peers, and gather more documentation; extend the discussion to other health professionals; recruit others who recognize the problem; discuss possible solutions; map strategies; rally community leaders around the cause; form speakers bureau; talk to any and all interested groups to generate grass-roots support; arrange formal public meetings which result in action; continue to talk-talk-talk to others, alerting them to the problem; be willing to put your money where your mouth is when the occasion arises; establish an organization to take an active role in meeting the need.

ADVOCACY

An organization will generally define its role in clear cut terms in its Constitution and Bylaws. Hopefully, the agency's Board of Directors will accept the role of advocate whether or not this is spelled out. Matters which call for advocacy may arise frequently and at different levels of government and private groups. If a handicapped organization plans to express its concerns regarding transportation in the city, it is fitting that all other organizations with interests in this area join the sponsoring group. In unity there is strength, so each group should invite participation by others when unity might accomplish similar goals. However, when an organization finds it is duplicating services offered elsewhere, one or the other should instigate discussions to find a way to extend these services to additional areas rather than duplicate them.

Voluntary health agencies have traditionally interpreted their role as provider, not lobbyist. Lobbying cannot be the major role of tax-exempt health agencies, but the law does permit expression of opinions on proposed legislation. Many health professionals are invited to State Capitols or Washington to express an opinion based on the experience of the individual or agency. Since government at various levels is taking a larger role in providing services and advice, legislators increasingly depend on the expertise of the professional. Because of this, organizations should include patients who are in a unique position to offer knowledgeable insights on their boards and committees.

Remember that the agency should be well-organized and capable of changing to meet new needs in the community. Organization members, from the Board of Directors Chairperson to the newest volunteer should be utilized to the fullest. All organization members should be oriented toward the agency's goals, and all members should follow existing procedures and policies to attain these goals.

Team Care

The director of the team care unit may be a rheumatologist in an outpatient or private physician setting. In a hospital or clinic where physicians rotate, the social worker or counselor may implement the process. It is the coordinator's responsibility to ensure the most practical use of both patient's and health professionals' time by scheduling to get the most out of each patient visit. The coordinator not only schedules appointments with various consultants, but also insures that appointments have been kept and appropriate reports are circulated to the team, and that a copy of the report is placed in the patient's chart.

THE STAFFING

The team approach revolves around the staffing, where the group gathers and develops plans to overcome present problems and prevent future ones. The patient is a valued member of the team, and it is generally accepted that an educated patient will respond to treatment better than an uneducated one. Education is a cornerstone in the pyramid of arthritis care. When available, it is advisable to involve an education specialist in presenting informative materials in workshop or symposium settings for patients.

The physician's office staff will set up a procedure to follow-up on referrals. A referral will serve no purpose if the patient fails to keep an appointment, or does not make an appointment for the indicated services.

Unless someone conducts follow-up, valuable time may be lost in obtaining needed services. Failure to complete a referral may be due to finances or a misunderstanding. It is not uncommon to learn that a patient did not have a prescription filled. When a doctor discovers financial limitations that prevent a patient from obtaining needed services, the office staff should be able to refer the client to a potential source of funds. Locating needed services can be time-consuming, sometines even frustrating, but the patient's welfare dictates that the effort be made.

THE PHYSICIAN

As community organizations proliferate, practicing physicians face an increasingly difficult task in keeping up with a community's expanding services. Since the physician will frequently serve as coordinator of the total medical care appropriate for the patient, both doctor and staff must continually educate themselves about available services. Holistic health care has become an accepted approach in matters of health, although the appropriateness of particular segments may still be open to question. Totality includes preventive and diagnostic care as well as therapeutic and rehabilitative treatments. The doctor owes it to the patient to know how to find those modalities that can augment his own services. Physicians are generally aware of the many and varied social, emotional, and environmental factors that can influence the patient's overall health.

PHYSICAL THERAPIST

Most patients see a physical therapist at an early stage, shortly after the initial visit to the primary care doctor. The therapist may put the patient through range of motion tests to serve as a base for future test comparisons. The physical therapist should develop and start the patient on a set of exercises to minimize the disease's destructive forces, and eventually maintain and even restore range of motion. The therapist must also be a motivator since daily range of motion exercises are boring and the patient needs constant encouragement to remain faithful to the exercise program.

Occasionally a physical therapist will be called upon to make rest casts for wrists or legs to slow down or reverse flexion contractures or relieve stress on involved joints. The therapist may stretch joints, use water or heat treatments, or use electric stimulation to improve a patient's condition.

It is not unusual for the patient to use the therapist to unload worries, concerns, and frustrations which in turn may result in referrals to a counselor. If a patient is concerned that the inability to abduct hips is interfering with an enjoyable sex life, counseling from the therapist may be necessary (if the therapist is comfortable in this role).

COUNSELOR

Due to pain, actual or feared, and due to the chronic nature of rheumatoid disease, many patients experience psychological symptoms ranging from mild depression to severe psychosis. The busy practitioner cannot always take the time to render the psychological support indicated for the troubled arthritis patient. Indeed, many physicians do not feel competent in this area. If patient and doctor are fortunate enough to live in a community where clinics and staff to care for the mental health needs of the arthritis patient are available, a mere referral may start in motion the necessary ancillary treatment. Even here though, the primary care physician should keep abreast of the counselor's approach. The primary physician should be aware of any prescribed drugs and may want to make appropriate notes in the patient's chart.

The team leader may automatically involve a counselor even if signs of emotional distress have not become evident. The rheumatologist may do this by recommending the patient join a counseling group. If sexual or family problems (related to the disease) manifest themselves, the social worker's role will grow in the team approach.

NURSE

The nurse acts as the physician's right hand and is the person the patient will turn to first, after the doctor. She is the one who is told those things the patient may feel too shy to confide to the doctor. Knowledgable about drugs, dosages, and side effects, the nurse may be the one who spots drug reactions and, if the patient is not scheduled to see the doctor, she will bring the condition to his attention. In some communities, the nurse practitioner is the sole contact for the patient.

OCCUPATIONAL THERAPIST

When the need for self-help devices become evident, an occupational therapist may make a home visit to see first-hand how the patient functions. An evaluation of problems shared with the team may lead to new goals in the treatment process.

EDUCATION SPECIALIST

The education specialist can answer questions such as: 1. Should aspirin be continued when the pain diminishes or disappears? 2. Why is aspirin prescribed when the patient does not have a headache? 3. What are the latest drugs? 4. The newest surgical procedures? 5. When are they appropriate? 6. What does the ANA test indicate? 7. Why does the sedimentation rate fluctuate? 8. Can arthritis be fatal? 9. What part does heredity play? 10. Are copper bracelets really helpful? 11. What is there to the latest cure reported in the tabloid newspaper at the supermarket?

Even the intelligent, well-educated patient wants to understand better his or her disease. All these questions and more can be addressed at a workshop or patient seminar. In team care many of these questions, fears, and concerns may surface during interactions with one team member or another.

More and more, insurance programs will fund the additional services required for well-rounded treatment programs. Even patient education services may soon be covered for the arthritis patient.

PODIATRIST

The podiatrist is an integral part of the team. With the large number of bones in the foot, weight-bearing stresses frequently lead to foot problems.

ORTHOPEDIC SURGEON

An orthopedic surgeon should be consulted since a surgical procedure at an early stage in the disease's development may prevent damage to other joints. It must be remembered that there is a right time for surgery if it is to achieve maximum results. A hand surgeon with particular expertise in this area is often a team member.

PEDIATRICIAN

Referrals to the team frequently come from the pediatrician who makes the initial diagnosis. The holistic health approach demands that the pediatrician be kept fully informed of the patient's progress and where possible be involved in the staffing. Other health problems can influence the course of the arthritis and, conversely, changes in the treatment modalities should be passed on to the child's primary care physician.

OPHTHALMOLOGISTS

Because regular slit lamp exams are important when treating juvenile rheumatoid arthritis as well as some adult forms of the disease, an ophthalmologist trained in possible ocular involvements is also a team member.

PARENTS AND TEACHERS

When a child is the patient the parents become team members. The counselor may also talk to the classroom teacher, gym teacher, or the school administration to clarify the child's special problems and particular needs. Due consideration without coddling is the goal of a well-rounded team approach. With the help of the team the child may live as normally as possible.

COMMUNITY AGENCIES

Community agencies serve the team in a variety of ways. Just knowing where to find existing services is time-saving, and a local information and referral organization can often facilitate this process. As an example of agency usefulness, the Red Cross, Easter Seal Society, and various church groups may all provide transportation for the handicapped. The patient who lives 120 miles from available treatment and cannot drive to it is in the same boat as the patient who is 4 miles away in a wheelchair and cannot get to doctor or therapy. In addition, Vocational Rehabilitation can on occasion provide funding for transportation.

VOCATIONAL REHABILITATION

A vocational counselor can be an important team member for a variety of input. The counselor may believe a patient's depression revolves around feelings of worthlessness generated by an inability to put bread and butter on the table as well as before the disease caused him to give up work. A referral to Vocational Rehabilitation may result in a new vocational goal, which all the team members are made aware of and can work toward.

TEAM APPROACH

The team approach can help in finding and meeting unmet needs in the community. For example, a physician may wonder why a newly prescribed drug is not having the desired and expected results. The counselor may learn the prescription was never filled due to a lack of finances on the part of the client. The physician is alerted, and if the community has an organization which can assist in providing prescription drugs, this group then becomes part of the team. If there is not such an agency, a new unmet need has been found and perhaps another agency will be formed, or an existing organization will take on an additional function. Occasionally a women's club or service club will sponsor such a service for a few years while endeavoring to build a group which will sustain the activity. Junior Leagues are noted for starting needed services and then passing them on to other groups for continued operation.

Fund-raising

When a new organization is wrestling with the question of how best to raise needed funds, consideration should be given to membership in a federated campaign. While not always feasible, a federated campaign does have several advantages over independent campaigns. The fewer separate requests the community receives, the easier it is to allocate limited philanthropic dollars. Therefore, pressures may be brought to bear on an organization to join an umbrella group. Usually community leaders prefer that an organization such as the United Way represent as many legitimate agencies as possible.

If the decision is to seek funding independently, an organization must have the volunteers and leadership necessary to succeed. A strong organization with program appeal can utilize the independent campaign to solidify volunteers' interest and the community's awareness of the agency. (This also strengthens the agency's bargaining position if and when it seeks United Way monies.)

A considerable percentage of any fund-raising effort should be in the form of advanced corporate gifts. If early support is not received, other potentially large donors may hold back or reduce their contributions. Failure this year will decrease the expectations for next year's campaign.

With the realization that the first years of independent campaigning are the most expensive, the agency can estimate the net income for the immediate future and compare that figure with what the United Way is offering. Staff members of a federated fund agency can devote time to serving clients during the fund drive, negating the need to add additional staff. Independent fund-raising can be costly as well as time-consuming (see Table 15.3).

As part of the initial planning of the organization, a decision should be considered about participation in the local United Way. This decision is not an easy one. It must be preceded by full discussion with the board of the United Way as to their estimation of the need for the organization and the parts of the program they may be willing to fund. While United Way may not provide funding the first year, it may after a track record has been established. Sometimes it is necessary to show the amount of community interest in the program. This interest can be measured by the dollars raised through the organization's own efforts.

Generally speaking, United Ways are not very interested in research, national dues, or fellowships. They prefer people-oriented programs. Direct services that do not duplicate existing programs and fulfill a recognized need are likely to be accepted for funding. Many United Ways will fund particular services and suggest alternative means for funding others.

United Way is usually a deficit funding agency. Special money received this year may be deducted from next year's allocation. Remember that in the long run, the manner in which United Way treats an agency at budget time will reflect its ability to interpret its services and goals.

The decision to join the United Way may hinge in some respects on restrictions placed on supplementary fund-raising efforts. Special events, membership drives, and soliciting bequests may be taboo. It would be a good idea, before making a decision to find out if the fund is well supported by local media and business leaders. Independent fund-raising allows much more flexibility and a greater freedom to pick types and times of campaigning. Many agencies believe independent campaigns give greater agency visibility.

TABLE 15.3. *Fund-raising Statistics*

	United Way	Independent Campaign
Total funding	\$50,000	\$50,000
Fund-raising costs	100	20,000
Programable funds	\$49,900	\$30,000

DONATIONS

When organizations think of fund raising, they may think of the big contributor, the angel who will give thousands of unrestricted dollars at a time. This makes fun thinking, but it is the small, regular donors that make on-going programs possible. If the agency is lucky enough to attract the large contributor; take the money with caution. Large bequests can ruin a successful organization by destroying a volunteer's sense of urgency. The big legacy will eventually dissipate, and the organization will falter if the board has not been functioning in the area of fund-raising. Large, unexpected windfalls should be used to augment and enrich on-going projects, not to replace existing sources.

Many bequests come from strangers to the organization. Something done in the past may have generated an interest. Perhaps it was the courtesy shown when someone came in for a pamphlet, or stopped to see an exhibit at a fair. Perhaps it was the story in the evening paper with the picture of the child being helped. The author's agency received $20,000 after one class presentation in a local high school. It is urgent that all staff and volunteers realize that they are the agency's representatives and their conduct of agency affairs will affect the way others view the organization.

A well-run agency will have a wish list, written out to supply any potential donor who asks, "What do you need?" This list can have projects for $200 or $1,000,000 with many stops in between. Perhaps a donor would like to endow a chair in the agency's special interest at the local university. By attracting the endowment, the organization will have some input into the direction of research or programs.

A valid suggestion is to not underestimate the capabilities of a potential donor. Very rich people can afford to ignore dress codes, and being comfortable may take precedence over someone else's sense of propriety. It is easier to downgrade a request for support than it is to upgrade it. A potential donor may be flattered that you thought him capable of giving a thousand dollars when he was thinking of $200. He may give $500. On the other hand, if Mrs. Jones is thinking in terms of $500 and you ask for $100, that is probably all the organization will get.

It has already been noted that large bequests can wreak havoc with a board. This does not mean they should be avoided or refused, but rather that the dangers should be recognized, and the pitfalls avoided.

For the typical United Way agency, endowed income can make the organization less dependent on United Way budget allocations. These often vary with priorities of that year's committee, individual committee member's understanding of programs, and their personal perceptions of the community's needs. Some years the agency may make a good presentation of its programs and goals for the coming year which hits right on target. Another year a well-planned approach leaves the allocations committee with many unanswered questions. When the United Way falls short of its goal, the member agency suffers and has little recourse.

SPECIAL EVENTS

Special events run the gamut from an educational forum for 25, 250, or 2,500 people, to fund-raisers aimed at bringing in $200, $2,000 or $20,000. Fund-raising events should also be programed to obtain the highest educational yield, acquaint new potential supporters with the program, and promote deferred giving programs. Like every aspect of community organization, if a special event is planned carefully and realistically, and alternate actions are planned in case of unforeseen events, success can be expected.

Almost any event can be programed for additional benefits. The important concept is programed or planned. A newsletter that does not contain an article about bequests or estate planning is not complete. A speech to a service club that has no reference to possible sponsorship is unfinished.

Special events generally fall into two categories: educational, or fund-raising. As was pointed out earlier, each should have a bit of the other. A few fund-raisers are: fashion shows; golf tournaments; coffee days; auctions; film openings; department store openings; bike-a-thons; telethons; horse shows; flower days; hotel openings; dinners; walk-a-thons; radio-thons; art sales; candle sales; and dances.

A very successful telethon may result in large cash pledges. If planned correctly, it may also plant the seed of deferred giving, which in time may flower into additional thousands of dollars.

On occasion, outside organizations will conduct an event with the agency as beneficiary. Expect to take part in the planning, offer help in publicizing, and insure that the event is conducted according to the highest ethical standards. After any special event, thanks and appreciation should flow down the chain of command. The lowest person on the totem pole may work harder the next year if his or her efforts are recognized. And, from the lower echelon comes the chairperson of future years.

Since special events can be very time consuming, it is recommended that great care be taken not to ask the chairperson of a highly successful program to immediately chair the next big event. Overworked volunteers may become disenchanted by growing demands. If a chairperson wants to do the same special event year after year, accept, but be sure to find an assistant chairperson who accepts important roles and could, if necessary step in as chairperson in a succeeding year.

It might be appropriate to caution against special events which cheapen the character of the sponsoring organization. Occasionally a transient promoter wants only to use the agency's name to sell tickets, and will operate a boiler room type sales campaign. When the transient leaves town the agency has to deal with people who have been antagonized and think the agency is the culprit. Anyone who allows the use of the agency's name in a manner that will bring the organization a bad image is the culprit. The few dollars picked up must be balanced against the resulting loss of stature. Stay completely within the law. When tempted to do otherwise, envision the headlines, look at clients who will suffer, and fellow board members in whose society the agency will continue to operate. Dishonest techniques and questionable activities just do not pay off in the long run.

When undertaking any special event, seek out knowledgeable, experienced volunteers. Research the historical success of similar events in the community. And, do not forget that a continuing appeal to the same constituency on a monthly basis will soon wear out the agency's welcome.

Organizations may take several different routes to obtain funds. Since dollars they obtain are distributed for services to clients, physicians should be aware of the different methods of obtaining funds, as well as the services for which these monies can be used.

Arthritis Foundation

The Arthritis Foundation is a voluntary health agency seeking the total answer—cause and cure in the field of rheumatological disease. Established in 1948 and now numbering 71 chapters around the country, its varied programs touch on many facets of the disease. Though research, basic and clinical, is a primary concern of the national group, many local chapters have programs (i.e., clinics, patient education) which community health professionals utilize. The Arthritis Foundation is the only voluntary health agency solely concerned with arthritis. The Foundation can provide services and also mobilize health professionals to support legislative efforts.

SERVICES

A listing of services provided by a local chapter of the Arthritis Foundation may include the following.

1. Funding of direct patient treatment through existing universities or hospitals.

2. Establishment of fellowships for physicians, allied health personnel, and researchers.

3. Operation of its own diagnostic and treatment clinics.

4. Funding of research, basic and clinical, on a local or national level.

5. Education of physicians, allied health personnel, patients and public on symptom recognition (what can be done and where to get help).

6. Printed brochures (Fig. 15.2) provided by the Arthritis Foundation include: *Basic Facts about Arthritis*, a down-to-earth booklet on important facets of the disease; a *Self-Help Manual for Arthritis Patients* which contains hundreds of suggestions to make daily living easier; and *Home Care Programs in Arthritis* listing exercises and self-help devices.

7. Handbooks for patients who have *Rheumatoid Arthritis* or *Osteoarthritis*.

8. Smaller brochures on *Gout*, *Lupus*, *Arthritis in Children*, *Diet*, and *Aspirin* may answer patients' questions.

9. In 1979 quack arthritis remedies and devices cost patients $940 million.

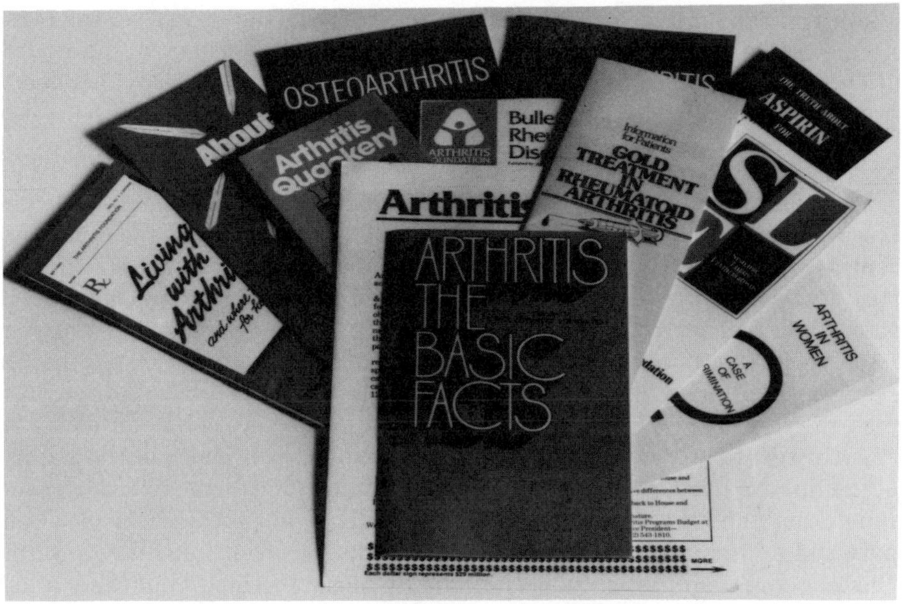

Fig. 15.2. Publications of the Arthritis Foundation.

The Foundation published a brochure on *Quackery*, warning potential victims to steer clear of the unscrupulous who prey on those in pain.

Arthritis Foundation Chapters sponsor forums, seminars, speakers bureaus, and television and radio shows to educate the public about arthritis. Chapters can be called upon to provide speakers or entire programs. Local chapters may have physical therapists, counselors, or other staff who can be brought in to work as part of a team.

Chapters are often involved in a plethora of services including vocational rehabilitation, manufacturing self-help devices, and home modification. Occasionally, the Foundation may be the source of funds for drugs, surgery or other components of a patient's program. Since these programs vary from year-to-year according to available funding, close contact should be maintained with the chapter in your area.

A well-known problem encountered in motivating handicapped to consider employment is their concern that if they try and fail, the red tape involved in obtaining reinstatement of a monthly SSI check can take months. A nationally endorsed campaign by the Arthritis Foundation to rectify this problem, if supported by other national health agencies, could precipitate changes in the bureaucratic environment.

Since governmental agencies show an increasing concern with health, the Arthritis Foundation may eventually be encouraged to assume an increasing role in recommending program funding or revising procedures. A quick phone call can familiarize any doctor or patient with the services of the local Arthritis Foundation. Or, a call may trigger action on the part of the Board of Directors or staff to initiate a program to meet a newly discovered need.

Quackery

For every dollar spent by responsible organizations in legitimate arthritis research, more than $25 will be spent for useless "quack cures" and unproven remedies. These run the gamut from the copper bracelet to the month-long stay at the desert spa with its dietary regimen, physical therapy and special waters. Obviously, if the first month doesn't have the desired effect, another month's stay certainly will bring the promised relief, and $475.00 per month seems a small price to pay for blessed relief. And, if this isn't effective, just read the tabloid newspapers. They list a new "cure" every 3 months.

Arthritis victims are susceptible to quack's claims because of the nature of the disease itself. A patient faced with crippled joints will anxiously await relief from pain. If the pain grows, or at least does not subside, the constant pain and apprehension of future pain can soften a client's attitude towards "instant cures" and "miraculous new discoveries." Victims of quackery often find it difficult to discuss their experiences with their physicians. Fear of disapproval or rejection can impede the client-doctor communication that is critical to the success of the legitimate treatment program.

It is important that a doctor know about a patient's treatment by a quack. If the patient feels betrayed because of negative effects from illegitimate treatments, he or she may cut off all treatments, including potentially beneficial ones. It is quite conceivable that a quack treatment can have harmful side effects. This can be complicated by clinics outside the United States prescribing medication with numbers instead of names.

Perhaps the most effective method of combating quackery is education. It is important to keep abreast of legitimate new research developments and communicate them to health practitioners and the public. This necessitates a coordinated, active, and responsible communication network among community agencies, volunteers, and physicians.

Health professionals themselves rarely have time to deal with general quackery problems, or become knowledgeable in specific examples of quackery. These professionals can, however, advise their clients that quackery does exist and that it is a glaring problem. They can also advise patients of sources that can be checked to determine the trustworthiness of advertised cures and remedies. The Better Business Bureau, Federal Food and Drug Administration, local Consumer Fraud Agencies, and the Arthritis Foundation are all potential sources for substantiating advertising claims. In Canada, the Canadian Arthritis and Rheumatism Society maintains a file on misrepresented treatments.

A knowledge of local, as well as national, deceptive practices and practitioners is a first step in protecting clients from quackery. Material describing these practices can be printed and distributed to the public, communications media, and clients. This allows patients to perceive the shortcomings of certain treatments and allows them to decide on the wisdom of undertaking certain treatments.

Quackery should not be confused with overzealous advertising, although the line dividing the two is often blurry. An example is aspirin, a drug originally developed to combat rheumatoid arthritis. Today's consumer is confronted by an overwhelming number of aspirin substitutes and derivatives, each acclaimed as better than its competitors. It is important that the patient be able to sort through the ads and choose the most beneficial product. Physicians can assist their clients, and the Arthritis Foundation can furnish pertinent information.

A related field which approaches the quackery subject is the "health food" fads of today. The problem arises when someone claims that a special diet or specific organic food can cure whatever ails the body and mind. After trying chemicals and other treatments, the ailing patient may feel that "natural" is right.

In the rheumatic diseases, no special diet or specific ingredient causes or cures. A sound, well-balanced diet is always helpful, and patients should avoid being overweight because of the extra strain on weight-bearing joints. This is the type of information that can and should be disseminated to clients in the clearest terms possible.

The Arthritis Foundation through its national office is kept apprised of the latest flim-flam. Health personnel will do well to keep in touch with the Foundation for the latest in quackery, be it "moon dust" or the latest juicerator guaranteed to relieve all aches and pains. The Foundation is frequently able to provide printed materials to patients and health personnel, and is also a source for speakers at health symposium or other educational affairs.

Quackery can best be dealt with through education, research, and open communication. It can be dealt with most effectively through a coordinated effort of allied health professionals. Professionals involved directly with patients who remember that their clients are in pain and accordingly susceptible to quack's claims can approach the problem with a clear mind and deal with it most effectively.

Summary

In this chapter various topics concerned with community organizations have been covered. Certainly, not everything discussed is applicable in all areas, but much may be relevant to many organizations.

The concept of the friendly family doctor in his horse and buggy being the sole purveyor of health services has no place in the practice of modern day medicine. Team care and the utilization of services provided by private and public agencies can improve the lot of many a patient suffering with arthritis.

Though finding the source of the needed extra modalities may be a problem, it need not be overwhelming. The satisfaction provided by the improvement in the patient's condition will make the time and efforts expended well worthwhile.

Arthritis is a disease which costs the nation over $13 billion a year in medical expenditures, lost taxes, welfare, Social Security and Veterans Administration benefits among others. Four billion dollars are lost in wages alone. The human costs include five million people in daily pain, and the break-up of marriages and families. In 1976, 70,000,000 days were spent in bed due to arthritis, 500,000 people required hospitalization, and 1,000,000 people were totally disabled. The efforts health professionals can bring to bear to alleviate the myriad of problems faced by patients and their families are invaluable.

16

Epidemiology and Statistics: An Introduction to Progress-Oriented Information Processing

JEAN PORTA

Progress in medicine is undoubtedly difficult to measure, and surely more difficult to obtain. In a climate of cost containment and rising consumer demands, to accomplish and document medical progress cannot be called a challenge—it is a requirement.

Under the pressure of this requirement the body of medical research activities separates into three areas of endeavor. These have different objectives, hence contribute in different ways to overall progress. The areas are model development, intervention assessment, and a third area which can be called persuasion. If epidemiology and statistics, are expected to advance the disciplines they serve, there must be an understanding as well as an explicit incorporation into studies of the different research objectives in these three areas.

Model Development

The first area, that of model development, includes what is ordinarily thought of as basic research. The objectives in modeling studies can range from an increased understanding of the nature of a biological system, through the determination of the scope of a medical problem, to the development of a therapeutic intervention.

Progress through model development cannot be expected unless testable hypothesis are put forth, for "Hypotheses are nets: only he who casts will catch." (1). If an experiment will not lead to a choice between different actions, there can be nothing gained in carrying it out. Specifically to be avoided in this context of progress-oriented information is the Baconian experiment of the sort that answers only the question, "I wonder what would happen if . . . ?" This Medawar (2) labels "not a critical activity but a kind of creative play."

Thus in a modeling process aimed at progress, an investigation results in a decision of whether or not to reject a specific hypothesis. This decision, since it determines a strategy to be followed in subsequent research, should be based on a study which has as its goal not the saving of lives of candidate hypotheses, but, as was pointed out by Popper (1), "to select the one which is by comparison the fittest, by exposing them all to the fiercest struggle for survival." An experiment, therefore, ought not be an attempt to prove a hypothesis, but rather must include the strongest possible efforts to disprove it.

Intervention Assessment

The second area to be considered within the research process is that of assessment of therapeutic interventions, such as pharmacological agents and physical modalities. An appointment system or an encounter form may also require assessment. It is in the area of assessment that one finds the controlled clinical trial, which attempts to answer the question, "Is the effect of a particular intervention such that its use is justified?"

In medicine, assessment implies the additional responsibility of action, so that if one modality can be shown to be clearly superior to another, in the future that modality should be used. This decision to use the superior of two treatments is coupled with the hope on the parts of both patient and physician that there does in fact exist a better treatment. Herein lies a potential source of bias so important that what is practically a controlled clinical trial industry has developed in an attempt to remove the bias from assessment studies. Even with this bias effectively removed, the superiority of one modality over another can be less than clear, since undesirable effects such as harmful side effects or low patient compliance must be taken into account. This dilemma may lead to only a tentative decision, but a decision nonetheless, as to whether or not to accept or reject a new modality. It is important in the assessment study that the strongest possible efforts be made to observe an effect. However, it is also important to control the study so that an observed difference in treatment effects is not likely to be due to any factor other than the treatments.

Persuasion

The third area of research is the persuasive study, which asks the question, "Is the benefit of a program substantial enough that it will be supported by others." The evaluation studies sometimes required of federally funded projects are perhaps the most important example of this kind of study. The persuasive aspect has been recognized by some statisticians and has even been incorporated into research design (3). While it could be argued, perhaps convincingly, that this persuasive type of study is not truly research, such a study can be both a product and a producer of research funds. It is carried out by research professionals, including statisticians and epidemiologists, and is expected to incorporate scientific methodology. Moreover, if there is to be an opportunity for progress through means such as management programs, support for those programs must be obtained. Decisions regarding that support require the results of factual studies. It is for these reasons that persuasive studies, even those which may not be research in the strictest sense, are included in this discussion.

Persuasion plays a more formal research role in debates between competing theories or paradigms, as discussed by Kuhn (4) in The *Nature of Scientific Revolutions.* There Kuhn maintains that "the emergence of a new candidate for paradigm . . . and the subsequent battle over its acceptance" arise in the situation where there are "recognized anomalies whose characteristic feature is their stubborn refusal to be assimilated by existing paradigms." The histories of physics and medicine provide examples of such debates and subsequent shifts of thought. It may be that a resolution of the apparent paradoxes in the area of associations between histocompatibility antigens and disease will require some sort of theory upheaval.

The differences which exist between persuasion and the assessment and modeling processes are due to the nature of the postexperimental decision. If the time of that decision is fixed, perhaps for administrative reasons, the persuasive study must be conducted not when it is convenient or after supporting research has pointed the way to experimental success, but at a time when its results can influence the decision-making process. Furthermore, the decision following an assessment or modeling study can usually be taken by the researcher, whereas in the persuasive process that decision is in the hands of another party. The deciding party, like the jury in a courtroom proceeding, does not itself collect the evidence—the statistical information. Here to tell the truth is not enough: one must also convince the jury that it is the truth.

Planning for Progress

Research programs in the areas of modeling, assessment, and persuasion may have different objectives, but the system rewards the factual experiment. That experiment must satisfy certain standards of reproducibility and clarity and should be described in such a way that anyone familiar with the relevant techniques can repeat it. The successful experiment must be effective as well as factual, hence must be approached with an eye on the research objectives which constrain it at various stages. Thus the plans for a research study for each stage need to be discussed separately for the three research areas. Although we could discuss research study stages in the order

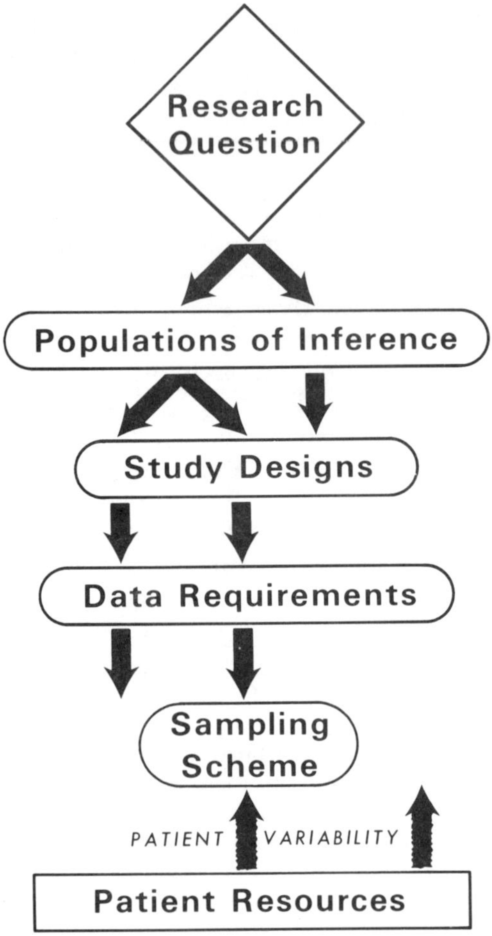

Fig. 16.1. A model for planning progress-oriented medical research.

of their implementation—sampling, data collection, analysis and inference—that may not be the best way to plan.

Planning is a sequence of decisions, each of which limits the choices that are available at the next decision point. Starting this decision sequence with the most critical decision narrows the choices at each point to a set which includes only those which can support the earlier more critical choices. This top-to-bottom method of planning starts with the choices of research objectives and the conclusions one hopes to be able to draw. These choices determine populations that would be of interest and the study designs which permit an answer to the research question. What is to be measured and how—the data and its means of collection—can then be determined. It is at this point that the researcher, before shooting for the stars, places both feet firmly on the ground and identifies the available groups in which data can be reliably obtained. The amount of variability in those groups determines the sample size necessary to answer the research question. This in turn calls for a bridging from resources to data via a sampling scheme.

Figure 16.1 depicts a planning model in which some choices cannot be supported, e.g., the two paths which do not continue through to a sampling scheme, and not all data sources are useful.

Planning in Model Development

In the modeling situation one wishes to subject an a priori hypothesis to the strongest possible attempts to disprove it. In addition, one wishes to know the range of the model, that is, under what circumstances, if any, the model is adequate. In order to meet these objectives, the population to be studied should include subpopulations in which the model can be most severely tested, hence from which the strongest conclusions can be drawn. In a study to develop diagnostic criteria, for instance, the population should include patients in whom the diagnosis is particularly difficult. The next decision point is that of study design, where the choices, which depend on the research question, are between case-control and cohort study, for instance. It is never easy to determine the designs which can be used to answer the question at hand.

Statistical methods to be used and subgroups to be analyzed should be enumerated along with the choices of design. This is a far better time than in the flood of data acquisition, when the only decision sometimes is which straw to grasp. In the modeling situation relatively sophisticated techniques, such as discriminant analysis or analysis of variance can sometimes be used. However, with rheumatic disease studies, the data are not usually suitable.

If choices of relevant and useful measurements are available for at least one of the designs, the research planner moves on to the decision of selection of patients on whom the measurements are to be made. In the modeling situation it is particularly important that patient material comes from a clearly enumerable source, such as a roster of clinic patients or a listing of households. Otherwise, it is altogether too easy, consciously or not, to converge on a suitable matching of patients and hypothesis. Such an inductive procedure may win applause, but it is likely to be unreproducible and may lead to a study from which no reliable conclusions can be drawn. It is worthwhile here to return to the example of a differential diagnosis study in which the objective is to select criteria with which to discriminate between diagnostic groups. In order for the criteria to be useful in practice, patients must be selected from diagnostic groups defined by a mechanism external to the study, such as a previously determined diagnosis. Also to be avoided is the self-selected sample in which subjects from a poorly defined population volunteer in response to some form of invitation, perhaps a lay publication. Frequency of clinic visitation can be a source of selection bias if a group of sequential patients is to be studied, since those persons who visit frequently are most likely to be included in the study. Their higher visitation rate may be associated with higher or lower values of a relevant variable, hence results can be misleading. Therefore, unless the research question is one about visits, such as their average cost or duration, rather than a question about patients, the subjects should be selected from a listing of patients, not from a log of their clinic visits.

The choice of a study group, with its inherent variability in the response variables, determines how large a sample is necessary for adequate testing of the hypothesis. (See for instance Fleiss (5) on the matter of sample size determination.) If not all eligible patients are to be included in the study, then a random sampling scheme needs to be devised. The choice of a random sample avoids the shortcomings of a sample in which the selection is left to the researcher. Hill (6) points out that the haphazard method "is very unlikely to be truly haphazard." This situation is particularly likely to occur when data are collected at the time of a clinic visit on a form which is additional to the routine encounter form. Completion of any such form, no matter how brief, requires a break in the routine and an increase in the work. Hence clinicians almost invariably will include only a portion of their patients. It is therefore preferable to obtain a random sample of manageable size, from which less biased information is to be expected.

It is frequently the case in rheumatic disease studies that no single clinic population of eligible patients is large enough to convincingly test the hypothesis. In that case, collaboration between institutions can be sought and the research process implemented with the strictest possible attention to standardization of procedures.

A sampling method commonly used is that of systematic sampling, where, say, every 10th patient is selected. It is recommended for its simplicity but should not be used if there are important trends in patient order. In a prevalence study using emergency room encounter forms, for instance, similar problems were filed together in clusters, so that whole groups of problems were likely to be missed. To guard against this, forms could be sampled in sequential groups of 10, with a single form selected at random from each group.

If an experiment is feasible, the final choices of sampling schemes will yield at least one complete decision sequence to serve as the research protocol. The selection among several protocols, should that be necessary, would aim for the most strenuous test of the hypothesis through a combination of low patient variability, large sample size, and powerful study design.

Planning in Intervention Assessment

An assessment study to answer a question of the form, "Is the effect of a particular intervention such that its use is justified?" can be planned by the same process as the modeling study and has many of the same requirements. It is essentially the same, for instance, to require that the population of inference should be one in which an effect, if it exists, is most likely to be observed. This implies that a population of patients with treatable disease should be the one of inference.

Differences in the two study designs arise mainly from the objective that the assessment study be one in which an effect, if it is observed, is unlikely to be due to any factor other than the treatment. Therefore every choice of design, sample, etc. which is included in the planning model must be unbiased with respect to the treatments under consideration. In the face of strong possibilities of bias in treatment selection and posttreatment assessment, this objective can be met adequately only by a controlled clinical trial in which patients are randomly allocated to treatment groups. In an uncontrolled trial the inherent lack of comparability between groups of dissimilarly treated patients cannot be compensated for by study size, for, as Merrell is quoted by Hill (6) as having observed, "large numbers in themselves are worse than useless if the groups are not comparable, since they encourage confidence in erroneous opinion."

Within the confines of the controlled clinical trial there are several commonly used designs from which to choose. A trial which is completely randomized may be used, but is likely to yield noncomparable treatment groups. Also an option is a design in which the patients are first divided into subgroups on the basis of what are thought to be relevant variables, and then in each subgroup patients are randomly allocated to treatment groups. With this design a smaller total sample size is required to obtain the same power as with a completely randomized trial. In a chronic disease such as rheumatoid arthritis, a cross-over design is sometimes used. Here each patient is treated for a period with one drug, then for a second period with the other, with a wash-out period in between. The random allocation in the cross-over design is to treatment sequence AB or BA, rather than to treatment groups A or B. Another possibility is a matched pairs design, in which patients are first paired on the basis of relevant variables. Then there is a random assignment of members of a pair to the two treatment groups. The method has the shortcoming that since only pairs of patients rather than single patients are entered into the study, eligible patients who cannot be paired must be omitted. Another choice which can sometimes be used to advantage in studies of physical modalities is a design in which a pair of observations is made within the same patient. For instance, among patients with bilateral joint involvement, a topical ointment can be applied to one joint, selected at random, and a placebo ointment applied to the opposite joint.

The choices of analytical techniques should be simple in assessment studies so that the results are as understandable as possible. Further, the data collected should be extensive in order that a wide variety of disease processes and side effects can be assessed.

When choices are established down to the point of data to be collected and the available patient resources are identified, an appropriate sampling scheme can be devised for sequences which are possible to complete. Hence the feasible assessment protocols are determined. If more than one protocol is possible, then selection between them should be an attempt to give the treatment difference, if it exists, the highest possible chance of appearing.

Planning in Persuasive Studies

As was pointed out in the earlier discussion describing the persuasive research study, the overall objective of persuading must be sought with two primary concerns: one is timeliness, the other credibility. Study results must be available prior to the decision. Further, results which are not understandable or believable must be avoided, for they have the potential of setting indelible stains of distrust and disillusionment. The public may have come to expect such practices from its politicians or industries, but not from its medical community.

What is proposed here is a model for planning which forces a pair of studies designed to show the program in both better-than-average and worse-than-average light.

The planning begins by ordering the choices at each decision point according to how strongly they favor the research program. For instance, three possible populations of inference may be known to be affected adversely, not affected, and benefitted by the program. Just as choices which were unbiased were the only ones allowable in assessment planning, here only those choices which meet the timing requirements need to be included. This could exclude, for instance, data sources from which individual patient information would have to be collected de novo. In acute situations, in fact, it could restrict data sources to only routinely collected summary data on groups of patients.

Planning proceeds through the various steps as in the modeling and assessment situations until the complete decision sequences are determined. It is from these that one is expected to choose according to the following rule. At each decision point two choices are selected, one being more favorable than average, and the other choice being equally less favorable. (The reader is referred to Fig. 16.2, which illustrates the rule at the first decision point.) This rule, while based on admittedly subjective rankings, serves the function of selecting two protocols with some spread of favorability between them. Subsequent study results will give a credible range of the performance of the program aspect under study.

Summary

The planning of a successful research study is by no means a simple task. The widest possible range of alternatives must be considered and difficult tradeoffs made between them. Valuable assistance in broadening that range and predicting the consequences of the various tradeoffs can often be gained

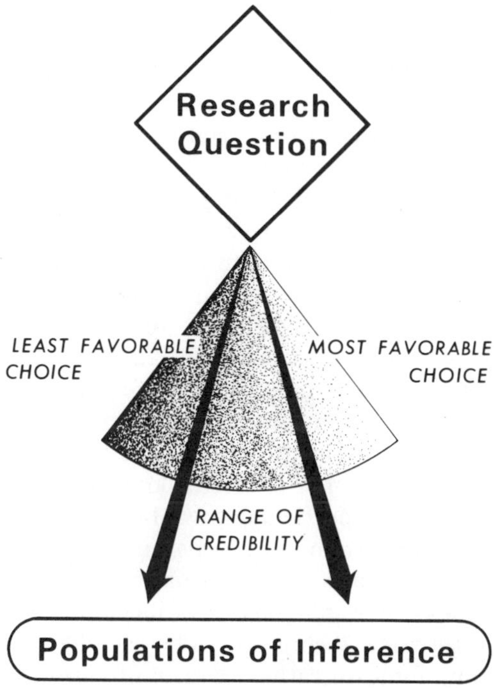

Fig. 16.2. A decision model for achieving credible persuasive research.

by obtaining the services of a statistician with experience in one's particular research field.

Implementation and Analysis

If all objections must first be overcome, nothing will ever be done. Recognizing that studies are never perfect—even if plans appear to be—one must at some point begin. At that point, when the protocol is determined, the researcher faces the often sizeable task of form design. While general tools are available to help, the problem is somewhat easier to solve in the rheumatic diseases than in most other fields. Here, one can begin with the Time-Oriented Data form (7), which displays measurements included in the Uniform Database for the Rheumatic Diseases. It can serve as a valuable guide to the requirements of a data collection form. This is a crucial element in a research study since its proper development requires a thorough understanding of the research protocol. Very often one doesn't realize just what has been decided or overlooked until commiting the protocol to paper in a data collection form.

The most careful planning cannot anticipate or prevent all of the multitude of ways in which study objectives can unconsciously be compromised or information devalued as the research plans are implemented. Repeated occurrences of untoward events, such as patients removing themselves from the study or not all measuring instruments operating equally well, if not corrected or accounted for, may not only weaken a study; they can in fact invalidate it. A pilot trial may point out some of the pitfalls, but during the actual study performance the involvement of a statistician who pays occasional unannounced visits is probably the best insurance.

There are points in study implementation at which blind assessments—those made on individual patients without knowledge of other diagnostic, treatment, or laboratory variables—can noticeably increase the validity of a study. Without this precaution in such procedures as the reading of x-rays or the assessment of a patient's response to treatment, there may be a tendency towards treatment bias or circular reasoning. Hill (6) recommends that "if any judgements or interpretations are required of the data recorded for each patient, then those judgements or interpretations should be made *before* the treatments are decoded." The double-blind procedure in clinical trials, where neither patients nor clinicians know the identity of the treatments during the trial, has a particular advantage in the rheumatic diseases. The double-blind procedure allows the physician's assessment to be used as an objective, rather than subjective, measurement in the analysis, hence is recommended whenever possible in spite of its cumbersome nature.

In selecting the statistical techniques to be used in the data analysis, one should strive to communicate rather than to obscure the meanings in the data. Any statistical procedure which reduces a set of data to only a number and its degrees of freedom introduces some distortion. Since different statistics distort reality in different ways, the selections one makes should be in keeping with the objectives of strenuous testing, unbiasedness, and credibility.

While post hoc hypothesis testing is strongly discouraged, this is not to say that the compiled data are not to be thoroughly examined. On the contrary, patients who did and did not respond well to treatment should be compared to learn more about both the treatments and the disease. Extreme outliers in the modeling study should be investigated. Trends in performance found from a persuasive study should be examined to see if program improvements can be made. These tasks require the simultaneous examination of a number of variables, hence are a major reason for recommending the use of a computer in all but very small studies.

The successful implementation and analysis of research studies is admittedly difficult. Since every study has some of its own unique ingredients, no cookbook could completely solve all the problems. However, the reader is referred to references by Fleiss (5) and Hill (6) for accessible presentations that may prove helpful.

Summary and Conclusions

What has been proposed here is a plan for retrieving progress-oriented information from epidemiological and statistical investigations. The focus has been on different objectives in three areas of research. In model development every effort must be made to meet the objective of testing the hypothetical model in the most strenuous way. In intervention assessment one strives for the objective of insuring that if there is observed to be a better response in a group of patients given one intervention rather than another, that difference in response will be unlikely to be due to any factor other than the interventions. In persuasive research the objectives of timeliness and credibility are stressed. It is proposed that plans for processing progress-oriented information be a sequence of decisions made from the top down, starting with the decisions most critical to the research objectives and selecting for implementation a decision sequence which can be supported by the available patient resources. It is further proposed that in persuasive research fairness can be demonstrated by providing what is in fact a pair of studies designed to cover a range of credibility.

Although the methods discussed here could lead to an increased number of technically successful experiments, the value of those experiments is limited by the questions which they answer. The selection of those questions is almost exclusively in the hands of medical leaders. Medicine benefits, however, when that process is opened to the quantitative sciences.

REFERENCES

1. Popper, K. R. *The Logic of Scientific Discovery*, Ed. 5. Hutchinson, London, 1965.
2. Medawar, P. B. *The Art of the Soluble*. Methuen and Co., Ltd., London, 1967.
3. Novick, M. R. A course in Bayesian statistics. *Am. Statis., 29:* 94, 1975.
4. Kuhn, T. S. *The Structure of Scientific Revolutions*. University of Chicago, Chicago, 1962.
5. Fleiss, J. L. *Statistical Methods for Rates and Proportions*. John Wiley and Sons, New York, 1973.
6. Hill, A. B. *A Short Textbook of Medical Statistics*, Ed. 10. J. B. Lippincott Co., London, 1977.
7. Fries, J. F. Alternatives in medical record formats. *Med. Care, 12:* 871; 1974.

appendix

1

Section 504 of the United States Rehabilitation Act of 1973

STEVEN L. ABRAMS

Affirmative action for those suffering from various types of disabilities has been the subject of legislation, in one form or another, in many parts of the world. Switzerland, for example, has long had a "law against arthritis," i.e., those with that disorder are covered for their expenses and rehabilitation. The legislative history of the appropriate law in the United States is instructive to study. It came about without full consideration of the implications, chiefly because it seemed a worthwhile cause that one could not oppose. Perhaps more precise wording would have helped achieve the aims without the distortion that now seems inevitable.

Section 504 of the Rehabilitation Act of 1973 (Public Law 93-112), signed by President Richard M. Nixon on September 26, 1973, prohibits discrimination against the handicapped. The law simply provides that "no otherwise qualified handicapped individual in the United States, as defined in section 7(6), shall, solely by reason of his handicap, be excluded from the participation in, be denied the benefits of, or be subjected to discrimination under any program or activity receiving Federal financial assistance." The regulation of this law by the then Department of Health, Education and Welfare (HEW now Health and Human Services), 5 years later, posed a "classical regulatory dilemma," pitting the high costs of implementation against good will (1).

Groups required to effect the law were not opposed to the regulations because of insensitivity to the needs of the disabled; as a practical matter, the unique character of these institutions made it impossible for them to implement the regulations. Institutions of higher education, for example, had many problems, including the compliance deadlines, affirmative action requirements, provision of services, and costs. Regarding affirmative action, an admissions officer at Tufts University stated: "We were ordered to discriminate in admissions policy on the basis of a physical or psychological handicap. . . . I recall the mentally retarded were also candidates for affirmative action. Only a lout would joke about the mentally retarded. . . . The point is that the committee which designed these guidelines seemed blissfully unaware that, in an educational environment, rules reasonably applicable to, say, AT & T or General Motors, would be absurd" (2).

HEW has estimated that of the $400 million in capital investments that will be required to meet the regulations, most of the cost will be borne by educational institutions. But in the area of public transportation, a staffer on the House Education and Labor Committee found, in 1979: "The potential cost of implementing Section 504 is unknown. Two years ago, HEW conservatively estimated the cost to be $2.4 billion. The Department of Transportation estimated several billion dollars for buses alone" (3). In fact, a more recent study by the Congressional Budget Office reported that the total cost of making mass transit vehicles accessible to handicapped riders could cost $6.8 billion—a sum equal to $38 per trip. In general, because the act does not require any kind of goals, timetables, or cost-benefit analyses, it will be nearly impossible to measure progress or costs in a meaningful way.

Plainly, Congress failed to consider carefully the implications of Section 504. Section 504, which was not adopted in the committees of Congress with jurisdiction over civil rights matters (the Committees on the Judiciary), was not even the subject of hearings or debate in any committee. The 43 word law eventually resulted in 51 pages of federal regulations and billions of dollars in compliance costs, even though the problem of discrimination against the handicapped had never been studied as a question of public policy. Although the Senate gave birth to the provision, Section 504 was conceived by a congressman from Ohio, Charles A. Vanik. In 1971, he met with members of the Council of Parents of Handicapped Children, who expressed their legitimate concern over the lack of government involvement in areas related to rehabilitation that limited a handicapped person's ability to function in society. He promised to take some type of action and instructed his staff to "do something." His chief legislative assistant then devised two antidiscrimination measures, relating to recipients of federal contracts and grants (and copied from Section 601 of the Civil Rights Act of 1964, which prohibits discrimination on the basis of race). As the congressman was not a member of the Judiciary Committee or of the Select Committee on Education (with jurisdiction over rehabilitation programs), he consequently asked a colleague, Senator Hubert H. Humphrey, to use his influence to secure passage of the measures.

The Senator introduced Senate bills 3044 and 3458, dealing with discrimination against handicapped persons in employment and federally subsidized activities, respectively, which were referred to the Judiciary Committee since they amended Titles VI and VII of the Civil Rights Act.

Amending the Civil Rights Act to include handicapped persons probably would have resulted in the act's emasculation, since conservatives, who did not have an expansive view of civil rights, controlled the committee. The vocational rehabilitation program, however, was 53 years old and, as its scope had been enlarged over that time, never faced opposition. Hearings were being held in the Senate Labor and Public Welfare Committee on the Vocational Rehabilitation bill, H.R. 8395, which the House Committee on Education and Labor had reported on March 16, 1972, and the full body passed on March 22. They did not focus on problems of discrimination against handicapped persons; rather, testimony dealt with the operation of the basic state-federal rehabilitation program and ancillary grant programs for research, training and special projects in rehabilitation. However, during the subsequent mark-up, a routine proposal of Senate bills 3044 and 3458 as amendments to the bill was made, as these bills were making no progress in the Judiciary Committee. The amendments did not meet any objections from the members of the subcommittee (many of whom had handicapped relatives themselves). These amendments subsequently were adopted in the Senate and by the House conferees on October 4.

As described by a staffer: "Very tough negotiations took place [on the entire bill]. As the conferees concluded, there were a few items left. The very last was Section 504. Although members were tired, they all agreed there should not be any discrimination against the handicapped. Section stayed in the final version and became law" (4). The conference report was agreed to unanimously be the Senate on October 13, and by the House the next day. But on October 27, President Richard M. Nixon announced his pocket veto of H.R. 8395.

Following the veto, the Subcommittee on the Handicapped held hearings on a new bill, Senate bill 7, in early 1973, and no reference at all was made to the antidiscrimination provisions, which had not been objected to in the President's Memorandum of Disapproval issued after his veto. In addition, the House Education Select Subcommittee held a day of hearings on the Rehabilitation bill in February. On February 28, Senate bill 7 passed the Senate by a vote of 86 to 2. Eight days later, the House substituted H.R. 17. The Senate agreed to the bill with an amendment, and on March 15, the House agreed to the Senate version, thereby clearing the measure for the President once more. But once again, on March 27, the President vetoed the bill. Again, the President deemed the bill too expensive, and while he made no mention of the antidiscrimination provisions, stated that the bill "masked bad legislation beneath alluring labels." Although the President's veto was sustained in the Senate by a vote of 60 to 36, the sensitivity of the issue was clear: "The rehabilitation bill struck a sympathetic note in most members of Congress. During Senate debate on the veto April 3, many crippled and blind persons, representing thirty organizations for the handicapped, crowded Senate corridors . . . [Senator Robert Taft portrayed the President as a man] 'callously drawing a line through programs for the handicapped with the heartless pen of parsimony.' " (5).

Following the second veto, members of the two committees met with Administration officials to discuss a compromise version of the bill. The two vetoes had delayed the reauthorization of rehabilitation legislation, and the existing programs were due to expire shortly, so a compromise bill, H.R. 8070, which preserved the antidiscrimination provisions, was reported from committee the day after it was introduced. On June 5, the House considered the bill under a suspension of the rules (where debate is limited to forty minutes, no floor amendments are permitted, and a vote by two-thirds of those present is required for passage), and it passed overwhelmingly, 384–13. Opponents objected to its hasty and superficial consideration under the suspension calendar. Only Mr. Vanik, their author, mentioned the antidiscrimination provisions, but even he in passing.

In the Senate there was no opposition and just as perfunctory an acknowledgement of Section 504. Senator Taft was the only senator to do more than just list Section 504 in a recitation of the bill's provisions: " . . . if we are to assure that all handicapped persons may participate fully in the rewards made possible by the vocational rehabilitation program, we must devote more of our energy toward the elimination of the most disgraceful barrier of all—discrimination." Section 504 was also treated perfunctorily in the conference committee.

On September 13, the Senate agreed to the conference report. Senator Alan Cranston, cited Section 504 in the debate as one of "several major new programs" in the bill, even though it had not even been mentioned in the Joint Explanatory Statement of the Committee of Conference. Similarly, without discussion of it, other senators referred to Section 504 as a "significant provision." In any case, the conference report passed unanimously. The House of Representatives followed suit on September 18, and the President signed the bill into law 8 days later. Some observers believe that the Senate Labor and Public Works Committee knew what it was doing by interpolating Section 504 into the massive rehabilitation bill. Lobbyists for groups of handicapped individuals did not request hearings on the subject, and Congress did not provide such a forum for views on the matter. Staffers on the committee sympathetic to rights for handicapped individuals (one of whom was a paraplegic herself) may have realized that if the implications of Section 504 were to be subjected to scrutiny, it ultimately would be opposed by Congress. Others generally agreed that if Section 504 had gone through as a single bill (as it was originally introduced by Senator Humphrey), then it would have been controversial and probably would not have passed. In fact, a member of Mr. Vanik's staff was "amazed" at its passage: "I did not think it would be passed. Clearly, people didn't realize the enormity [sic] of its potential." (6).

Except perhaps for a handful of staffers and handicapped-rights lobbyists, it is clear that no one realized the full implications of Section 504. Even Mr. Vanik, its author, has stated: "We never had any concept that it would involve such tremendous costs" (7). The Senate Subcommittee on Handicaps did not consider the long-range implications of Section 504 because they were caught up in the sensitivity of the issue. Initial support for the measure rested on unstated abstract sentiments. Only after its vague content had been applied specifically through regulations could reasonable arguments be marshalled against the mandate. But these pragmatic arguments did not prove effective: "When we raised issues of costs and other problems with [the Chairman of the House Subcommittee on Select Education, which oversees Section 504's implementation], he simply turned around and asked us: 'Don't you believe in equal opportunity?' It's awfully hard for someone to come in and oppose the issue, because immediately you're in the posture of somehow being anti-handicapped people." (8). There really were no politics involved in the passage of Section 504. Everybody had to vote for it, even if they were aware of its existence in the Rehabilitation bill (and its implications).

There existed no mandate for regulations nor were there enforcement guidelines, and HEW was slow in implementing the law. Questions were raised by its author as to whether "the strong language on non-discrimination and program participation [will] actually be enforced, or . . . molder in the law books, unused and forgotten" -in November, 1973, Mr. Vanik asked thirty-five federal agencies "how they intended to implement, in particular, title V of law," which included Section 504 (9). After continued delay, a Senate report to the Rehabilitation Amendments of 1974 (which did not alter Section 504) stated that regulations were intended to be enforced by HEW after the pattern of the Civil Rights Act and Title IX of the Education Amendments of 1972 (prohibiting sex discrimination in education). Finally, in 1976, President Gerald R. Ford issued an executive order requiring the issuance of regulations for Section 504 by HEW and, subsequently, other federal agencies.

The regulations were then written by HEW's Office of Civil Rights, but Congress was unable to review them ("the ranking member of the House Education and Labor Committee . . . suggested that one page of general regulations be promulgated and then all questions HEW may have had about the provision be sent in a communication to the Congress and have Congress vote on the matter. Unfortunately, there was a Presidential election and a change in Administration . . . and no such communication was sent to Congress until January 19, 1977. It promptly got lost in the shuffle.") (4).

In the first few months of the Administration of President Jimmy Carter, the handicapped movement, which had become better represented in Washington since 1973, pressured the new Secretary of HEW to issue the regulations. In consultation with the Senate subcommittee staff and the groups representing the handicapped population (but not groups representing the recipients of federal funds, such as higher education associations), preliminary regulations were drawn up. Afterwards, education groups had an opportunity to comment, and they basically agreed with their intent, although they objected to their cost. On May 4, 1977, HEW issued 26 pages of regulations, covering schools, colleges, hospitals, and employment, among other areas receiving government subsidies.

Numerous court cases have decided unclear issues in each of these areas. However, in Davis V. Southeastern Community College, the first major ruling on Section 504 by the United States Supreme Court (June 1979), substantial ambiguity was created. The Court ruled against a registered nurse denied admission to a college's nursing program because she had a hearing disability, in deference to the objectives of institutions of higher learning. Many saw the decision as unfavorable to the rights of the handicapped but others viewed the decision as not being damaging (10). The same month, the Court refused to review a case brought under Section 504 of a nurse fired from her job because she was losing her eyesight.

Despite the ambiguity surrounding the implementation of the law, Congress has only clarified Section 504 twice. In the 1974 Rehabilitation Amendments, Congress changed the definition of a handicapped person to read: "For the purpose of Titles IV and V of this Act, such term means any person who (A) has a physical or mental impairment which substantially limits one or more major life activities; (B) has a record of such an impairment; or (C) is regarded as having such an impairment." The Senate Report also included the first congressional discussion of Section 504: "It was clearly the intent of the Congress in adopting . . . section 504 (nondiscrimination) that the term "handicapped individual" in those sections was not to be narrowly limited to employment (in the case of section 504), nor to the individual's potential benefit from vocational rehabilitation services under titles I and III (in the case of both sections 503 and 504) of the Act. . . . Section 504 was enacted to prevent discrimination against all handicapped individuals regardless of their need for, or ability to benefit from, vocational rehabilitation services, in relation to Federal assistance in employment, housing, transportation, education, health services, or any other federally-aided programs."

In the Rehabilitation Comprehensive Services and Developmental Disabilities Amendments of 1978, Section 504 was amended, without detailed discussion, with respect to the application of rights, remedies and procedures, and its coverage of drug addicts and alchoholics. The law's other troublesome aspects were still not clarified. Once more in the 1978 Amendments, the Rehabilitation Act's provisions were formulated without the participation of most members: "Contrary to what the textbooks say, the laws that Congress passes are rarely the result of deliberation in committees and debate on the House and Senate floors. More often they are born in the backrooms of the Capitol with arm-twisting and back-scratching as midwives. . . . Using the threat of a veto, [the Assistant to the President for Congressional Liaison] persuaded five senators to support severe cuts in rehabilitation budget. . . . Thus assured of a flipflop by the five—all of whom spoke eloquently for the original authorization—the President signed the bill November 6." (11). Most of the other questions about Section 504, particularly those involving the bearing of costs, were never addressed by Congress beyond oversight hearings. Even though the Senate Report for the 1974 Amendments commented on whether Section 504 required affirmative action and the debate on 1978 amendments contained a statement that Section 504 should extend to the activities of federal agencies, the Supreme Court in the *Davis* decision held that " . . . isolated statements by individual Members of Congress or its committees, all made after the enactment of the statute under consideration, cannot substitute for a clear expression of legislative intent at the time of enactment."

As a result of all of the above, Congress is trapped between groups who oppose the high costs imposed by Section 504 and groups fighting for rights for the handicapped exerting pressure for Congress to reverse the Davis decision. According to Education and Labor Committee counsel: "The problem facing the Congress is that in order to modify Section 504, Congress has to address itself to the regulations as promulgated, which were issued by non-elected officials of Agencies. The Congress would have to, in effect, change the law because of regulations, which although they have the force of law, were not passed or approved by law makers." (13). Thus, in approaching the controversy, Congress, ironically, is coming full circle. With the Judiciary committees now more disposed towards rights for handicapped individuals, some members of Congress (with handicapped group support) are pushing for inclusion of handicapped persons as a protected class under the Civil Rights Act. A bill to amend Title VII of the Act to prohibit discrimination against individuals who are handicapped was pending in the House Committee on Education and Labor at the end of 1979, and garnering support.

Obviously, arthritis falls under the provision when it produces disabilities. Architectural barriers in public buildings, schools, and other institutions receiving federal funds obviously come under the provision; so would transportation design and development, hospitals, and other aspects discussed in this book.

REFERENCES

1. LABICH, K., ET AL. Now, wheelchair rights. *Newsweek*, January 11, 1979, p. 26.
2. Quoted in ROCHE, J. P. The court, HEW and the handicapped. *The Washington Star*, June 25, 1979, p. A-17.
3. LAVOR, M. L. Senior Legislative Associate, Committee on Education and Labor, United States House of Representatives. "Section 504 of the Vocational Rehabilitation Act" Memorandum to All Minority Members, House Education and Labor Committee, June 14, 1979, p. 3.

4. LaVor, M. L. "Section 504 of the Vocational Rehabilitation Act" Memorandum to All Minority Members, House Education and Labor Committee, June 14, 1979, p. 2.
5. Senate sustains President on spending priorities. *Congressional Quarterly Weekly Report*, April 7, 1973, p. 3–4.
6. Interview with William Vaughan, former Legislative Assistant to the Honorable Charles A. Vanik. United States House of Representatives, Washington, D.C., August 3, 1979.
7. Quoted in Peirce, N. R. The great wheelchair flap. *The Washington Post*, December 29, 1978.
8. Interview with John Phillips, President, National Association of Independent Colleges and Universities, Washington, D.C., August 7, 1979.
9. Vanik, C. A. A law isn't enough. *Hearing Speech News*, March–April, 1974, pp. 27, 13.
10. No fatal blow for disabled. *The Philadelphia Inquirer*, June 25, 1979.
11. Anderson, J. Carter's deal to gut aid program. *The Washington Post*, January 21, 1979, p. B13.

Index